FLEX
REVIEW

FLEX

REVIEW

PREPARATION FOR
THE FEDERATION LICENSING EXAMINATION

810 MULTIPLE-CHOICE QUESTIONS WITH
REFERENCED EXPLANATORY ANSWERS
PLUS PATIENT MANAGEMENT PROBLEMS

THIRD EDITION

Michael A. Baker, M.D.
Alfonse A. Cinnoti, M.D.
Sidney A. Cohn, Ph.D
Daniel L. Coury, M.D.
Thomas J. DeKornfeld, M.D.
Joseph R. DiPalma, M.D.
Stanley N. Farb, M.D.
A. Olusegun Fayemi, M.D.
Count D. Gibson, Jr., M.D.
Kalman Greenspan, Ph.D.
Nancy B. Hansen, M.D.
John Eric Holmes, M.D.
Stephen N. Joffe, M.D.
Irving I. Kessler, M.D.

Charles W. Kim, Ph.D.
Edward H. Liston, M.D.
James J. Mathews, M.D.
Alan E. Oestreich, M.D.
Raymond E. Probst, M.D.
M.D. Ram, M.D., Ph.D.
Raymond M. Russo, M.D.
Lawrence R. Shapiro, M.D.
John E. Verby, M.D.
Bruce H. Weber, Ph.D.
Raymond O. West, M.D.
Larry D. Young, Ph.D.
Jared B. Zelman, M.D.
David Zull, M.D.

MEDICAL EXAMINATION PUBLISHING COMPANY

Notice

The authors and the publisher of this book have made every effort to ensure that all therapeutic modalities that are recommended are in accordance with accepted standards at the time of publication.

The drugs specified within this book may not have specific approval by the Food and Drug Administration in regard to the indications and dosages that are recommended by the authors. The manufacturer's package insert is the best source of current prescribing information.

Medical Examination Publishing Company
A Division of Elsevier Science Publishing Co., Inc.
655 Avenue of the Americas, New York, New York 10010

Library of Congress Cataloging in Publication Data

Medical examination review.—Flushing, N.Y. : Medical Examination Pub. Co.,
1960-<1981   >
      v.<1-9,12-32, 34-37   > : ill. ; 22 cm.
   Includes various editions of some volumes.
   Published 1960-1980 as: Medical examination review book.
   Includes bibliographical references.
   1. Medicine—Examinations, questions, etc.
RC58.M4   610'.76—dc19   61-66847   AACR 2 MARC
ISBN 0-444-01141-2

Current printing (last digit)
10   9   8   7   6   5

Manufactured in the United States of America

Contents

Contributors   ix
Preface   xiii
Acknowledgments   xv

Part I
BASIC SCIENCES

1 Anatomy   3
2 Behavioral Sciences   12
3 Biochemistry   23
4 Biostatistics/Epidemiology   33
5 Genetics   43
6 Microbiology   49
7 Pathology   60
8 Pharmacology   68
9 Physiology   77

Answers and Comments   85
References   127

Part II
CLINICAL SCIENCES

10 Anesthesiology 135
11 Emergency Medicine 141
12 Family Medicine 150
13 Internal Medicine 158
14 Medical Ethics 176
15 Neurology 179
16 Obstetrics and Gynecology 192
17 Ophthalmology 210
18 Otorhinolaryngology 218
19 Pediatrics 224
20 Public Health and Preventive Medicine 235
21 Psychiatry 246
22 Radiology 254
23 Surgery 284

Answers and Comments 309
References 383

Part III
CLINICAL COMPETENCE

24 Therapeutics 393
25 Pictorial 399

Answers and Comments 416
References 421

26   Patient Management Problems   423

Instructions   423
Problems   425
Scoring System   449
Scoring and Discussion   449

Responses   471

Contributors

Michael A. Baker, M.D., F.R.C.P.(C), F.A.C.P., Professor of Medicine, University of Toronto Faculty of Medicine, Director of Oncology and Hematology, Toronto General Hospital, Toronto, Ontario, Canada

Alfonse A. Cinotti, M.D., F.A.C.S., Professor and Chairman, Department of Ophthalmology, University of Medicine and Dentistry of New Jersey, New Jersey Medical School, Medical Director, Eye Institute of New Jersey, Newark, New Jersey

Sidney A. Cohn, Ph.D., Emeritus Professor, Department of Anatomy, The University of Tennessee, Memphis, The Health Science Center, Memphis, Tennessee

Daniel L. Coury, M.D., Assistant Professor of Pediatrics, Ohio State University, Attending Pediatrician, The Children's Hospital, Columbus, Ohio

Thomas J. DeKornfeld, M.D., Professor of Postgraduate Medicine and Health Professions Education, and Chairman, Department of Anesthesiology, University Hospital, University of Michigan School of Medicine, Ann Arbor, Michigan

Department of Epidemiology and Preventive Medicine, University of Maryland School of Medicine, Baltimore, Maryland, Irving I. Kessler, M.D., Chairman. Faculty members: J.R. Hebel, Ph.D.; M.S. Levine, M.D.; J. Magaziner, Ph.D.; M.J. Sexton, Ph.D; and R.W. Sherwin, M.B.

Joseph R. DiPalma, M.D., Emeritus Professor of Pharmacology and Medicine, Hahnemann University, School of Medicine, Philadelphia, Pennsylvania

Stanley N. Farb, M.D., Chief of Otolaryngology, Montgomery Hospital and Sacred Heart Hospital, Norristown, Pennsylvania

A. Olusegun Fayemi, M.D., Attending Pathologist, St. Joseph's Hospital and Medical Center, Patterson, New Jersey

Count D. Gibson, Jr., M.D., Professor and Chairman, Department of Family, Community, and Preventive Medicine, Stanford University School of Medicine, Stanford University Medical Center, Stanford, California

Kalman Greenspan, Ph.D., F.A.C.C., Professor of Medicine and Physiology, Indiana University School of Medicine, Indianapolis, Chief, Section of Physiology, Terre Haute Center for Medical Education, Terre Haute, Indiana

Nancy B. Hansen, M.D., Associate Professor of Pediatrics, Ohio State University, Attending Neonatologist, The Children's Hospital, Columbus, Ohio

John Eric Holmes, M.D. Emeritus Associate Professor of Neurology, University of Southern California, Los Angeles, California, and Visiting Scientist, Department of Human Anatomy, Oxford University, Oxford, England

Stephen N. Joffe, M.D., Professor of Surgery, University of Cincinnati, Medical Center, College of Medicine, Cincinnati, Ohio

Charles W. Kim, M.S.P.H., Ph.D., Associate Professor of Microbiology and Clinical Medicine, School of Medicine, Health Sciences Center, State University of New York at Stony Brook, Stony Brook, New York

Edward H. Liston, M.D., Professor of Psychiatry, Neuropsychiatric Institute and Hospital, University of California, Los Angeles, Center for the Health Sciences, Los Angeles, California

James J. Mathews, M.D., Chief, Section of Emergency Medicine, Northwestern University, School of Medicine, Chicago, Illinois

Alan E. Oestreich, M.D., Professor of Radiology and Pediatrics, Division of Radiology, Children's Hospital Medical Center, Cincinnati, Ohio

Raymond E. Probst, M.D., Clinical Professor of Obstetrics and Gynecology, St. Louis University School of Medicine, St. Louis, Missouri

M. D. Ram, M.D., M.S. (Surg), **Ph.D., F.R.C.S.** (England, Edinburgh, and Canada) **F.A.C.S.,** Professor of Surgery, University of Kentucky Medical Center, Chief, Surgical Service, Veterans Administration Medical Center, Lexington, Kentucky

Raymond M. Russo, M.D., F.A.A.P., Associate Professor of Pediatrics, University of Medicine and Dentistry of New Jersey, Rutgers Medical School, Piscataway, New Jersey

Lawrence R. Shapiro, M.D., Director, Department of Medical Genetics, Westchester County Medical Center, Professor of Pediatrics and Pathology, New York Medical College, Valhalla, New York, Director of Genetics at Letchworth Village, Thiells, New York

John E. Verby, M.D., Director, Rural Physician Associate Program, Professor, Department of Family Practice and Community Health, University of Minnesota, Medical School, Minneapolis, Minnesota

Bruce H. Weber, Ph.D., Professor of Chemistry and Biochemistry, California State University, Fullerton, Fullerton, California

Raymond O. West, M.D., Adjunct Professor, Loma Linda University School of Health, Section of Epidemiology, Loma Linda, California

Larry D. Young, Ph.D., Assistant Professor of Psychology, Bowman Gray School of Medicine, Winston-Salem, North Carolina

Jared B. Zelman, M.D., F.A.A.F.P., Attending Physician in Emergency Medicine, Union Memorial Hospital, Clinical Assistant Professor, Department of Family Medicine, University of Maryland, School of Medicine, Baltimore, Maryland

David Zull, M.D., Associate Professor of Clinical Medicine, Northwestern University, School of Medicine, Chicago, Illinois

Preface

The Federation Licensing Examination (FLEX) is the gateway for licensure to practice medicine in every state in the United States, the District of Columbia, the Virgin Islands, Guam, and Saskatchewan. This Third Edition of *FLEX Review* offers the FLEX candidate an up-to-date, comprehensive review of all of the disciplines in which he/she will be tested. The book's structure mirrors that of the actual examination, with three distinct parts corresponding to Days I, II and III of FLEX. The questions presented are similar in format to actual exam questions and cover the content prescribed by the Federation of State Medical Boards of the United States. In each chapter, the questions are arranged by type to prepare you for the variety of question formats in current use.

Part I of this book contains 235 board-type questions, in each of the required basic science disciplines: anatomy, behavioral sciences, biochemistry, biostatistics/epidemiology, genetics, microbiology, pathology, pharmacology, and physiology. The answers, with explanatory comments and references to major textbooks, begin on page 85.

Part II includes 520 board-type questions, distributed across the clinical subjects of anesthesiology, emergency medicine, family medicine, internal medicine, medical ethics, neurology, obstetrics/gynecology, ophthalmology, otorhinolaryngology, pediatrics, preventive medicine, psychiatry, radiology, and surgery. Answers, explanations, and references for these chapters begin on page 309. Many of the questions in the clinical sciences are based on case histories and/or illustrative material.

Part III, like Day III — the clinical competence segment of FLEX—is divided into three sections: therapeutics, a multidisciplinary review of drug therapy comprising 25 multiple-choice questions; pictorial, a compilation of 30 practice questions based on a variety of illustrative materials intended to exercise clinical interpretive skills; and patient management problems. Explanatory answers and references for the first two sections begin on page 416. There are ten patient management problems: two each in medicine, obstetrics and gynecology, pediatrics, and surgery, and one each in psychiatry and radiology. Scoring, discussions, and references appear after the problems. A response section for marking the selected management steps appears at the back of the book. A special pen is included to reveal the information printed by a latent image process.

It is our hope that the candidate will find this material both informative and challenging, and that its use will render the familiarity with both subject and format needed to facilitate the path to licensure.

Acknowledgments

The Publisher would like to extend a special thank you to all of this volume's contributors. For this edition, a number of additional changes were required of those who had contributed to the second edition, and the new authors were given more detailed guidelines for preparation of material. Each author's enthusiasm and conscientiousness for his/her work was a great source of encouragement. A thank you, however, would not be complete without one being extended to the numerous educators who reviewed each section and rendered detailed, constructive criticisms. They, too, share in the joy of the finished product.

The Publisher would like to acknowledge the contributions of the following authors to previous editions of this volume:

Robert Abrams, M.D.	*Cornell University*
Majid Ali, M.D.	*Columbia University*
Craig W. Clarkson, Ph.D.	*University of California*
James E. Nininger, M.D.	*Cornell University*
Merwyn Peskin, M.D.	*Cornell University*
Robert E. Pieroni, M.D.	*University of Alabama*
Mary Katherine Shear, M.D.	*Cornell University*
John A. Talbott, M.D.	*Cornell University*
Robert E. Ten Eick, Ph.D.	*Northwestern University*

disclaimer

The authors have made every effort to thoroughly verify the answers to the questions which appear on the following pages. However, as in any text, some inaccuracies and ambiguities may occur; therefore, if in doubt, please consult your references.

The Publisher

FLEX
REVIEW

PART I

The material on the following pages is designed to help you prepare for Day I of the Federation Licensing Examination (FLEX). It includes a total of 235 board-type questions distributed over the required basic science subjects: anatomy, behavioral sciences, biochemistry, biostatistics/epidemiology, genetics, microbiology, pathology, pharmacology, and physiology. The answers with accompanying comments and page references to major textbooks begin on page 85. The reference list for Part I appears at the end of the answer section. The questions are a representative sampling of the topics in the Federation's content for Day I. They are grouped by question types to familiarize you with the variety of question formats you will see on the actual examination.

1

Anatomy
Sidney A. Cohn, Ph.D.

DIRECTIONS: Each of the questions or incomplete statements below is followed by five suggested answers or completions. Select the **one** that is best in each case.

1. The submandibular gland receives its parasympathetic innervation from a branch of which one of the following nerves?
   A. Maxillary
   B. Lingual
   C. Glossopharyngeal
   D. Facial
   E. Vagus

2. Each of the following structures traverses the adductor canal EXCEPT the
   A. femoral vein
   B. obturator nerve
   C. lower nerve to vastus medialis muscle
   D. femoral artery
   E. saphenous nerve

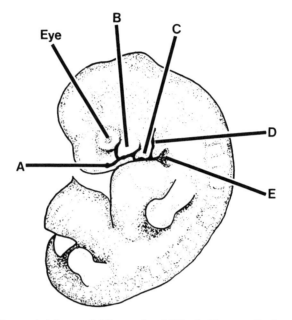

Figure 1.1 Lateral View of a 6-Week Human Embryo

3. Each of the lettered items in Fig. 1.1 is correctly associated with the following parts of a 6-week human embryo EXCEPT the
   A. nasal pit
   B. maxillary prominence
   C. third branchial arch
   D. hyomandibular cleft
   E. cervical sinus

4. The blood supply to the spleen is usually a *direct* branch of which one of the following arteries?
   A. Celiac
   B. Left gastric
   C. Common hepatic
   D. Superior mesenteric
   E. Abdominal aorta

5. The descending efferent fiber tracts of the hypothalamus contribute to the regulation of all the following EXCEPT
   A. rectal reflexes
   B. blood pressure
   C. proprioception
   D. body temperature
   E. sweating

6. Lesions involving lower motor neurons of the spinal cord result in all of the following skeletal muscle deficits EXCEPT
   A. loss of superficial abdominal reflexes
   B. loss of muscle tone
   C. loss of reflex activity
   D. muscle paralysis
   E. muscle atrophy

7. Each of the following functions is performed by the smooth endoplasmic reticulum EXCEPT
   A. lipid metabolism
   B. cholesterol synthesis
   C. secretion of chloride ions
   D. storage of calcium ions
   E. intercellular digestion

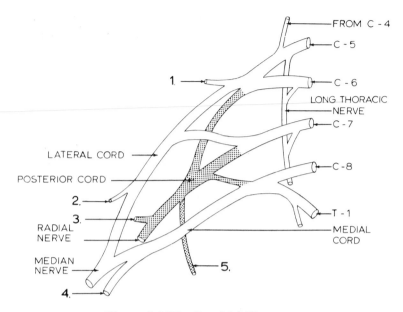

Figure 1.2 The Brachial Plexus

8. A lesion involving which one of the numbered structures in Fig. 1.2 of the brachial plexus would be expected to result in a paralysis of the deltoid and teres minor muscle?
   A. 1
   B. 2
   C. 3
   D. 4
   E. 5

DIRECTIONS: Each group of questions below consists of five lettered headings or a diagram with lettered components followed by a list of numbered words or statements. For **each** numbered word or statement, select the **one** lettered heading that is most closely associated with it. Each lettered heading may be selected once, more than once, or not at all.

Questions 9–11: For each organ, identify the type of epithelium associated with it.

  A. Pseudostratified columnar ciliated
  B. Simple cuboidal
  C. Simple columnar
  D. Transitional
  E. Stratified squamous

9. Urinary bladder

10. Esophagus

11. Cecum

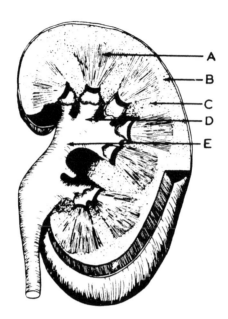

Figure 1.3

Questions 12–16 (refer to Fig. 1.3):

12. Major calyx

13. Medullary pyramid

14. Cortex

15. Renal column

16. Renal pelvis

DIRECTIONS: Each set of lettered headings below is followed by a list of numbered words or phrases. For each numbered word or phrase select

    A. if the item is associated with A *only*
    B. if the item is associated with B *only*
    C. if the item is associated with *both* A and B
    D. if the item is associated with *neither* A nor B

Questions 17–20:

    A. Ulnar nerve
    B. Median nerve
    C. Both
    D. Neither

17. Innervation of flexor carpi ulnaris muscle

18. Innervation of brachioradialis muscle

19. Innervation of flexor digitorum profundus muscle

20. Innervation of coracobrachialis muscle

DIRECTIONS: For each of the questions or incomplete statements below, **one or more** of the answers or completions given is correct. Select

    A. if only *1, 2, and 3* are correct
    B. if only *1 and 3* are correct
    C. if only *2 and 4* are correct
    D. if only *4* is correct
    E. if *all* are correct

Questions 21–23:

21. The superior cerebellar peduncle is formed by efferent axons that arise in the
    1. emboliform nucleus
    2. anterior spinocerebellar tract
    3. dentate nucleus
    4. pontine nucleus

22. Pseudostratified columnar ciliated epithelium can be found in the
    1. trachea
    2. larynx
    3. nose
    4. bronchus

23. Important mechanisms in the transport of materials across the placental membrane consist of
    1. pinocytosis
    2. facilitated diffusion
    3. active transport
    4. simple diffusion

DIRECTIONS: This section of the test consists of situations, each followed by a series of questions. Study each situation and select the **one** best answer to each question following it.

Questions 24 and 25: While doing a self-examination, a 52-year-old woman felt a lump in the lower lateral quadrant of her left breast. The woman's physician had her admitted to the hospital, where the lump was surgically removed. A frozen section showed it to be malignant.

24. The most likely pathway for the spread of this malignancy would first be to the
    A. pectoral group of axillary nodes
    B. supraclavicular nodes
    C. internal thoracic nodes
    D. apical axillary nodes
    E. lymph nodes in the anterior mediastinum

25. In doing a radical mastectomy the surgeon must identify and preserve two important motor nerves that are in the surgical field. One of these nerves is the thoracodorsal; the other is the
    A. second intercostal
    B. radial
    C. ulnar
    D. long thoracic
    E. intercostobrachial

2

Behavioral Sciences
Larry D. Young, Ph.D.

DIRECTIONS: Each of the questions or incomplete statements below is followed by five suggested answers or completions. Select the **one** that is best in each case.

---

26. Which of the following is detectable by the Guthrie test?
    A. Tay–Sachs disease
    B. Maple sugar urine disease
    C. Glycogen storage disease
    D. Gangliosidosis
    E. Phenylketonuria

27. At the end of which year of life is gender identity firmly established and not easily changed?
    A. First
    B. Second
    C. Third
    D. Fourth
    E. Fifth

28. Which of the following statements is NOT true of the narcolepsy syndrome?

A. It is also known as sleep paralysis and sleep attacks

B. It responds well to treatment with amphetamines

C. Hypnagogic hallucinations may occur

D. It has been found to be associated with an abnormally slow transition from the waking state to rapid eye movement sleep

E. It is also known as cataplexy

29. The person with an obsessive-compulsive personality would NOT be

A. irrational in his or her approach to life and its problems

B. cautious and deliberate

C. objective and honest

D. neat, orderly, and punctual

E. conscientious and reliable

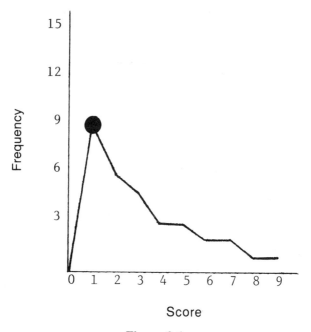

Figure 2.1

30. The point circled on the graph in Fig. 2.1 is known as the
    A. median
    B. mean
    C. mode
    D. range
    E. standard deviation

31. Individuals from low socioeconomic conditions
    A. have a low incidence of psychotic illness
    B. have a low probability of institutionalization
    C. tend to view most authority figures in the dominant society as agents of the established order
    D. have a lower incidence of a wide range of diseases
    E. are more likely to emphasize acceptance and equality than order and obedience in childrearing

32. Which of the following statements concerning extrapyramidal effects is NOT true?

A. Thioridazine produces fewer extrapyramidal effects than the other phenothiazines

B. Extrapyramidal effects are usually classified into three categories: Parkinsonian syndrome, dyskinesias, and akathisia

C. Bizarre involuntary motor movement is found

D. Extrapyramidal effects are peripheral nervous system effects

E. Haloperidol would cause more extrapyramidal effects than chlorpromazine

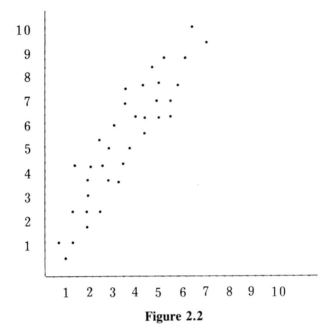

Figure 2.2

33. A study was done to test the hypothesis that abused children become child abusers. The findings were then plotted on the graph in Fig. 2.2. This graph shows
    A. low negative correlation
    B. low positive correlation
    C. no correlation
    D. high negative correlation
    E. high positive correlation

34. A patient is undergoing cancer chemotherapy that reliably produces nausea and vomiting. The patient encountered the nurse who administers his chemotherapy while at the post office and experienced nausea and emesis. In learning-theory terms, the nurse serves the function of
    A. an unconditioned stimulus
    B. a discriminative stimulus
    C. an operant
    D. a conditioned stimulus
    E. a neutral stimulus

35. All of the following effects are associated with amphetamines EXCEPT
A. mood elevation
B. increase in alertness
C. decreased sense of fatigue
D. an increase in motor and speech activity
E. poor performance of simple mental and physical tasks

36. Several clinical investigations have reported positive results in the treatment of alcoholic patients using chemical aversion procedures to produce a conditioned response of nausea and vomiting to the stimulus of alcohol. These studies have reported that the proportion of patients who remained abstinent for 1 year after treatment was
A. 85%
B. 75%
C. 60%
D. 35%
E. 10%

DIRECTIONS: Each group of questions below consists of lettered headings or a diagram with lettered components followed by a list of numbered words or statements. For **each** numbered word or statement, select the **one** lettered heading that is most closely associated with it. Each lettered heading may be selected once, more than once, or not at all.

Questions 37 and 38: A pooled sample of core schizophrenic patients was examined to determine their most frequently observed symptoms. Three of the reported symptoms are charted on the graph in Fig. 2.3. Match the numbered symptoms with the lettered frequency at which it would be expected to occur.

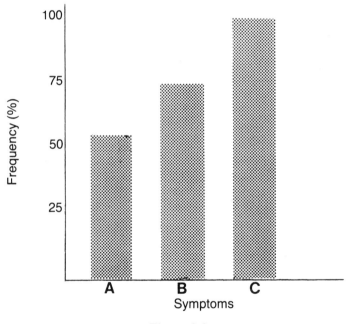

Figure 2.3

37. Auditory hallucinations

38. Thoughts spoken aloud

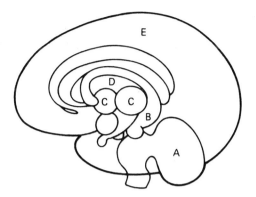

Figure 2.4

Questions 39–43 (refer to Fig. 2.4):

39. Cerebellum

40. Caudate nucleus

41. Thalamus

42. Hippocampus

43. Motor cortex

Questions 44 and 45:

    A. Sinequan
    B. Compazine

44. Doxepin

45. Prochlorperazine

20 / Part I

Questions 46–48:

    A. The perception of pain characteristic of Jews and Italians
    B. The perception of pain characteristic of the Irish
    C. The perception of pain characteristic of "Old Americans"

46. More often deny the existence of pain

47. Tend more often to express anxiety and other emotions and to be less precise in indicating the anatomic sites of the pain

48. Tend to be more matter of fact about the pain and describe its primary and secondary sites in intricate detail

---

DIRECTIONS: For each of the questions or incomplete statements below, **one or more** of the answers or completions given is correct. Select
    A if only *1, 2, and 3* are correct
    B if only *1 and 3* are correct
    C if only *2 and 4* are correct
    D if only *4* is correct
    E if *all* are correct

Questions 49–55:

49. Both the American Association of Mental Deficiency and DSM-III require the following for a definition of mental retardation:
    1. Subaverage intellectual functioning
    2. Onset occurring during or prior to adolescence
    3. Deficits or impairments in adaptive behavior
    4. Identifiable etiologic factors

50. Which of the following would NOT be characteristic of a patient suffering from a major affective episode?
    1. The subjective feeling of being slowed down, with the absence of observable psychomotor changes
    2. Marked changes in sleep pattern
    3. Long-lasting affective disorders with a gradual onset
    4. Fatigue

51. The factors that are associated with increased risk for suicide attempts and increased risk for completed suicides are slightly different. Statistically, which of the following groups would be at greatest risk for committing suicide?
    1. Men rather than women
    2. Blacks rather than whites
    3. Elderly rather than young adult
    4. Widowed rather than divorced

52. Experimental as well as clinical evidence indicates that fear
    1. is a slowly learned response
    2. can motivate the learning of new habits
    3. is extremely susceptible to extinction
    4. can be reduced by drugs

53. Which of the following would NOT be true regarding the behavior therapy technique of systematic desensitization?
    1. It involves repeatedly confronting the patient with the unconscious conflict that originally increased his/her anxiety
    2. It has been used successfully in the treatment of a variety of psychophysiologic disorders, such as dysmenorrhea and asthma
    3. It entails having the patient confront anxiety-provoking situations in full intensity for prolonged periods of time until the anxiety reaction is "extinguished"
    4. It involves the repeated, gradual exposure to anxiety-eliciting circumstances while in a psychophysiologic state of relaxation, a state that inhibits the experience of anxiety

54. Strategies proven useful in increasing compliance of patients with prescribed medical regimens include which of the following?

1. Providing written as well as verbal instructions
2. Reducing the complexity of the treatment regimen
3. Using special reminders and other behavior modification procedures
4. Using child-resistant pill containers

55. In some humans, REM-state deprivation leads to

1. increased anxiety
2. improved memory
3. increased hostility and irritability
4. decreased appetite

3

Biochemistry
Bruce H. Weber, Ph.D.

DIRECTIONS: Each of the questions or incomplete statements below is followed by five suggested answers or completions. Select the **one** that is best in each case.

---

56. Which of the following statements about aspartate transcarbamoylase, an allosteric enzyme, is FALSE?
    A. CTP shifts the enzyme toward an inactive conformation
    B. CTP has no effect on V_{max} of the enzyme
    C. CTP lowers the apparent K_m of the enzyme for aspartate
    D. The catalytic subunit binds the regulatory subunit in a 1:1 ratio
    E. ATP reverses the effects of CTP

57. Met-enkephalin and Leu-enkephalin have the following amino acid sequences:

    ^+H_3N-Tyr-Gly-Gly-Phe-Met-COO$^-$ Met-enkephalin
    H_3^+N-Try-Gly-Gly-Phe-Leu-COO$^-$ Leu-enkephalin

    Which of the following methods would separate the two?
    A. Sodium dodecyl sulfate–polyacrylamide gel electrophoresis
    B. Paper electrophoresis at pH 6
    C. Butanol–acetic acid–water paper chromatography
    D. Ammonium sulfate precipitation
    E. Gel filtration

58. Cyclic AMP affects glycogen metabolism in muscle by stimulating
   A. phosphorylation of glycogen synthetase and glycogen phosphorylase
   B. dephosphorylation of a glycogen synthetase and glycogen phosphorylase
   C. phosphorylation of glycogen synthetase and dephosphorylation of glycogen phosphorylase
   D. dephosphorylation of glycogen synthetase and phosphorylation of glycogen synthetase
   E. glucose-6-phosphatase

59. The chemiosmotic theory of oxidative phosphorylation uniquely explains how
   A. the mitochondrial protein F_1 has ATPase activity
   B. three ATP molecules are synthesized for each molecule of NADH that reduces $\frac{1}{2}$ O_2
   C. 2,4-dinitrophenol prevents phosphorylation by dissipating the protein gradient across the mitochondrial inner membrane
   D. a phosphate residue on a mitochondrial protein F_1 is transferred to ADP
   E. mitochondria couple fatty acid oxidation to electron transport

60. Which of the following mixtures for the assay of ATP is NOT appropriate? All the listed components are present in excess. Each assay is based on the increase in reduced pyridine nucleotide.
   A. Glucose-6-phosphate dehydrogenase, hexokinase, glucose, NADP
   B. Hexokinase, lactate dehydrogenase, pyruvate kinase, glucose, phosphoenolpyruvate, NAD
   C. Acetyl-coenzyme A synthetase, aconitase, citrate synthetase, isocitrate dehydrogenase, acetate, coenzyme A, oxaloacetate, NADP
   D. Glycerol phosphate dehydrogenase, glycerokinase, glycerol, NAD
   E. Aldolase, glyceraldehyde phosphate dehydrogenase, phosphofructokinase, phosphoglycerate kinase, fructose-6-phosphate, NAD

61. The enzymes that synthesize oxaloacetate from pyruvate and malonyl-CoA from acetyl-CoA are both
    A. pyridoxal phosphate dependent
    B. biotin dependent
    C. flavoproteins
    D. metalloproteins
    E. tetrahydrofolate dependent

62. Which of the following statements is NOT true about enzymes that exhibit Michaelis–Menten kinetics?
    A. The rate of breakdown of ES equals the rate of formation of ES
    B. K_m is equal to K_d (the dissociation constant for ES)
    C. Initial velocities are used, so that the back reaction ($P \rightarrow S$) can be ignored
    D. V_{max} depends both on k_{cat} and on the concentration of the enzyme
    E. The conversion of substrate to product is assumed to be the rate-limiting step

63. Both pH and the concentration of 2,3-diphosphoglycerate (DPG) affect the oxygen affinity as measured by P_{50} of hemoglobin. The pH effect is due to the Bohr effect and the DPG effect involves stabilization of the T or deoxy form of hemoglobin. Which of the following statements is true?
    A. An increase in pH would increase P_{50} and an increase in [DPG] would increase P_{50}
    B. An increase in pH would increase P_{50} and an increase in [DPG] would decrease P_{50}
    C. An increase in pH would decrease P_{50} and an increase in [DPG] would increase P_{50}
    D. An increase in pH would decrease P_{50} and an increase in [DPG] would decrease P_{50}
    E. An increase in pH would increase P_{50}, but an increase in [DPG] would not affect P_{50}

64. The molecular defect in most cases of familial hypercholesterolemia is
  A. deficiency of functional LDL receptors
  B. deficiency of functional LDL
  C. deficiency of functional 3-hydroxy-3-methylglutaryl reductase
  D. deficiency of functional acyl-CoA cholesterol acyltransferase
  E. deficiency of functional HDL

65. Net synthesis of glucose can occur in mammalian liver from which of the following?
  A. Ethanol
  B. Even-numbered-carbon fatty acids
  C. Odd-numbered-carbon fatty acids
  D. Acetate
  E. Acetyl-CoA

66. Which of the following statements is NOT true about phosphofructokinase (PFK)?
  A. ATP serves both as a substrate and an inhibitor
  B. A decrease in energy charge will increase PFK activity
  C. Citrate is an inhibitor of PFK activity
  D. Changes in PFK activity are reflected by changes in [NADH]
  E. The reaction catalyzed by PFK can be reversed by high [AMP] during gluconeogenesis

67. Under which of the following conditions does the pentose shunt NOT produce any CO_2 in the conversion of glucose-6-phosphate to ribose-5-phosphate?

A. Much more ribose-5-phosphate than NADPH is required

B. There is a nearly equal need for ribose-5-phosphate and NADPH

C. Much more NADPH is required than ribose-5-phosphate, but no ATP is needed

D. Much more NADPH is required than ribose-5-phosphate and ATP is needed

E. None of the above, since CO_2 must always be produced when glucose-6-phosphate is converted to ribose-5-phosphate

68. At what point, and how much, label will appear in CO_2 from pyruvate labeled with ^{14}C in the third carbon,

$$\overset{\displaystyle O}{\overset{\displaystyle ||}{^{14}CH_3\,C\text{-}COO^-}}$$

provided as the sole carbon source to a suspension of mitochondria?

A. All the ^{14}C appears as CO_2 from the pyruvate dehydrodrogenase reaction before any resulting acetyl-CoA can enter the Krebs cycle

B. All the ^{14}C appears as CO_2 during the first turn of the Krebs cycle

C. No ^{14}C appears as CO_2 during the first turn of the Krebs cycle, but all of the ^{14}C appears as CO_2 during the second turn of the Krebs cycle

D. No ^{14}C appears as CO_2 during the first turn of the Krebs cycle and only 50% of the ^{14}C appears as CO_2 during the second turn of the cycle

E. No ^{14}C appears as CO_2 during either the first or the second turn of the Krebs cycle

69. Uniformly ^{14}C-labeled histidine is provided in the diet of guinea pigs and the appearance of ^{14}C label in Pro, Phe, GTP, and CTP is monitored. Label will appear in
  A. Pro, Phe, GTP, and CTP
  B. Pro, GTP, and CTP, but not in Phe
  C. GTP and CTP, but not in Pro or Phe
  D. Pro, Phe, and GTP, but not in CTP
  E. Pro and ATP, but not in Phe or CTP

70. The inborn error of metabolism known as branched-chain ketoaciduria, or "maple syrup disease," involves a defect in the metabolism in
  A. isoleucine
  B. isoleucine, methionine, threonine, and valine
  C. isoleucine, leucine, and valine
  D. leucine
  E. phenylalanine

71. Which of the following statements describes the course of some β-thalassemias?
  A. There is a point mutation in the $β_6$ position that converts Glu to Val
  B. There is a point mutation in one of the intron or splice function regions of the β-hemoglobin gene
  C. There is a point mutation in one of the exon regions of the β-hemoglobin gene
  D. There is a point mutation in the β-hemoglobin repressor
  E. There is an insertion of 21 codons in the β-hemoglobin gene

DIRECTIONS: The group of questions below consists of five lettered headings followed by a list of numbered words or statements. For **each** numbered word or statement, select the **one** lettered heading that is most closely associated with it. Each lettered heading may be selected once, more than once, or not at all.

Questions 72–76:

    A. Pyridoxamine
    B. Coenzyme Q
    C. Glucose-1-phosphate
    D. Thiamine pyrophosphate
    E. Geranyl pyrophosphate

72. Glycogen metabolism

73. Cholesterol biosynthesis

74. Transamination reactions

75. Electron transport

76. Pyruvate dehydrogenase

DIRECTIONS: For each of the questions or incomplete statements below, **one or more** of the answers or completions given is correct. Select

    A if only *1, 2, and 3* are correct
    B if only *1 and 3* are correct
    C if only *2 and 4* are correct
    D if only *4* is correct
    E if *all* are correct

Questions 77–80:

77.   Below is a representation of a segment of double-stranded DNA molecule:

    $...$C A T^{1}G G^2 A C G T C C G A T T$...$
    $...$G T A C C T$_3$G C A$_4$ G G C T A A$...$

    Restriction endonucleases have a specificity that allows them to attack the bonds at
    1. position 1
    2. position 2
    3. position 3
    4. position 4

78.   Figure 3.1 gives two representations of Michaelis–Menten enzyme kinetics, showing the dependence of rate v on substrate concentration S. The relations among the characteristics of these representations are such that
    1. $a = 1/e$
    2. $d = -1/c$
    3. $f = c/a$
    4. $e = 2b$

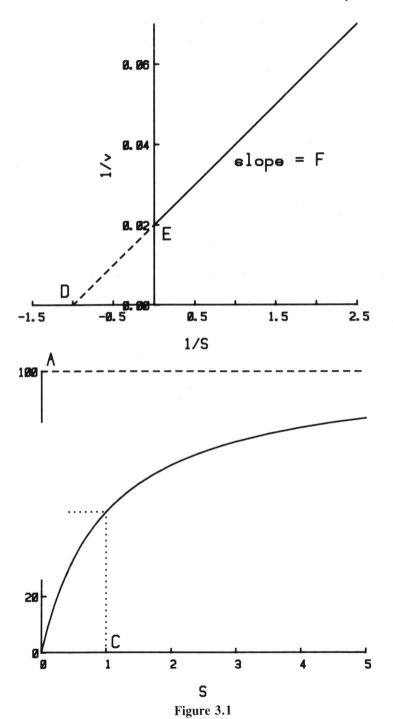

Figure 3.1

79. The differences between fatty acid oxidation and fatty acid synthesis include:
1. Oxidation occurs in the mitochondria, and synthesis in the cytosol
2. Synthesis depends upon carnitine and oxidation does not
3. Oxidation uses a flavine-linked dehydrogenase, and synthesis uses a triphosphopyridine nucleotide-linked dehydrogenase
4. In oxidation the γ,β-unsaturated fatty acyl thioester has the *cis* configuration, but in synthesis it has the *trans* configuration

80. Prostaglandins
1. are derived from arachidonic acid
2. have short half-lives *in vivo*
3. are catabolized in the lung
4. exert effects through cAMP

4

Biostatistics/Epidemiology

Department of Epidemiology and Preventive Medicine
University of Maryland School of Medicine

Irving I. Kessler, M.D.
Chairman

DIRECTIONS: Each of the questions or incomplete statements below is followed by five suggested answers or completions. Select the **one** that is best in each case.

81. An investigator plans to estimate the proportion of elderly women in a retirement community who take estrogen. It is determined that a sample of 100 will be required to be accurate to within 10 percentage points with 95% confidence. To be accurate to within 5 percentage points with 95% confidence would require a sample size of
   A. 25
   B. 50
   C. 100
   D. 200
   E. 400

82. A blood pressure screening program refers for further evaluation anyone whose diastolic blood pressure is above the 90th percentile for people of the same age and sex. If five people are screened, what is the probability that at least one will be referred for further evaluation?
   A. 0.10
   B. 0.90
   C. $(0.10)^5$
   D. $(0.90)^5$
   E. $1 - (0.90)^5$

83. During any given year, 10% of those with Disease X will die from it. In the population, ten in 100,000 will have Disease X during a given year. What is the probability that a person, chosen at random from the population, will die of Disease X in a given year?
   A. One in 100,000
   B. Ten in 100,000
   C. One hundred in 100,000
   D. One thousand in 100,000
   E. Ten thousand in 100,000

84. People with high levels of plasma high-density lipoprotein (HDL) cholesterol have been found to be at low risk for coronary heart disease. Factors associated with plasma HDL cholesterol were sought in a study of 293 healthy men. The following table shows the correlation coefficient and the p value associated with a test of zero correlation for plasma HDL cholesterol and each of the variables listed. All observations were taken at the same time for each of 293 participants.

	r	p
Plasma triglyceride	−0.42	<.001
Alcohol intake	0.24	<.001
Serum glucose	−0.19	<.001
Body mass index	−0.11	<.05
Diastolic blood pressure	0.04	>.05

Of the variables studied, the best apparent predictor of plasma HDL cholesterol level is
A. plasma triglyceride
B. alcohol intake
C. serum glucose
D. body mass index
E. diastolic blood pressure

85. Investigators would like to know whether air pollution is more difficult to control in coastal regions or in regions farther inland. Ten urban areas, five classified as coastal and five as inland, were monitored closely during a recent year. Of the five coastal areas, two were found to be within standards set by the Environmental Protection Agency (EPA); of the five inland areas, four were within EPA standards. The following table gives exact probabilities of various chance outcomes in this study:

Coastal areas		Inland areas		Probability of chance occurrence
Within EPA standards	Not within standards	Within EPA standards	Not within standards	
1	4	5	0	0.0238
2	3	4	1	0.2381
3	2	3	2	0.4762
4	1	2	3	0.2381
5	0	1	4	0.0238

The exact P-value for a two-tailed test would be reported as
A. 0.0238
B. 0.0476
C. 0.2381
D. 0.4762
E. 0.5238

86. A pharmaceutical company is developing a screening program for new drugs. First, the efficacy of each new drug is to be compared with that of a standard drug in a small-scale animal experiment. At the end of this experiment one of two actions will be taken; either (1) the new drug will be discarded, or (2) the new drug will be submitted for more extensive evaluation. Action 2 is to be taken when the improvement in efficacy over the standard drug is statistically significant at the 10% level (one-tailed); action 1 will be taken otherwise. The experiments will be large enough to enable the detection of a 15% increase in efficacy with 80% power at the 10% significance level using a one-tailed test. In the long run, of the new drugs that provide a 15% increase in efficacy over the standard drug, the proportion that are discarded will be

A. 10%
B. 15%
C. 20%
D. 80%
E. unknown

87. A 47-year-old construction worker has been involved in the demolition of painted steel structures. He has been cutting sections with a blow torch for disposal. For the past several weeks he has complained of fatigue, headache, sleeplessness, and muscle and joint pain: He most likely

A. has a severe case of the "flu"
B. is suffering from nervous tension and stress
C. has been exposed to lead
D. exhibits classical symptoms of mercury intoxication
E. is malingering

88. Aplastic anemias occur infrequently (0.5–1.0 case per 10,000 population per year). Approximately one-half of these cases are idiopathic and half are secondary. Of the latter, over 40% are due to the use of chloramphenicol. Three other agents have been shown to cause aplasia on a dose-dependent basis. These are ionizing radiation, alkylating agents, and
   A. *bis*-chloromethyl ether
   B. benzene
   C. toluene
   D. ethylene oxide
   E. polychlorinated biphenyls (PCBs)

89. Chlorinated hydrocarbons such as DDT, dieldrin, and chlordane have frequently been used as pesticides. These compounds affect the central nervous system, and may also affect the liver in that they tend to be mixed-function oxidase inducers. These compounds
   A. are easily degradable in the environment
   B. tend to be acutely toxic
   C. are preferentially stored in body fat
   D. are well-absorbed through the skin
   E. are of little environmental consequence

90. Hearing loss results from long-term exposure to industrial noise. The pathologic changes occur slowly, depending on intensity, frequency, and duration of exposure. A temporary threshold shift or loss of hearing is greatest shortly after exposure and improves gradually if the noise has not been too loud or lasted too long. With repeated exposure, hearing acuity does not return to its original level and a permanent threshold shift results. Which of the following statements is true?

   A. This hearing loss affects a frequency range centering around 4000 Hz
   B. This loss is noticed by the worker soon after onset
   C. This hearing loss "notch" varies according to the nature of the noise exposure
   D. Mechanical forces affecting the middle ear ossicles result in noise-induced hearing loss
   E. As hearing loss develops, the worker is unable to hear speech, but retains the ability to discriminate consonants

91. A proportional mortality study of four fatal cases of angiosarcoma of the liver provided the link to vinyl chloride production. Proportional mortality ratios (PMR) allow comparisons to be made when death certificates are available, but complete information on the population at risk is not. One potential problem with PMR is incomplete ascertainment of death certificates. Which of the following statements is true?

   A. Another potential problem is the known poor quality of death certificates
   B. A high ratio of observed to expected deaths may be due to an excess of one cause of death or a deficit of another
   C. PMRs are relatively easy and inexpensive to perform
   D. PMRs are based upon a comparison of ratios
   E. Case–control studies are more effective than prospective studies

92. A classification scheme for interpreting x-rays of occupational lung diseases has been developed and revised by the ILO. This classification was originally intended for use only in epidemiologic studies, but has evolved to provide assistance in clinical evaluation and compensation. This classification
   A. is intended as a diagnostic tool for asbestosis
   B. is intended only to codify opacities and not to define pathologic changes
   C. is intended for use without comparison to standard films
   D. classifies by profusion, but not shape, size, or extent of opacities
   E. uses the notation 0/1 or 1/0 to diagnose silicosis

93. Which of the following attributes best distinguishes an experimental study from an observational study?
   A. The inclusion of treated patients
   B. The inclusion of untreated patients
   C. Blind evaluation of endpoints
   D. Adjustment for covariables
   E. Intervention by the investigator

94. Which one of the following is not regarded as a criterion for the assessment of causality?
   A. Consistency
   B. Strength
   C. Sensitivity
   D. Temporal relationship
   E. Coherence

DIRECTIONS: For each of the questions or incomplete statements below, **one or more** of the answers or completions given is correct. Select

    A   if only *1, 2, and 3* are correct
    B   if only *1 and 3* are correct
    C   if only *2 and 4* are correct
    D   if only *4* is correct
    E   if *all* are correct

Questions 95–105:

95. The health situation of the aged population is characterized by
    1. decrease in acute conditions
    2. increase in chronic conditions
    3. increase in disability resulting from illness
    4. increase in acute conditions

96. The psychiatric status of the older population (aged 65 +) is best described by which of the following?
    1. The most prevalent psychiatric conditions are dementia and schizophrenia
    2. The most prevalent conditions are dementia and depression
    3. The prevalence of dementia in community-resident aged is on the order of 25%
    4. The prevalence of dementia in community-resident aged is on the order of 5%

97. The situation of the aged with regard to nursing home utilization is accurately described by which of the following?
    1. Twenty-five percent of the aged are institutionalized in nursing homes at any given time
    2. Minorities are overrepresented in nursing homes
    3. The elderly prefer nursing homes to all other forms of care
    4. Five percent of the aged are institutionalized in nursing homes at any given time

98. The inverse relationship between socioeconomic status and psychiatric disorder is well established. The explanation for this is less clear. Which of the following explanations would be likely?
   1. Child-rearing practices associated with lower socioeconomic conditions may contribute to mental disorder
   2. Stresses related to lower socioeconomic conditions may lead to mental disorder
   3. Individuals may move downward in socioeconomic status after an episode of psychiatric disorder
   4. Mental impairment hinders one's ability to attain higher socioeconomic status

99. A comprehensive health-behavior change program will include which of the following aspects?
   1. An external support system from disinterested individuals
   2. Analysis of the behavioral sequence
   3. Development of a negative feedback system
   4. Self-monitoring

100. Federal regulatory approaches for containment of health costs included which of the following?
   1. Generic Drug Program
   2. Economic Stabilization Program
   3. Prospective Medicaid Physician Requirement
   4. Certificate of Need (CON) Requirement

101. Smokers have an increased relative risk of
   1. Parkinson's disease
   2. coronary heart disease
   3. endometrial cancer
   4. bladder cancer

Directions Summarized

A	B	C	D	E
1, 2, 3	1, 3	2, 4	4	All are
only	only	only	only	correct

102. Which of the following pieces of information is necessary to calculate the positive predictive value of a screening test for a given disease?
    1. Sensitivity
    2. Specificity
    3. Prevalence
    4. Incidence

103. Advantages of cohort (prospective) studies over case–control (retrospective) studies include
    1. direct measurement of incidence
    2. elimination of recall bias
    3. concurrent study of a number of diseases
    4. applicability to all diseases

104. Which of the following will increase the prevalence of a given chronic disease (other things being equal)?
    1. Increased incidence
    2. Reduced case-fatality
    3. Increased duration of the disease
    4. Reduced incidence

105. The primary prevention of a disease may entail intervention
    1. before the disease occurs
    2. after risk factors develop
    3. before the risk factors develop
    4. after the disease occurs

5

Genetics

Lawrence R. Shapiro, M.D.

DIRECTIONS: Each of the questions or incomplete statements below is followed by four or five suggested answers or completions. Select the **one** that is best in each case.

---

106. Neural tube defects are inherited according to which mode of inheritance?
  A. Autosomal dominant
  B. Autosomal recessive
  C. X-linked recessive
  D. Polygenic/multifactorial
  E. Not inherited

107. A buccal smear reveals three sex-chromatin masses. One can conclude that this individual
  A. is 48,XXXX
  B. is 49,XXXXY
  C. is a male
  D. is female
  E. has four X chromosomes

108. The procedure of amniocentesis for prenatal diagnosis has
A. no risks
B. a risk of 1/4–1/2%
C. a risk of 1%
D. a risk of 3–5%

109. An individual has ambiguous genitalia, ovo-testes on gonadal biopsy, and a 46,XX chromosome constitution. This patient
A. is a female pseudohermaphrodite
B. is a male pseudohermaphrodite
C. is a true hermaphrodite
D. has testicular feminization syndrome

DIRECTIONS: Each of the following incomplete statements is followed by two suggested completions. Select one
A if the statement is completed by A *only*
B if the statement is completed by B *only*
C if the statement is completed by *both* A and B
D if the statement is completed by *neither* A nor B

Questions 110–117:

110. Mitotic nondisjunction
A. can account for a 45,X/46,XY mosaic
B. occurs with increasing frequency with advancing maternal age
C. both
D. neither

111. A 25-year-old woman gives birth to a child with trisomy 21 Down's syndrome. Her risk for recurrence for another child with Down's syndrome is
A. 1:5 (20%)
B. 1:100 (1%)
C. both
D. neither

112. A ring chromosome results in phenotypic abnormality because of
   A. duplication of genetic material
   B. deletion of genetic material
   C. both
   D. neither

113. A point mutation with amino acid substitution accounts for
   A. hemoglobin S disease
   B. β-thalassemia
   C. both
   D. neither

114. Criteria for X-linked recessive disorders include:
   A. The incidence of the disorder is much higher in males than females
   B. The disorder is never transmitted directly from father to son
   C. Both
   D. Neither

115. Criteria for autosomal recessive inheritance include:
   A. On the average, autosomal recessive disorders are transmitted by an affected person to half his or her children
   B. Males and females are equally likely to have autosomal recessive disorders
   C. Both
   D. Neither

116. Criteria for polygenic inheritance include:
   A. The incidence of a polygenic disorder may be higher in one sex than the other
   B. The risk of recurrence is higher when more than one member of a family is affected
   C. Both
   D. Neither

117. Two genetic loci are linked if
    A. each genetic locus is on the same chromosome
    B. recombination of alleles at each locus is less than 50%
    C. both
    D. neither

DIRECTIONS: For each of the incomplete statements below, **one or more** of the completions given is correct. Select

    A   if only *1, 2, and 3* are correct
    B   if only *1 and 3* are correct
    C   if only *2 and 4* are correct
    D   if only *4* is correct
    E   if *all* are correct

Questions 118–129:

118. The Philadelphia chromosome
    1. is present at birth
    2. is found in myelocytes
    3. persists in remission
    4. results from a t(9q;22q)

119. A newborn female with lymphedema would most likely have
    1. mental retardation
    2. normal external genitalia
    3. ultimate normal stature
    4. 45,X

120. For an individual with a 45,X/47,XYY mosaicism
    1. the external genitalia could be male or female
    2. the gonads could contain testicular elements and should be removed if intra-abdominal
    3. the cause is mitotic nondysjunction
    4. the cause is anaphase lag

121. The fragile X chromosome is associated with
    1. induction of the fragile site by a folate-deficient tissue culture medium
    2. mental retardation
    3. characteristic face and ear appearance in affected males
    4. X-linked recessive inheritance with an unexplained excess of affected females

122. Lyonization
    1. occurs at 16–19 days of embryogenesis
    2. is random
    3. accounts for the sex-chromatin mass
    4. accounts for the interphase Y body

123. A restriction nuclease is
    1. an enzyme that can be used in prenatal diagnosis of hemoglobinopathies
    2. an enzyme that cleaves DNA at specific sites
    3. an enzyme that produces restriction length fragment polymorphisms
    4. bacterial in origin

124. Stable gene and genotype frequencies result from
    1. selection favoring heterozygotes
    2. genetic isolation
    3. Hardy–Weinberg equilibrium
    4. migration

125. Somatic cell hybrids are useful for
    1. gene mapping studies
    2. complementation studies
    3. studies of mutations in cell culture
    4. studies of differentiated cell function

126. Thalassemia screening is appropriate for
    1. Italians
    2. Asians
    3. Mexicans
    4. Greeks

127. Amniocentesis for prenatal diagnosis is indicated by
  1. advanced maternal age
  2. a previous child with hydrocephaly
  3. a previous child with anencephaly
  4. consanguineous parents

128. Prenatal chromosome diagnosis reveals a fetus with an abnormal long arm of number 3 chromosome. Chromosome analysis of either parent could reveal
  1. normal results
  2. a balanced reciprocal translocation
  3. a paracentric inversion
  4. a balanced centric fusion translocation

129. Conjoined twins
  1. are monozygotic
  2. result from the fusion of dizygotic twins
  3. result from very late cleavage
  4. result from uterine abnormalities

130. In *monozygotic* twins concordant for Down's syndrome
  1. both parents could be normal
  2. meiotic nondisjunction could be responsible
  3. either parent could be a balanced translocation carrier
  4. mitotic nondisjunction could be responsible

6

Microbiology
Charles W. Kim, Ph.D.

DIRECTIONS: Each of the questions or incomplete statements below is followed by five suggested answers or completions. Select the **one** that is best in each case.

---

131. Which of the following statements does NOT describe the production of monoclonal hybridoma antibodies?
    A. Splenic B lymphocytes from immunized mouse or rat are used for fusion
    B. Cells from a mutant plasmacytoma lacking the gene for hypoxanthine-guanine phosphoribosyltransferase (HGPRT) are used for fusion
    C. The unfused splenocytes continue to live in the culture
    D. Fused cells express the HGPRT gene
    E. Fused cells also express products of the immunoglobulin genes of B lymphocytes

132. Which of the following statements is true of babesiosis?
    A. It is a flea-borne protozoan infection
    B. It is exclusively a human infection
    C. It has been observed only in splenectomized individuals
    D. The etiologic agent is a small protozoan
    E. Most of the recognized infections have occurred on the West Coast of the United States

133. Which of the following classes of antibody is formed nearly always early and at low levels in an immune response?
A. IgA
B. IgG
C. IgM
D. IgD
E. IgE

134. Interferons
A. are virus-specific
B. are cell-specific
C. are produced in large amounts
D. consist of highly unstable proteins at low pH
E. are highly sensitive to heat

135. In terms of timing, with which of the following types of reaction can delayed skin-type reactions be confused?
A. Cutaneous anaphylaxis
B. Generalized anaphylaxis
C. Prausnitz-Küstner (PK)
D. Arthus
E. Serum sickness

136. All of the following statements referring to hepatitis virus A (HAV) infection are correct EXCEPT
A. distribution of hepatitis A is worldwide
B. HAV infection appears to be spread by fecal–oral route
C. HAV infection is never transmitted parenterally
D. jaundice may be the first sign of HAV infection
E. antibody level rises quickly and remains elevated for at least 10 years after recovery

137. Which of the following statements concerning *Chlamydia psittaci* infection is correct?
    A. Psittacosis refers to all human infections caused by *C. psittaci*
    B. Ornithosis refers to animal infections caused by *C. psittaci*
    C. Psittacosis is clinically distinguishable from ornithosis
    D. Respiratory tract is the main portal of entry
    E. All cases give a clear history of exposure to psittacine birds

138. Which of the following stages of syphilitic lesions contains large numbers of spirochetes (especially in the mucous membranes) and when located on exposed surfaces is highly infectious?
    A. Primary
    B. Secondary
    C. Tertiary
    D. Congenital
    E. Late

139. Transplants from one region to another in the same individual are known as
    A. heterografts
    B. autografts
    C. isografts
    D. allografts
    E. xenografts

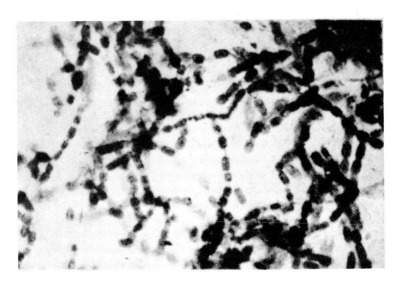

Figure 6.1

140. Figure 6.1 shows a microscopic examination of cultures in which the hyphae of *Coccidioides immitis* broaden and break up into numerous thick-walled, rectangular or ellipsoidal
   A. blastospores
   B. chlamydospores
   C. arthrospores
   D. sporangiospores
   E. ascospores

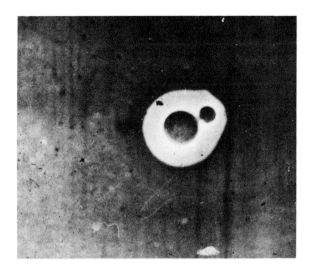

Figure 6.2

141. The yeastlike organism shown in Fig. 6.2 reproduces by budding in culture and in tissue, and is surrounded by a wide, gelatinous capsule. It is
    A. *Paracoccidioides brasiliensis*
    B. *Cryptococcus neoformans*
    C. *Sporothrix schenckii*
    D. *Blastomyces dermatitidis*
    E. *Histoplasma capsulatum*

142. Which of the following statements concerning IgA is correct?
    A. It accounts for about 50% of total immunoglobulins in human serum
    B. It is the principal immunoglobulin in exocrine secretions
    C. It occurs only as monomers
    D. Its molecular weight is about 900,000 daltons
    E. None of the above

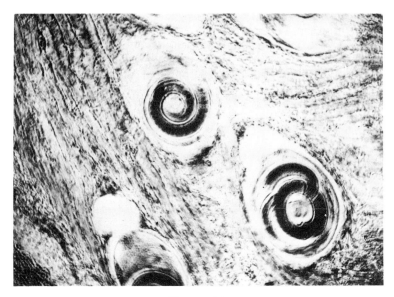

Figure 6.3

143. The larvae of a nematode shown in Fig. 6.3 encyst only in striated muscles. They are the larvae of
    A. *Strongyloides stercoralis*
    B. *Trichinella spiralis*
    C. *Ascaris lumbricoides*
    D. *Taenia solium*
    E. *Necator americanus*

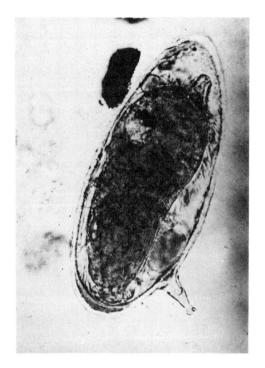

Figure 6.4

144. The egg of a bloodfluke shown in Fig. 6.4 measues 115–174 μm × 45–70 μm and is characterized by a prominent lateral spine. It is recovered from patients infected with
   A. *Schistosoma haematobium*
   B. *Schistosoma mansoni*
   C. *Schistosoma japonicum*
   D. *Fasciola hepatica*
   E. *Fasciolopsis buski*

145. *Campylobacter*
   A. are gram-negative and curved
   B. are nonmotile
   C. comprise many human pathogens
   D. infections are rare in animals
   E. are difficult to isolate due to lack of selective media

DIRECTIONS: The group of questions below consists of five lettered headings followed by a list of numbered words or statements. For **each** numbered word or statement, select the **one** lettered heading that is most closely associated with it. Each lettered heading may be selected once, more than once, or not at all.

Questions 146–150:

    A. *Clostridium tetani*
    B. *Haemophilus influenzae*
    C. *Proteus vulgaris*
    D. *Pseudomonas aeruginosa*
    E. *Bacillus anthracis*

146. V and X factors

147. "Swarming"

148. Spore with "drumstick" appearance

149. "String-of-pearls" reaction

150. Pyocyanin

DIRECTIONS: For each of the questions or incomplete statements below, **one or more** of the answers or completions given is correct. Select

A   if only *1, 2, and 3* are correct
B   if only *1 and 3* are correct
C   if only *2 and 4* are correct
D   if only *4* is correct
E   if *all* are correct

Questions 151–160:

151.   Immunologic abnormalities found in AIDS include
1. absence of delayed hypersensitivity
2. absolute lymphopenia
3. reduction in T helper cells
4. increased lymphocyte responses to mitogens

152.   Cryptosporidiosis
1. is caused by *Cryptosporidium* sp., a coccidium
2. is a self-limiting gastrointestinal infection in normal individuals
3. can be severe in immunocompromised patients with chronic, profuse, watery diarrhea
4. can be diagnosed by demonstrating the oocysts in the stool

153.   With regard to retroviruses,
1. their genome consists of two identical plus-stranded RNA molecules
2. their genome consists of single-stranded DNA molecules
3. glycoproteins make up the envelope spikes
4. they are all morphologically identical

Directions Summarized

A	B	C	D	E
1, 2, 3	1, 3	2, 4	4	All are
only	only	only	only	correct

154. With regard to *Pneumocystis* pneumonia,
1. the usual mode of acquisition of *Pneumocystis carinii* is airborne
2. there is a definite correlation between immunoglobulin levels and infection in infants and adults
3. the sporadic form is five times more common in the first year of life than at any other age
4. *Pneumocystis carinii* can be easily cultivated *in vitro*

155. Herpes simplex virus type 2 (HSV-2)
1. is morphologically indistinguishable from HSV-1
2. can be distinguished from HSV-1 on an antigenic basis
3. infections do not generally occur before puberty
4. infection is a function of sexual activity

156. In Legionnaires' disease
1. there is an incubation period of 2–10 days
2. fever is absent
3. cough, dyspnea, and chest pain are present
4. diarrhea is not present

157. Concerning influenza A,
1. it is the least virulent of types A, B, and C
2. periodically, one or both of its surface antigens changes subtype
3. it occurs exclusively in humans
4. influenza A strains in animals may provide a source of new antigenic subtypes for human influenza A viruses

158. Herpes zoster
1. is a generalized disease
2. occurs most frequently in the older age group
3. is a primary exogenous VZV infection
4. is caused by the varicella-zoster virus

159. *Klebsiella pneumoniae*
1. is never found in the respiratory tract of healthy individuals
2. causes approximately 3% of all acute bacterial pneumonias
3. has virulent unencapsulated (R) strains
4. is found in the feces of 5–10% of healthy individuals

160. Cytomegalovirus (CMV)
1. is the most common cause of congenital viral infection
2. is seasonal in its prevalence
3. is an important pathogen in post-bone marrow-transplant patients
4. is not likely to be venereally transmitted

7
Pathology
A. Olusegun Fayemi, M.D.

DIRECTIONS: Each of the questions or incomplete statements below is followed by five suggested answers or completions. Select the **one** that is best in each case.

161. Amyloid deposits may be encountered in all of the following EXCEPT
    A. familial Mediterranean fever
    B. multiple myeloma
    C. medullary carcinoma of the thyroid
    D. medullary carcinoma of the breast
    E. rheumatoid arthritis

162. During the early stages of the inflammatory process, which of the following chemical mediators most probably is responsible for vasodilatation and fever?
    A. Kinnins
    B. C3a and C5
    C. Leukotriene B4
    D. Prostaglandins
    E. Histamine

163. Which of the following features is NOT associated with Klinefelter's syndrome?
    A. 47,XXY or 46XY/47,XXY karyotype
    B. Elevated serum follicle-stimulating hormone
    C. Low serum testosterone
    D. Severe mental retardation
    E. Hypogonadism

164. Which of the following histocompatibility antigens has un-equivocally been associated with ankylosing spondylitis and postinfectious arthropathies?
    A. HLA-D/DR
    B. HLA-B8
    C. HLA-A1
    D. HLA-B27
    E. HLA-B5

165. Enteroinvasion is the primary pathogenesis of gastrointes-tinal disease caused by all of the following organisms EXCEPT
    A. *Campylobacter enteritis*
    B. *Vibrio cholerae*
    C. *Yersinia enteritis*
    D. *Salmonella typhi*
    E. *Shigella sonnei*

166. The microscopic demonstration of a granulomatous lesion containing thick-walled, nonbudding spherules filled with endospores is characteristic of
    A. histoplasmosis
    B. tuberculosis
    C. pneumocystosis (*Pneumocystis carinii*)
    D. coccidiodomycosis
    E. ecchinococcosis

167. Typical clinicopathologic features of lead poisoning include all of the following EXCEPT
  A. anemia with basophilic stipling of red blood cells
  B. membranous nephropathy with nephrotic syndrome
  C. increased urinary excretion of aminolevulinic acid and coproporphyrin
  D. lethargy, stupor, mental retardation, and encephalopathy
  E. peculiar radiodensity along epiphyseal lines of the long bones in children

168. Which of the following statements does NOT characterize chronic myelogenous leukemia?
  A. Approximately 95% of cases show the presence of Philadelphia chromosome
  B. Leukemic cells show elevated alkaline phosphatase levels
  C. It produces the most striking splenic enlargement of all leukemias
  D. Deoxynucleotidyl transferase is identifiable in some leukemic cells during "blast crisis"
  E. When the liver is involved, both the portal tracts and sinusoids show leukemic infiltration

169. Liver injury that may be caused by alpha-methyl dopa (Aldomet) includes all of the following EXCEPT
  A. massive hepatic necrosis
  B. chronic active hepatitis
  C. chronic persistent hepatitis
  D. granulomatous hepatitis
  E. hepatic steatosis

170. Which of the following does NOT characterize nephrotoxic acute tubular necrosis?
    A. Lesions involve multiple parts of the nephron with large skip areas in between
    B. The kidneys are swollen and pale
    C. The tubular basement membranes are preserved
    D. The lumina of the distal tubules and collecting ducts contain casts
    E. The lesions may be caused by ingestion of ethylene glycol

171. The most common histologic type of thyroid cancer associated with irradiation is
    A. medullary carcinoma
    B. undifferentiated small-cell carcinoma
    C. undifferentiated large-cell carcinoma
    D. papillary carcinoma
    E. follicular carcinoma

172. The finding of Negri bodies in sections of the brain is diagnostic of
    A. arthropod-borne encephalitis
    B. rabies encephalitis
    C. eastern equine encephalitis
    D. herpes simplex I encephalitis
    E. herpes zoster encephalitis

DIRECTIONS: The set of lettered headings below is followed by
a list of numbered phrases. For each numbered phrase select

    A   if the item is associated with A *only*
    B   if the item is associated with B *only*
    C   if the item is associated with *both* A and B
    D   if the item is associated with *neither* A nor B

Questions 173–177:

    A. Adenomatous polyp (tubular adenoma) of colon
    B. Villous adenoma (papillary adenoma) of colon
    C. Both
    D. Neither

173. Composed of well-formed glands and crypts lined by colonic
epithelium, most of which show differentiation toward absorptive or mature goblet cells

174. Associated with familial multiple polyposis

175. Carcinoma-in-situ may be expected to occur in about 10%
of these

176. Prevalent in the rectosigmoid

177. Histologically similar to juvenile polyps

Questions 178–185:

178. Conditions characterized by type III hypersensitivity (immune complex-mediated) reaction include
    1. tuberculosis
    2. serum sickness
    3. bronchial asthma
    4. Arthus reaction

179. Small and/or medium-sized muscular artery is the principal site of involvement in
    1. polyarteritis nodosa
    2. temporal (giant cell) arteritis
    3. allergic granulomatosis and angiitis (Churg–Strauss syndrome)
    4. Takayashu's disease (arteritis)

180. Malignant lymphomas NOT derived from follicular center cells include
    1. malignant lymphoma, large cleaved cell type
    2. Burkitt's lymphoma
    3. B-cell immunoblastic sarcoma
    4. mycosis fungoides

Directions Summarized				
A	**B**	**C**	**D**	**E**
1, 2, 3	1, 3	2, 4	4	All are
only	only	only	only	correct

181. Familial multiple polyposis is characterized by
1. autosomal dominant transmission
2. involvement of not only the colon, but also the small intestine and sometimes the stomach
3. tendency to malignant transformation of the polyps
4. the fact that histologic examination of most of the polyps shows villous adenomas

182. HBeAg (e antigen of the hepatitis B virus)
1. is immunologically distinct from HBsAg (surface antigen)
2. is a subset of HBcAg (core antigen)
3. shows similar physicochemical properties to that of an immunoglobulin
4. has been used to produce a vaccine against hepatitis B virus

183. Characteristic renal lesions in systemic lupus erythematosus include
1. diffuse proliferative glomerulonephritis
2. diffuse membranous nephropathy
3. demonstration of Cl_q and C_4 in the glomeruli
4. nodular glomerulosclerosis

184. Young women whose mothers were treated with diethylstilbestero (DES) to prevent abortion have an increased frequency of lesions of the genital tract. These lesions include
1. vaginal adenosis
2. vaginal sarcoma botryoides
3. clear cell adenocarcinoma of the vagina
4. clear cell adenocarcinoma of the ovary

185. Pseudomembranous enterocolitis has been unequivocally associated with
1. broad-spectrum antibiotic therapy
2. the enterotoxin of *Clostridium difficile*
3. recurrent attacks of ulcerative colitis
4. ischemic cardiovascular disease

8

Pharmacology
Joseph R. DiPalma, M.D.

DIRECTIONS: Each of the questions or incomplete statements below is followed by five suggested answers or completions. Select the **one** that is best in each case.

---

186. The hepatic microsomal mixed-function oxidase system can carry out all of the following drug biotransformation reactions EXCEPT
    A. aromatic hydroxylation
    B. *N*-methylation
    C. deamination of amines
    D. sulfoxide formation
    E. *N*-oxidation

187. An investigational drug was evaluated for its safety by performing a number of quantal dose–response curves. From these curves, the following values were taken:

    $ED_{50} = 10$ mg $ED_1 = 1$ mg $ED_{99} = 50$ mg
    $LD_{50} = 100$ mg $LD_1 = 10$ mg $LD_{99} = 500$ mg

What is the calculated median therapeutic index?
A. 0.1
B. 10
C. 100
D. 1.0
E. 0.01

188. Which of the following is NOT a common symptom of acute salicylate poisoning?
A. Nausea and vomiting
B. Hepatic injury
C. Gastrointestinal bleeding
D. Hyperventilation
E. Tinnitus and deafness

189. Which of the following agents will be able to both dilate the pupil and inhibit accommodation when topically applied to the eye?
A. Pilocarpine
B. Neostigmine
C. Atropine
D. Epinephrine
E. Acetazolamide

190. Each of the following is typical of acute opioid intoxication EXCEPT
A. coma
B. depressed respiration
C. cold and clammy skin
D. hypertension
E. reversal can be rapidly effected with naloxone

191. Which of the following statements concerning carbon monoxide poisoning is FALSE?

A. The pathophysiologic reactions that follow the inhalation of CO are primarily the result of tissue hypoxia

B. The binding of CO to one or more of the heme groups of hemoglobin will increase the affinity of the remaining heme sites for oxygen

C. Inhalation of 100% oxygen will not reduce the blood half-life of carboxyhemoglobin

D. Anemic individuals are more susceptible to CO intoxication than are individuals with normal amounts of hemoglobin

E. Dizziness and weakness may be the only premonitory warnings prior to unconsciousness during CO poisoning

192. A patient enters the emergency room with the following symptoms: dry, flushed skin, xerostomia, tachycardia, blurred vision, fever, and delirium. Treatment should include

A. atropine

B. bethanechol

C. trihexyphenidyl

D. physostigmine

E. neostigmine

DIRECTIONS: Each group of questions below consists of five lettered headings followed by a list of numbered statements. For **each** numbered statement, select the **one** lettered heading that is most closely associated with it. Each lettered heading may be selected once, more than once, or not at all.

Questions 193 and 194:

    A. 6-Mercaptopurine
    B. Methotrexate
    C. 5-Fluorouracil
    D. Cyclophosphamide
    E. Leucovorin calcium

193. An alkylating agent that cross-links DNA, RNA, and proteins

194. A folic acid antagonist that inhibits nucleic acid synthesis by blocking dihydrofolate reductase

Questions 195–197:

    A. Clonidine
    B. Hydralazine
    C. Minoxidil
    D. Prazosin
    E. Captopril

195. Its antihypertensive action depends upon the stimulation of alpha-adrenergic receptors in the medulla and the nucleus tractus solitarii

196. This drug's antihypertensive action depends upon the ability to block postsynaptic alpha$_1$ receptors with little action on presynaptic alpha$_2$ receptors

197. Inhibition of the enzyme peptidyl dipeptidase explains the antihypertensive action of this drug

DIRECTIONS: Each set of lettered headings below is followed by a list of numbered phrases. For each numbered phrase select

    A if the item is associated with A *only*
    B if the item is associated with B *only*
    C if the item is associated with *both* A and B
    D if the item is associated with *neither* A nor B

Questions 198 and 199:

    A. Trihexyphenidyl
    B. Bromocriptine
    C. Both
    D. Neither

198. Used to treat Parkinson's disease

199. This drug is a dopamine receptor agonist

Questions 200–202:

    A. Hydrochlorothiazide
    B. Metoprolol
    C. Both
    D. Neither

200. May be used to treat hypertension

201. May be used in hypertensive patients who also have asthma

202. This drug may cause potassium wasting

DIRECTIONS: For each of the questions or incomplete statements below, **one or more** of the answers or completions given is correct. Select

    A   if only *1, 2, and 3* are correct
    B   if only *1 and 3* are correct
    C   if only *2 and 4* are correct
    D   if only *4* is correct
    E   if *all* are correct

Questions 203–210:

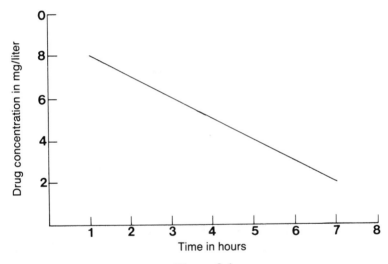

Figure 8.1

Directions Summarized				
A	**B**	**C**	**D**	**E**
1, 2, 3	1, 3	2, 4	4	All are
only	only	only	only	correct

203. Figure 8.1 represents an experiment where a relatively large amount of a drug was administered intravenously. The drug was known to be biotransformed to an inactive product by a single enzyme. When the results were plotted, as blood concentration versus time, the blood level was found to fall at the constant rate of 1.00 mg/liter per hour. Which of the following statements can be applied to this experiment?
   1. Elimination of the drug depends only upon renal excretion
   2. Zero-order kinetics is followed
   3. The one-compartment model is not valid in this experiment
   4. The enzyme was saturated by excess drug

204. Typical symptoms of digitalis toxicity are
   1. anorexia, nausea, and vomiting
   2. extrasystoles, both atrial and ventricular
   3. blurred vision and color distortion
   4. AV block and slow sinus rate

205. The general anesthetic nitrous oxide
   1. will not produce as profound a depth of anesthesia as will halothane
   2. is a highly explosive gas
   3. will produce analgesia prior to producing any significant anesthesia
   4. has a slower rate of induction than diethyl ether

206. With regard to isoniazid,
1. it is inactivated in the liver by acetylation, a function that is genetically controlled
2. patients who are phenotypic rapid acetylators are more prone to develop polyneuritis when treated with isoniazid than are slow acetylators
3. administration of pyridoxine (vitamin B_6) along with isoniazid can prevent isoniazid-induced polyneuritis, but will not appreciably affect isoniazid's antitubercular action
4. patients who are slow acetylators are more prone to develop hepatic toxicity when treated with isoniazid than are rapid acetylators

207. With regard to the effects of cortisol,
1. prolonged treatment with cortisol can cause gastric ulcers, produce osteoporosis, and result in adrenal atrophy
2. one of the major effects of cortisol is to increase the utilization of glucose by peripheral tissues
3. cortisol can inhibit inflammatory responses and increase glycogen deposition in the liver
4. prolonged treatment with cortisol will often result in hypoglycemia

208. Quinidine and procainamide are effective in the treatment of cardiac arrhythmias because they
1. increase membrane responsiveness and conduction velocity in ventricular muscle
2. suppress ectopic pacemaker sites more effectively than the normal sinus pacemaker
3. shorten the action potential duration of Purkinje fibers
4. increase the ratio of effective refractive period to action potential duration (ERP/APD)

Directions Summarized				
A	**B**	**C**	**D**	**E**
1, 2, 3	1, 3	2, 4	4	All are
only	only	only	only	correct

209. Agents that lower intraocular pressure in patients with glaucoma include
    1. epinephrine
    2. timolol
    3. physostigmine
    4. pilocarpine

210. Carbamazepine may be used to treat
    1. generalized tonic-clonic seizures
    2. mixed seizures
    3. complex partial seizures (psychomotor)
    4. tic douloureux (trigeminal neuralgia)

9

Physiology

Kalman Greenspan, Ph.D.

DIRECTIONS: Each of the questions or incomplete statements below is followed by five suggested answers or completions. Select the **one** that is best in each case.

---

211. Artificial respiration may be lifesaving in all of the following EXCEPT
   A. asphyxia due to drowning
   B. gas poisoning
   C. electrocution
   D. anesthetic overdose
   E. air embolism

212. The menstrual cycle is characterized by
   A. high estrogen secretion from day 1 to day 14 and high estrogen and high progesterone secretion from day 14 to day 28
   B. high progesterone secretion from day 1 to day 14, with high estrogen and high progesterone secretion from day 14 to day 28
   C. high estrogen and high progesterone from day 1 to day 14, with high estrogen secretion from day 14 to day 28
   D. high estrogen and high progesterone through the entire cycle of 28 days
   E. none of the above

213. The parathyroid glands are extremely important in that they affect the metabolism of
    A. sodium
    B. potassium
    C. calcium
    D. catecholamines
    E. none of the above

DIRECTIONS: Each group of questions below consists of a diagram with lettered components followed by a list of numbered phrases or statements. For each numbered phrase or statement, select the **one** lettered heading that is most closely associated with it. Each lettered heading may be selected once, more than once, or not at all.

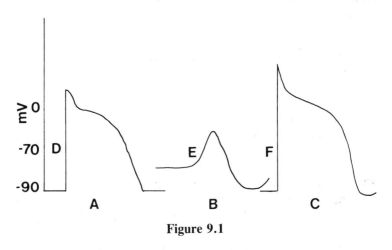

Figure 9.1

Questions 214–216   (refer to Fig. 9.1):

214. Pacemaker action potential configuration

215. Purkinje fiber action potential configuration

216. Voltage change responsible for, and associated temporally with, the QRS complex of the ECG

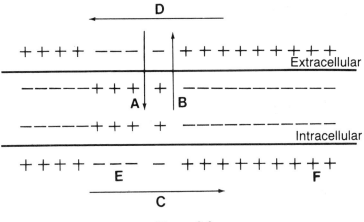

Figure 9.2

Questions 217–219   (refer to Fig. 9.2):

217. The direction of K$^+$ flux during repolarization

218. The direction of Na$^+$ flux during depolarization

219. The direction of impulse propagation

Questions 220–221   (refer to Fig. 9.3):

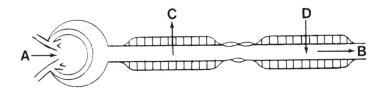

Figure 9.3

220. The site of glucose reabsorption

221. The site of H$^+$ secretion

DIRECTIONS: For each of the questions of incomplete statements below, **one or more** of the answers or completions given is correct. Select

    A   if only *1, 2, and 3* are correct
    B   if only *1 and 3* are correct
    C   if only *2 and 4* are correct
    D   if only *4* is correct
    E   if *all* are correct

Questions 222–235:

222. O_2 dissociation from hemoglobin at any level of capillary PO_2 is accelerated by
    1. increased organic phosphates in RBCs
    2. decreased pH
    3. increased PCO_2
    4. increased temperature

223. In a normal adult in the upright standing position, the lower region of the lung compared to the upper (apical) region has a
    1. greater ventilation
    2. higher blood flow (perfusion)
    3. lower ventilation/perfusion ratio
    4. lower alveolor PO_2

224. The below normal level of PO_2 in arterial blood is clinically referred to as hypoxemia, which can be caused by
    1. hypoventilation
    2. diffusion
    3. shunts
    4. ventilation–perfusion inequality

225. Skeletal muscle activity is normally dependent upon the presence of a baseline level of which of the following hormones?
   1. Insulin
   2. Epinephrine
   3. Glucosteroids
   4. Thyroid hormone

226. The clinical signs of type I diabetes mellitus include
   1. polyuria
   2. polydipsia
   3. polyphagia
   4. hyperglycemia

227. The first heart sounds consist of vibrations
   1. of the a.v. valves during and after their closure
   2. set up by eddy currents in the blood ejected through the aortic valve
   3. emanating from the heart muscle fibers themselves
   4. resulting from the closure of the semilunar valves

228. Extrinsic control of myocardial function may be exerted by the
   1. autonomic nervous system
   2. catecholamine content of the blood
   3. oxygen content of the myocardial blood
   4. carbon dioxide content of the myocardial blood

229. Gastric motility is affected by
   1. parasympathomimetic activity
   2. sympathetic activity
   3. gastrin
   4. liquid volume and content

Directions Summarized

A	B	C	D	E
1, 2, 3	1, 3	2, 4	4	All are
only	only	only	only	correct

230. Turbulent blood flow within the aorta occurs
    1. at high flow velocities when the streamline flow breaks down
    2. when the fluid particles move in irregular and varying paths forming eddies
    3. if and whenever the viscosity and density of the blood are altered
    4. following any change in blood vessel diameter

231. Gastric acid secretion is controlled by
    1. food
    2. nerve activity
    3. GI hormones
    4. fat

232. Pain perception occurs following
    1. chemical destruction of tissue
    2. mechanical irritation of tissue
    3. fluid distention of cells
    4. cell compression

233. Living organisms exist in sleep–wake cycles that are dependent upon
    1. an intact thalmus and reticular activating system
    2. norepinephrine
    3. dopamine
    4. serotonin

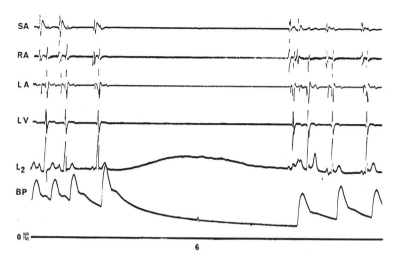

Figure 9.4

234. In Fig. 9.4 the electrical and mechanical activity of the heart were recorded by sewing electrodes over the sinoatrial node (SA), right atrium (RA), left atrium (LA), and left ventricle (LV), and L^2 was obtained by conventional surface lead II electrocardiogram. The blood pressure (BP) tracings were obtained following cannulation of the left femoral artery. Following the third beat, the effects of a physiologic and/ or pharmacologic "maneuver" may be observed. The initial response to this maneuver is a slowing of all electrical and mechanical activity followed by cardiac standstill. While the maneuver was continued during this cardiac standstill, the activity started spontaneously. The responses cited could be explained by the following maneuver(s):
1. Parasympathetic (vagal) nerve stimulation during which "ventricular" escape occurred
2. Sympathetic nerve stimulation during which "ventricular" escape occurred
3. Acetylcholine administration during which ventricular escape occurred
4. Catecholamine administration during which "ventricular or vagal" escape occurred

Directions Summarized

A	B	C	D	E
1, 2, 3	1, 3	2, 4	4	All are
only	only	only	only	correct

235. Exposure to heat necessitates body heat loss. This is usually accomplished by
    1. radiation
    2. convection
    3. evaporation
    4. urine and fecal loss

Answers and Comments

1. Anatomy

1. D. The submandibular gland receives its parasympathetic innervation by way of the chorda tympani nerve, a branch of the facial nerve. The preganglionic fibers of the chorda tympani nerve emerge from the skull through the petrotympanic fissure, travel with the lingual nerve, and synapse in the submandibular ganglion. (**REF.** 4—pp. 172–174)

2. B. The femoral vessels traverse the adductor canal through a fascial compartment in the middle one-third of the thigh. The canal begins at the crossing of the sortorius muscle over the adductor longus muscle and ends at the upper margin of the adductor hiatus. The canal contains the femoral artery and vein. The deep femoral vessels descend in the canal deep to the femoral artery and vein. The saphenous nerve and lower nerve to the vastus medialis also traverse the canal. The obturator nerve traverses the obturator foramen to reach the obturator canal. (**REF.** 4—pp. 468, 534–535)

3. C. The upper limb buds are prominent in a 6-week human embryo. One can identify the elbow and wrist. Digital rays indicate future digits. A groove that appears between the first two branchial arches will give rise to the external acoustic meatus. The adjacent swellings will form the auricle of the external ear. The eye is quite prominent due to the appearance of retinal pigment. The head is large in comparison to the trunk. Item C in Fig. 1.1 is the mandibular prominence. (**REF. 3**—pp. 84–85)

4. A. The spleen, a lymphatic organ, is situated posterior to the upper part of the stomach and between the stomach and diaphragm. The organ is in relation to the ninth, tenth, and 11th ribs, with the pleura and diaphragm intervening. Smooth muscle is found in the capsule of the spleen, which allows large quantities of blood to be expelled into the circulation. The splenic artery and vein are the blood vessels of the spleen. The artery is the largest branch of the celiac. The vein joins the superior mesenteric to form the portal vein. (**REF. 4**—pp. 404, 408–409)

5. C. The descending efferent fiber tracts of the hypothalamus, specifically the lateral and posterior hypothalamic regions, are involved in control of sympathetic responses. Stimulation of this area activates the thoracolumbar outflow, which results in increased metabolic and somatic activities related to emotional stress, combat, or flight. The responses are visualized in pupil dilation, increased heart rate, blood pressure elevation, increased respiration, sweating, and inhibition of gut and bladder. Proprioception is conveyed to the spinal cord by way of dorsal root afferent neurons and is projected to the cerebellum. (**REF. 1**—pp. 265, 571–573)

6. A. Striated muscle is innervated by anterior horn cells of the spinal cord. These cells form the final motor pathway for the lower motor neuron. Lower motor neuron lesions of the spinal cord result in weakness or paralysis, loss of muscle tone, muscle atrophy, and loss of reflex activity. All of these are localized in the affected muscles. Upper motor neuron lesions result in loss of superficial abdominal and cremasteric reflexes. (**REF. 1**—pp. 303–305)

7. E. The smooth endoplasmic reticulum is in the form of tubules which are closely packed and interconnected. Depending on the cell in which it is found, the smooth endoplasmic reticulum performs a number of functions. It functions in lipid and cholesterol metabolism in liver cells. In the corpus luteum, adrenal cortex, and testis, it participates in the production of steroid hormones and cholesterol synthesis. It is involved in the metabolism and transport of lipids absorbed from the mucosa of the intestines. It participates in the secretion of chloride ions in the parietal cells of the stomach. Intercellular digestion is one of the most important functions of the lysosome. (**REF.** 2—pp. 41–42, 47)

8. C. The brachial plexus is formed by the anterior primary rami of the fifth to the eighth cervical nerves and most of the anterior ramus of the first thoracic nerve. The fifth and sixth nerves join to form the superior trunk; the seventh continues as the middle trunk; and the eighth cervical and first thoracic unite to form the inferior trunk. Each trunk divides into an anterior and posterior division, and the divisions recombine in a definitive fashion to form the three cords of the plexus. The cords are closely associated with the second part of the axillary artery. The cords give rise to the definitive nerves of the upper extremity. The axillary nerve, a branch of the posterior cord, supplies the deltoid and teres minor muscles. (**REF.** 4—pp. 52, 54, 78–79)

9. D. Transitional epithelium is diagnostic for most of the urinary system and can be found in the renal pelvis, ureter, and the urinary bladder. This epithelium is stratified, but the shapes of cells and the number of layers vary with contraction and distension of the particular segment of the urinary tract. In the dilated state the epithelium consists of two or three layers of cells, while in the contracted state five or six layers of cells are visible. The surface cells are bulbous and project into the lumen. (**REF.** 2—pp. 115, 145–146, 677–678)

10. E. The oral cavity, pharynx, esophagus, and anus are lined by stratified squamous epithelium. This epithelium consists of many cell layers and forms the main protective epithelium of the body, either lining certain cavities or forming the covering of the skin. The number of layers varies in different sites, but the arrangement and shape of the cells are characteristic. Nuclei are seen in the luminal cells of stratified squamous epithelium that lines body cavities, but are lost in the surface cells of the skin. This epithelium is also found in the larynx, external auditory canal, conjunctiva, vagina, labia majora, and portions of the urethra. (**REF.** 2—pp. 143–145, 528)

11. C. Simple columnar epithelium lines most of the gastrointestinal tract as well as the gall bladder. It is also found in many glands, portions of the ducts of some glands, in the uterine tubes and uterus, small bronchi, and large bronchioles. This epithelium constitutes the primary absorptive and secretory tissue of the body. It consists of a single layer of tall cells, which rests on a continuous basal lamina. (**REF.** 2—pp. 141–143, 565–570)

12. D. The kidney consists of a cortex and medulla that partially surround a cavity called the renal sinus. The renal sinus consists of the upper, expanded part of the ureter known as the renal pelvis. Subdivisions of the pelvis form two or three major calcyces and about eight minor calcyces. (**REF.** 2—pp. 645, 677)

13. A. The main medullary component of the kidney is comprised of 8–18 medullary pyramids, the number corresponding to the number of lobes in the fetal kidney. The base of each pyramid contacts the cortex and the apex projects into a minor calyx. Usually, two or three pyramids unite to form a single papilla, which empties into the minor calyx. (**REF.** 2—p. 645)

14. B. The interior of the kidney consists almost entirely of parenchyma. The parenchyma is divisible into a cortex and a more centrally located medulla. The brownish cortex overlies the renal pyramids and dips down between them as the renal columns. The cortex contains the renal corpuscles, proximal convoluted tubules, distal convoluted tubules, arched collecting tubules, thick ascending and descending limbs of Henle, straight segments of proximal tubules, and straight collecting tubules. (**REF.** 2—pp. 645–646, 661)

15. C. The cortex of the kidney, in addition to forming the outer parenchymal zone, penetrates between the renal pyramids as the renal columns. The columns contain typical cortical tissue, consisting of renal corpuscles, proximal and distal convoluted tubules, arched collecting tubules, thick descending and ascending limbs of Henle's limb, and straight collecting tubules. (**REF.** 2—pp. 645–646, 661)

16. E. Sections of the kidney are seen to consist of a cortex and medulla. The medulla partially surrounds a cavity known as the renal sinus, which opens at the hilus of the kidney. The renal sinus contains the upper expanded portion of the ureter known as the renal pelvis, which is subdivided into two or three major calyces and about eight minor calcyces. (**REF.** 2—pp. 645–646, 661)

17. A. The ulnar nerve is the largest branch of the medial cord of the brachial plexus and is derived from the eighth cervical and first thoracic nerves. It has no branches in the arm. It enters the forearm behind the medial epicondyle of the humerus and supplies branches to the flexor carpi ulnaris and the medial portion of the flexor digitorum profundus. The nerve enters the palm and supplies the hypothenar muscles, the adductor pollicis, the medial two lumbricals, and all the interosseus muscles. (**REF.** 4—pp. 89, 106, 118–119)

18. D. The radial nerve, after spiraling around the humerus, enters the forearm in front of the lateral epicondyle, where it supplies the brachioradialis and extensor carpi radialis longus muscles. In the arm it supplies the triceps brachii and anconeus. In the forearm the deep branch of the radial nerve supplies all the extensors of the forearm as well as branches to the abductor pollicis longus and to extensor pollicis brevis and longus. (**REF.** 4—pp. 90–91, 107–108)

19. C. The median nerve has no branches in the arm. It leaves the cubital fossa by passing between the two heads of the pronator teres and descends deep to the flexor digitorum superficialis in the forearm to reach the hand at the distal border of the flexor retinaculum. Muscular branches in the forearm supply the pronator teres, flexor carpi radialis, palmaris longus, flexor digitorum superficialis, radial portion of flexor digitorum profundus, flexor pollicis longus, and pronator quadratus. In the hand it supplies the thenar muscles and the radial two lumbricals. The ulnar nerve supplies the medial half of flexor digitorum profundus. (**REF.** 4—pp. 105–106, 119)

20. D. The portion of the lateral cord that remains after this cord contributes to the median nerve forms the musculocutaneous nerve. This nerve is derived from the fifth and sixth cervical nerves. The musculocutaneous nerve supplies muscles in the preaxial compartment of the arm and becomes cutaneous to the lateral aspect of the forearm. In the arm it supplies muscular branches to the coracobrachialis, biceps brachii, and brachialis. The brachialis also receives a twig from the radial nerve. (**REF. 4**—pp. 89–91)

21. B. The deep cerebellar nuclei give rise to the largest and most widely distributed cerebellar efferent fibers. These are organized into two major systems, the superior cerebellar peduncle and the fastigial efferent projection. The superior cerebellar peduncle is the largest cerebellar efferent bundle. It is formed by the globose, dentate, and emboliform nuclei. The fibers of the cerebellar peduncle decussate at levels through the inferior colliculus. (**REF.** 1—pp. 480–481)

22. E. Pseudostratified columnar ciliated epithelium is diagnostic for the respiratory system. It lines the nasal passages, parts of the nosopharynx and larynx, the trachea, bronchii, and most of the bronchioles. This epithelium has a stratified appearance because the nuclei lie at different levels. However, all of the cells reach the basal lamina, although not all of them reach the luminal surface. (**REF. 2**—pp. 143, 619–634)

23. E. Four mechanisms are involved in the transport of all substances across the placental membrane. These are: active transport, simple diffusion, facilitated diffusion, and pinocytosis. The passage of carbon dioxide, oxygen, and carbon monoxide is by simple diffusion. This mechanism is also involved in the passage of water. The transfer of maternal antibodies is by pinocytosis. Simple diffusion also accounts for the passage of urea and uric acid, as well as most drugs and drug metabolites. (**REF.** 3— pp. 118–120)

24. A. In view of the frequent development of breast cancer and the subsequent spread of cancer cells from the gland through the lymphatic system, it is extremely important to know the lymphatic drainage of this organ. A cutaneous lymphatic network forms the subareolar lymphatic plexus, which drains into the circumareolar plexus. The lymphatics of the gland proper drain into the subareolar plexus. From the subareolar plexus a lateral and medial trunk form the principal axillary lymph paths. Both of these trunks terminate in the superior nodes of the pectoral group of axillary nodes. Other collecting vessels pass directly to the central and lateral groups of axillary nodes. (REF. 4—pp. 68–70)

25. D. Two very important motor nerves are in the surgical field and have to be identified. These are the long thoracic and thoracodorsal nerves. The thoracodorsal nerve is derived from the posterior cord of the brachial plexus by fibers from C–7 and C–8. This nerve reaches the latissimus dorsi in the axilla and divides into branches on the deep surface of the muscle. The long thoracic nerve arises from the roots of the fifth, sixth, and seventh cervical nerves, descends from the neck to pass deep to the brachial plexus, and enters the axilla to reach and supply the serratus anterior on its superficial surface. (REF. 4—pp. 51, 80–81, 83)

2. Behavioral Sciences

26. E. Of the diseases listed, only phenylketonuria can be detected by the Guthrie test. The other disorders listed are detectable by amniocentesis. (REF. 8—pp. 24, 25)

27. B. Excellent evidence now exists that by the end of the second year of life, gender identity is firmly established and cannot be changed easily. This does not mean that all the role attributes of masculinity or femininity are established at this age, but only that children by age 2 know in general that they are either boys or girls. (REF. 3—p. 214)

28. D. The narcolepsy syndrome has been found to be associated with the abnormal, rapid transition from the waking state to REM sleep. (REF. 3—p. 76)

29. A. Persons with an obsessive-compulsive personality are so cautious, deliberate, and rational in their approach to life and its problems that they may seem dry and narrow-minded at times. (REF. 4—p. 332)

30. C. The mode is the most frequent score. (REF. 7—p. 543)

31. C. Individuals from low socioeconomic conditions have a higher incidence of psychotic illness and institutionalization and suffer from a wider range of diseases. They are more likely to emphasize order and obedience in childrearing. (REF. 3—p. 271)

32. D. Extrapyramidal effects are central nervous system effects. Of the phenothiazines, thioridazine produces the fewest extrapyramidal effects; chlorpromazine, chlorprothixene, and acetophenazine produce an intermediate amount; and haloperidol, thiothixene, butaperazine, trifluoperazine, and fluphenazine produce the greatest amount of extrapyramidal effects. (**REF.** 4— p. 643)

33. E. The degree of correlation demonstrates the degree of association between the two events. If there were no correlation or association, the events would be statistically independent of one another; a negative correlation indicates that the two events are associated inversely. (**REF.** 6—pp. 545–546)

34. D. The nausea and vomiting responses described are typical of classical conditioning phenomena. Discriminative stimuli and operants are both terms associated with operant conditioning, the learning theory proposed by B. F. Skinner. The chemotherapeutic agent itself is the unconditioned stimulus, the stimulus that elicits a response (in this case nausea and vomiting) without training. The nurse in the example may originally have been a neutral stimulus; however, after repeated association, the nurse acquired the property of eliciting a response of nausea and vomiting. Thus, the nurse became a conditioned stimulus and the nausea and vomiting elicited at the post office could be considered conditioned responses. (**REF.** 4—p. 38ff)

35. E. Patients on amphetamines have an improved performance of simple mental and physical tasks. All other statements are true. (**REF.** 3—p. 48)

36. C. Early attempts to use behavior therapy procedures based upon classical conditioning in the treatment of alcoholism focused upon the use of electrical aversion. The literature convincingly demonstrates the ineffectiveness of electrical aversion procedures in the treatment of alcoholism. However, classically conditioned aversive reactions resulting from the administration of nausea-producing drugs have been remarkably successful in assisting patients to maintain abstinence. Long-term follow-up of these patients has resulted in estimates of abstinence of 50% at 2 years, 38% at 5 years, and 23% at 10 years posttreatment. In addition to the contribution of the behavior therapy procedures, it should be remembered that patients have to be extremely motivated to undergo this type of treatment regimen and this increased motivation may enhance the treatment's effectiveness. (**REF.** 7—p. 264)

37. B.
38. A. (Both in **REF.** 4—p. 219)

39. A.
40. D.
41. C.
42. B.
43. E. (All in **REF.** 5—p. 134)

44. A.
45. B. (Both in **REF.** 1—pp. 4, 5)

46. B.
47. A.
48. C. (All in **REF.** 9—p. 52)

49. A. The etiology in approximately 75% of the cases of mental retardation is unknown. These cases are usually referred to as cultural–familial and probably are caused by a combination of genetic and environmental factors. (**REF.** 4—p. 709)

50. B. Minor affective disorders (dysthymia or depressive neurosis) are clearly distinguishable from major disorders in that the latter present with clear and precise onset. Also, patients suffering from major affective disorders typically present with observable psychomotor retardation and not just subjective complaints. (**REF.** 4—p. 246ff)

51. B. Men commit suicide three times more frequently than women, although women are three times more likely to make suicide attempts. Approximately 65% of suicides are white males. Even though both widowed and divorced individuals have suicide rates that are greater than those of married individuals, the rate for the divorced is 50% greater than that for the widowed. The elderly make relatively few suicide attempts, but are successful at a more frequent rate; even though they comprise only 10% of the population, they constitute approximately 25% of suicides. (**REF.** 4—p. 575)

52. B. Fear is rapidly learned, but extremely resistant to extinction. Although fear can be reduced by drugs, a person taking such drugs may have difficulty differentiating between realistic and unrealistic fears and thus may endanger himself or herself and/or others. (**REF.** 4—p. 628–629)

53. C. Behavior therapy emphasizes objective, measurable behaviors and environmental factors rather than inferred mental processes, such as unconscious conflicts. The behavior therapy procedure involving exposure to anxiety-producing stimuli at full intensity for prolonged periods of time is known as flooding or implosion therapy. (**REF.** 4—p. 605)

54. A. The use of special pill containers has been found to improve compliance, probably because it serves as a salient reminding procedure. However, the use of child-resistant containers, which are more difficult to open, has been associated with poorer compliance. (**REF.** 2—p. 121ff)

55. B. In some humans, REM-state deprivation leads to increased anxiety, irritability, hostility, and appetite and to difficulty in remembering, concentrating, and motor coordinations. These deprived subjects have a heightened susceptibility to hallucinations after photic stimulation. (**REF.** 5—p. 167)

3. Biochemistry

56. D. The enzyme is the first metabolic step unique to pyrimidine biosynthesis. The end product of that pathway, CTP, regulates the rate of its own synthesis through regulatory subunits of the enzyme that, when bound to CTP, are inhibitory. (**REFS.** 1—pp. 237–240; 2—Vol I., pp. 678–679; 3—p. 523; 4—pp. 187–192, 729–730)

57. C. The methionine is more polar than leucine and hence the otherwise identical peptides can be separated by paper portion chromatography, since the Leu-enkephalin will be more hydrophobic and spend more time in the mobile phase. (**REFS.** 1— pp. 91, 96–98; 2—Vol. I, pp. 61, 162–167; 3—pp. 91–92)

58. C. Cyclic AMP activates a protein kinase, which phosphorylates glycogen synthetase, thus deactivating it, and phosphorylase kinase, which leads to phosphorylase activation. (**REFS.** 1— pp. 314–315; 2—Vol. I, pp. 430–442; 3—pp. 368, 371; 4—pp. 311–313)

59. C. DNP can cross the membrane in the protonated (neutral) form or as the phenolate ion. This collapses the proton gradient that, the chemiosmotic theory holds, is the energy store for ATP synthesis. (**REFS.** 1—pp. 524–529; 2—Vol. I, pp. 348–352; 3— pp. 325–326; 4—pp. 384–385, 387–393)

60. E. In this system the reduction of NAD is not proportional to ATP. (**REFS.** 1—pp. 422; 2—Vol. I, pp. 396–397, 415; 3— pp. 261–263; 4—pp. 295, 327)

61. B. They both fix CO_2 to biotin in an ATP-dependent reaction and subsequently transfer it to the other substrate, giving it a new carboxyl group. (**REFS.** 1—pp. 464, 662; 2—Vol. I, pp. 409, 524; 3—pp. 348–349, 396; 4—pp. 223–225, 344, 490–491)

62. B.

$$E + S \underset{k_{-1}}{\overset{k_1}{\rightleftharpoons}} ES \underset{k_{-2}}{\overset{k_2}{\rightleftharpoons}} EP \underset{k_{-3}}{\overset{k_3}{\rightleftharpoons}} E + P$$

It is assumed that k_2 is the rate-limiting step and that k_{-2} can be ignored, since there will be virtually no P present (initial velocity assumption). $V_{max} = k_2[E]$, where $k_2 = k_{cat}$, which is also called the turnover number. Further, the steady-state assumption $[d(ES)/dt = -d(ES)/dt]$ is made. However, $K_m = (k_{-1} + k_2)/k_1$, whereas $K_d = k_{-1}/k_2$. Thus, K_m can approximate K_d *only* when $k_2 \ll k_1$, k_{-1}.
(**REFS.** 1—pp. 189–194; 2—Vol. I, pp. 185–190; 3—pp. 110–114; 4—pp. 137–141)

63. C. P_{50} represents the partial pressure of oxygen necessary to achieve 50% saturation of hemoglobin. A lower P_{50} means greater oxygen affinity, whereas a higher P_{50} means less oxygen affinity. An increase in the pH means a reduction in $[H^+]$, thus shifting the following equilibrium to the right: $HHb^+ + O_2 \leftrightarrow HbO_2 + H^+$, thereby increasing oxygen affinity (decreasing P_{50}). An increase in [DPG] means more stabilization of the deoxy form and hence less oxygen affinity (increase in P_{50}). (**REFS.** 1—pp. 147–149; 2—Vol. II, pp. 117–118; 3—pp. 69–71; 4—pp. 111–113)

64. A. Homozygotes for familial hypercholesterolemia have virtually no LDL receptors and heterozygotes have approximately half the normal number. (**REFS.** 3—pp. 471–473; 4—pp. 558–560)

65. C. Animals lack the glyoxylate cycle; hence no net synthesis of glucose can occur from acetyl-CoA or from compounds converted to acetyl-CoA, such as acetate, ethanol, or even-numbered-carbon fatty acids. However, odd-numbered-carbon fatty acids will produce propionyl-CoA in addition to acetyl-CoA. The propionyl-CoA can be converted to succyl-CoA and hence to malate, where it enters gluconeogenesis. (**REFS.** 1—pp. 466–467, 555; 2—Vol. I, pp. 424–425, 520–522; 4—pp. 352–358, 484)

66. E. PFK catalyzes the first committed step of glycolysis and one of the three steps where $\Delta G' < O$; hence, reversal is not metabolically likely (a phosphatase is used to convert fructose diphosphate to fructose–6-phosphate during gluconeogenesis). All the other statements are true. Since PFK is the pacemaker of glycolysis, its activity determines how much glyceraldehyde-3-phosphate will be available for the glyceraldehyde-3-phosphate dehydrogenase and hence how much NADH is produced; this phenomenon gives rise to oscillation in [NADH] when a cell-free extract is provided a steady-state supply of glucose. (**REFS.** 1—pp. 251–252, 266–268; 2—Vol. I, pp. 414–417; 4—pp. 313–314)

67. A. Any mode of operation of the pentose shunt that produces NADPH will employ the oxidative branch that includes an oxidative decarboxylation catalyzed by 6-phosphogluconate dehydrogenase. Conversion of glucose-6-phosphate to fructose-6-phosphate and glyceraldehyde-3-phosphate allows conversion to ribose-5-phosphate via the nonoxidative branch. (**REFS.** 2—Vol. I, pp. 417–423; 3—pp. 333–340; 4—pp. 314–320)

68. E. $^{14}CH_3$-$\overset{\overset{\text{O}}{\|}}{C}$-COO$^-$ will be converted to $^{14}CH_3$-$\overset{\overset{\text{O}}{\|}}{C}$-SCoA and enter the Krebs cycle, where the carbons released are not the ones provided by acetyl-CoA. The label will appear in the two inner carbons of oxaloacetate (50% of the label each due to the scrambling at succinate). Since it is the carboxyl carbons of oxaloacetate that appear as CO_2, no label will show up in CO_2 during the second turn of the Krebs cycle either. Only during the third turn would label begin to show up in CO_2. (**REFS.**1—pp. 450–463; 2—Vol. I, pp. 319–331; 3—pp. 284–294; 4—pp. 325–338, esp. Fig. 9–7)

69. B. Histidine will be converted to α-ketoglutarate and N^5-formiminotetrahydrofolate. From α-ketoglutarate, proline can be made; α-ketoglutarate can be converted to oxaloacetate, the precursor of aspartate that is used for CTP biosynthesis. Also, α-ketoglutarate can be converted to malate and hence via the reactions of gluconeogenesis to 3-phosphoglycerate and thus to glycine via serine; glycine and N^5-formiminotetrahydrofolate are precursors of GTP. Phenylalanine is an essential amino acid and is not synthesized in mammalian liver. (**REFS.** 1—pp. 575, 695, 709, 729, 736; 2—Vol. I, pp. 584, 602, 607, 667; 3—pp. 415, 417, 488–490, 514, 519; 4—pp. 701, 705, 834, 872, 874)

70. C. The defective enzyme in "maple syrup disease" is the branched-chain keto acid dehydrogenase complex that acts on isoleucine, leucine, and valine. (**REFS.** 1—pp. 570, 576–578; 2—Vol. I, pp. 658–660, 830; 3—pp. 422–424; 4—pp. 900–901)

71. B. There are three main causes of β-thalassemias: loss of the gene for β-hemoglobin, lack of mRNA due to improper splicing caused by mutation in an intron or in a splice junction of the β-hemoglobin gene, or lack of translation of the mRNA. (**REFS.** 2—Vol. I, pp. 776, 786–787; 3—pp. 702–703, 709–710; 4—814–817)

72. C. Glucose-1-phosphate is the precursor to glycogen (via UDP-glucose) and the product of glycogen breakdown by phospharylure.

73. E. Geranyl pyrophosphate is an intermediate in the synthesis of cholesterol.

74. A. Pyridoxamine phosphate is an enzyme-bound intermediate in pyridoxal-phosphate-catalyzed transamination reactions of amino acids and keto acids.

75. B. Coenzyme Q (ubiquinone) is a component of the electron transport chain.

76. D. Thiamine pyrophosphate is the coenzyme of pyruvate decarboxylase that is one of the three enzymes of the pyruvate dehydrogenase complex. (**REFS.** 1—pp. 450–453, 493–496, 562–564, 645–646, 679–684; 2—Vol. 1, pp. 319–321, 337–344, 430–446, 558–560, 582–583; 3—pp. 290–294, 311–315, 359–366, 409–411, 464–468; 4—pp. 201–206, 310–312, 326–329, 369–374, 451–452, 547–554)

77. C. The enzymes cleave in palindromic sequences; i.e., where the sequence of one strand is the same as the other, each read in its 3′ to 5′ direction. (**REFS.** 1—pp. 882; 2—Vol. I, pp. 722–723; 3—p. 590; 4—pp. 766–767)

78. E. The identities are a $= V_{max}$; b $= V_{max}/2$; c $= K_m$; d $= -1/K_m$; e $= 1/V_{max}$; and f $= K_m/V_{max}$. (**REFS.** 1—pp. 189, 195; 2—Vol. I, pp. 186—189; 3—pp. 111, 113; 4—pp. 139–140)

79. B. Fatty acid synthesis occurs in the cytosol, where NADPH is available. For transport into the mitochondria for oxidation, the acyl-coenzyme A esters have to be transesterified with carnitine. Both oxidation and synthesis generate *trans* unsaturated fatty acid thioesters. (**REFS.** 1—pp. 545, 548, 659, 666; 2—Vol. I, pp. 513–517, 522–527; 3—pp. 395; 4—pp. 481–482, 488–490)

80. A. Prostaglandins are all derivatives of arachidonic acid and they are catabolized in the lung during a single pass. Although some prostaglandin effects are mediated by cAMP, many appear not to be. Different prostaglandins can have antagonistic effects or even the same prostaglandins can elicit different biological responses, depending upon concentration. (**REFS.** 1—pp. 300, 686–687; 2—Vol. II, pp. 397–411; 3—pp. 853–854; 4—pp. 535–542)

4. Biostatistics/Epidemiology

81. E. Since a sample size of 100 will make the half-width of the 95% confidence interval 10 percentage points, we have 1.96

$[p(1-p)/100]^{1/2} = 0.1$, where p is the population proportion. The n required to make the half-width 5 percentage points is given by $1.96\,[p(1-p)/n]^{1/2} = 0.05$. Dividing the first equation by the second and solving for n, we find n = 400. (**REF.** 6—p. 160)

82. E. The probability that a given person will not be referred is 0.90. Assuming independence, the probability that none of the five will be referred is $(0.90)^5$. The complement, $1 - (0.90)^5$, is thus the probability that at least one will be referred. (**REF.** 6—pp. 70–71)

83. A. From the case fatality and prevalence rates given for Disease X we have : P(Death|X) = 1/10 and P(X) = 10/100,000. Using the multiplication rule of probability, we have

$$P(X \text{ and Death}) = P(X)P(\text{Death}|X) = \frac{1}{10} \cdot \frac{10}{100,000} = \frac{1}{100,000}$$

(**REF.** 16—pp. 53–55)

84. A. The greater the absolute value of the correlation coefficient, the more precisely the dependent variable, plasma HDL cholesterol, can be predicted from the independent variable in question. The negative correlation between plasma HDL cholesterol and plasma triglyceride indicates that high levels of one variable are associated with low values of the other. (**REF.** 10—pp. 210–215)

85. E. The p value is the probability of the observed outcome or a more extreme one given that the null hypothesis is true. In this case the observed outcome and its probability are given in the second row of the table. Equivalent or more extreme outcomes and their probabilities are given in the first, fourth, and fifth rows. Summing the probabilities of these outcomes, we obtain the two-tailed p value. (**REF.** 2—pp. 135–137)

86. C. The proportion sought is equal to the probability of a type II error, i.e., the probability of accepting the null hypothesis when it is false. We are given that the power of the test is 80%. This is the probability of rejecting the null hypothesis when it is false and is then the complement of the probability we seek. (**REF.** 6—pp. 120–122)

87. C. Significant amounts of lead-containing paints remain on painted steel structures, bridges, and ships. Lead oxide fumes are released when these structures are burned or cut with blow torches. Lead oxide fume is rapidly absorbed through the respiratory tract and may result in biochemical abnormalities or vague nonspecific symptoms, as well as overt lead intoxication. (**REFS.** 12—pp. 649–651; 18—pp. 435–439)

88. B. Benzene exposure has been shown to result in aplastic anemia, of which 2–4% progress to acute nonlymphatic leukemia (ANLL). (**REF.** 14—pp. 367–370)

89. C. Chlorinated hydrocarbons tend to be lipophilic and are stored for long periods in body fat. (**REF.** 12—pp. 738–739)

90. A. Noise-induced hearing loss affects the organ of Corti, resulting in a typical "notch" at 4000 Hz, which may not be noticed until acuity at 2000 Hz is affected. The loss of the ability to discriminate consonants is an early feature. (**REF.** 18—pp. 708–709)

91. B. Although proportional mortality studies are relatively easy and inexpensive to perform, they are difficult to interpret due to the fact that a high proportion of deaths due to one cause may reflect either an excess of that cause of death or a deficit of deaths from other causes, and death certificate ascertainment can be incomplete (and possibly biased). (**REF.** 14—p. 59)

92. B. The ILO classification is intended to codify the extent of involvement, and not to indicate a specific diagnosis. Opacities are graded 0/1 or 1/0 for profusion, p,q,r, or s for size and shape, and by lung zone for extent. A set of comparison films is usually referred to. (**REF.** 18—pp. 114–115)

93. E. The key to an experimental study is the active intervention of the investigator for the purposes of the experiment. Intervention, such as the routine clinical treatment of disease, may occur during an observational study, but is not provided by the investigator for the purposes of the experiment. (**REF.** 9—pp. 50–51)

94. C. Sensitivity is not a property of associations and therefore cannot be a criterion for causality. The fifth criterion defined by the advisory committee to the Surgeon General (1964) was specificity—the degree to which one particular exposure produced one specific disease. If the biologic response to the exposure is variable, it is less likely to be causal. (**REF.** 16—pp. 120–121)

95. A. The incidence of acute conditions decreases with age. However, when the aged do experience acute conditions, they experience more days of bed disability or restricted activity. The proportion of the population with one or more chronic conditions increases steadily with age, from approximately 20% for those under 17 to about 85% for those over 65. Among those with chronic conditions, the resulting disabilities also increase with advancing age. (**REF.** 3—pp. 105–107)

96. C. Studies of community-resident aged indicate that organic brain syndromes or dementia occur in approximately 5–7% of the 65+ population, but that almost 20% of those over 80 are impaired. The most common functional psychiatric disorder in the aged is depression. (**REFS.** 4—pp. 34–56; 5—p. 70).

97. D. At any given time, 5% of the population over 65 are residing in a nursing home. Ninety percent of nursing home residents are white, and 60% of these are female. (**REF.** 1—p. 59)

98. E. Two alternative explanations have been proposed for the well-established inverse relationship between socioeconomic status and psychiatric disorder. The first is that of social causation, whereby the stresses and lifestyles associated with lower socioeconomic conditions lead to psychiatric disorders. The second explanation is the "selection–drift" hypothesis. This actually consists of two hypotheses (selection and drift). According to the drift hypothesis, individuals move downward in socioeconomic status after an episode of mental disorder. With regard to selection, the mental disorder hinders one's status attainment, so that the level of social status eventually reached is not as high as it might have been, had the disorder not developed. (**REF.** 7—pp. 146–160)

99. C. Building on principles of social learning, behavioral change programs require learning about the behavior and its circumstances by monitoring and analyzing it over a period of time. The control of the behavior is enhanced by a clear *positive* reward system, including social support from friends. (**REF.** 12—pp. 1095–1112)

100. C. In 1974, the federal government mandated through Public Law 93–641 that every state have a CON law. This was to control capital investments by hospitals and nursing homes. The 1971 Economic Stabilization Program instituted a price freeze on physician fees and hospital wages and prices. The other answers are non-existent approaches. (**REF.** 15—pp. 383–400)

101. C. Several studies have examined the relationship between cigarette smoking and endometrial cancer and others the relationship with Parkinson's disease. None have shown the risk for these two diseases to be as high as for nonsmokers. (**REFS.** 11—pp. 242–254; 13—pp. 593–596; 17—pp. 5–8)

102. A. The predictive value of a test is not a property of the test alone; it is determined by the sensitivity and specificity of the test and the prevalence of disease in the population being tested. Thus, the predictive value is not independent of the setting in which the test is used. (**REF.** 8—pp. 52–56)

103. A. Cohort studies allow the direct measurement of incidence, while case–control studies do not. There is no recall bias in information concerning risk factors between "cases" and "controls," since disease has not occurred at the time the information is collected. The incidence of more than one disease can be related to the risk factor information elicited. However, cohort studies are only applicable to relatively common diseases (e.g., coronary heart disease). The size of cohort needed to study a rare disease (e.g., carcinoma of the vagina) would be prohibitively expensive. (**REF.** 8—p. 100)

104. A. Both increased incidence and increased duration of a disease obviously increase prevalence, from the equation: Prevalence = Incidence × Duration. It is perhaps less obvious that a reduced case-fatality of a chronic disease will increase the duration of the disease, again resulting in increased prevalence. (**REF.** 16—pp. 27–29)

105. A. Primary prevention of a disease entails intervention at any time before the disease occurs and may therefore include intervention before or after the occurrence of risk factors for the disease. Intervention after the occurrence of the disease would fall into the domain of secondary prevention. (**REF.** 8—pp. 128–129)

5. Genetics

106. D. Neural tube defects (anencephaly and spina bifida) have a polygenic/multifactorial etiology. (**REFS.** 1—pp. 231–236; 2—pp. 210, 218)

107. E. Three sex-chromatin masses represent three inactivated X chromosomes; therefore, since the number of X chromosomes minus one is the number of sex chromatin masses, it can be concluded that the individual has four X chromosomes. There is no information on the absence or presence of a Y chromosome or the phenotypic sex. (**REFS.** 1—pp. 214–215; 2—pp. 137–140)

108. B. The risk associated with midtrimester amniocentesis is 1/4–1/2%. (**REFS.** 1—pp. 1460; 2—p. 292)

109. C. The finding of ovo-testes and ambiguous genitalia is indicative of true hermaphroditism. The great majority of true hermaphrodites are 46,XX. (**REFS.** 1—pp. 207–208; 2—p. 146)

110. D. 45,X/46,XY mosaicism is due to anaphase lag, and meiotic nondisjunction occurs with advancing maternal age. (**REF.** 2—pp. 110, 118)

111. B. The risk for recurrence for having a second child with trisomy 21 Down syndrome is 1% (1:100) regardless of age. (**REF.** 2—p. 122)

112. B. Chromosome material from both the short and long arms is lost in the formation of a ring chromosome because of chromosome breaks at both locations. (**REFS.** 1—p. 170; 2—p. 112)

113. A. A mutation resulting in the substitution of a valine for a glutamic acid in each of the two beta chains of the hemoglobin molecule results in sickle cell hemoglobin. (**REF.** 2—pp. 85–86)

114. C. Since males have only one X chromosome (XY), a single recessive gene that appears on their X chromosome will be expressed, whereas for a female, a single recessive gene that appears on one X chromosome is less likely to be expressed, since she has two X chromosomes (XX). In addition, since males give their sons only their Y chromosome, there is no male-to-male transmission. (**REFS.** 1—pp. 71–73; 2—pp. 58–61)

115. B. An affected person will transmit a disorder to half his or her children in an autosomal *dominant* disorder. Autosomal disorders affect both sexes equally. (**REFS.** 1—pp. 66–68, 69–71; 2—pp. 48, 53–54)

116. C. In polygenic/multifactorial inheritance, threshold traits may make the incidence of a disorder higher in one sex than the other. In addition, the recurrence risk is higher when more than one family member is affected, as compared to single-gene defects, in which the risk is the same regardless of the number of affected individuals. (**REF.** 2—p. 221)

117. B. Linkage occurs if two genes are on the same chromosome *but* not too far apart and are transmitted to the same gamete more than 50% of the time (recombination of alleles at each locus is less than 50%). (**REF.** 2—p. 193)

118. C. The Philadelphia chromosome occurs in chronic myelogenous leukemia and is found only in myelocytes. It results from a reciprocal translocation involving the long arm of one number 9 chromosome and the long arm of one number 22 chromosome. The deleted number 22 chromosome was discovered in Philadelphia and is referred to as the Philadelphia chromosome. (**REFS.** 1—pp. 1078–1079; 2—p. 131)

119. C. Lymphedema in a newborn female is usually caused by a 45,X chromosome constitution and clinically is known as the Turner syndrome. In the Turner syndrome, mental retardation is not anticipated and the external genitalia are normal, but the ultimate stature is short. (**REFS.** 1—pp. 193–196; 2—pp. 144–145)

120. A. Because of the mosaicism, the external genitalia could be male (47,XYY) or female (45,X), depending on distribution of the cell types in various tissues. The XYY cell line could produce testes, which should be removed if intra-abdominal, because of the increased risk of malignant degeneration. Mitotic nondisjunction is the responsible mechanism, since anaphase lag could not result in 47,XYY cells. (**REFS.** 1—pp. 198–199, 200–201; 2—p. 110)

121. E. The fragile X syndrome is due to an X-linked recessive gene that results in mental retardation and a characteristic clinical picture in males. There are unusual aspects not anticipated with X-linked recessive inheritance. The fragile X chromosome is a marker resulting from induction of a fragile site on the long arm of the X chromosome by culturing cells in medium deficient in folic acid. (**REF.** 2—pp. 63–65)

122. A. According to the hypothesis of Mary Lyon, at 16–19 days of embryogenesis, one X chromosome in a female is randomly inactivated and is represented by the sex-chromatin mass. (**REFS.** 1—pp. 57–58; 2—pp. 138–141)

123. E. A restriction nuclease is an enzyme of bacterial origin that cleaves DNA at specific sites, producing specific restriction length fragment polymorphisms (RLFP). Specific nucleases are used in the prenatal diagnosis of hemoglobinopathies. (**REF.** 2—pp. 35–36)

124. B. Heterozygote advantage can lead to the preservation of a gene even if it is detrimental when homozygous, as in the resistance to malaria associated with sickle cell trait. The Hardy–Weinberg equilibrium maintains stable gene frequency if there is random mating and no environmental influence. Migration and genetic isolation result in changes in gene frequencies. (**REF.** 1—pp. 255, 261, 269)

125. E. Somatic cell hybridization in human genetics refers to the fusion of human cells in culture with cultured cells from another species. Once hybrid cells have been formed and selected by survival, they can be grown as individual clones and used for linkage studies, complementation studies (to determine if two mutations are in the same gene), studies of mutagenesis in cell cultures, and studies of differentiated cell function. (**REF.** 2—pp. 187–191)

126. E. There is a band of distribution of thalassemia around the

Old World: the Mediterranean, the Middle East, parts of Africa, India, and the Orient. Migration patterns have resulted in extension to South America and the Caribbean. *Thalassa* is a Greek word for sea and pertains to the Mediterranean. (**REF.** 2—p. 88)

127. B. Advanced maternal age is associated with an increased risk for a pregnancy with a chromosome abnormality, which can be detected by prenatal chromosome analysis of amniotic fluid cells. Anencephaly can be detected by measuring alpha-fetoprotein (AFP) in the amniotic fluid. There is no test using amniotic fluid that can detect hydrocephaly or the nonspecific potential adverse effects of consanguinity. (**REF.** 2—pp. 291–296)

128. A. An abnormal long arm of one number 3 chromosome could result *de novo* and chromosome analysis of the parents would be normal. If either parent had a balanced reciprocal translocation, an abnormal long arm of one number 3 chromosome could result if one of the parents had a paracentric inversion of the long arm of a number 3 chromosome. A balanced centric fusion translocation would not apply, since it involves only acrocentric chromosomes, and chromosome number 3 is not acrocentric. (**REF.** 2—pp. 8, 113–116)

129. B. Conjoined (Siamese) twins are monozygotic twins resulting from late and incomplete cleavage after the eighth day. (**REF.** 2—pp. 280–281)

130. A. If both twins of a monozygotic (identical) pair have Down's syndrome, they could both have trisomy 21 or translocation Down's syndrome. If trisomy 21 was responsible, both parents would be normal and meiotic nondisjunction would be responsible. If translocation was responsible, either parent could be a balanced translocation carrier or both could be normal if the translocation arose *de novo*. Mitotic nondisjunction is a postfertilization event that would account for monozygotic twins *discordant* for Down's syndrome. (**REF.** 2—pp. 115–117, 119–120, 273, 280)

6. Microbiology

131. C. The unfused splenocytes die off in the culture system in which the parent cell line is unable to grow as a result of enzyme deficiency, while hybrid cells containing the HGPRT gene donated by the splenocyte grow continuously. (**REF.** 3—p. 287)

132. D. *Babesia* are small, malarialike protozoan parasites of red blood cells. (**REF.** 1—p. 1265)

133. C. The IgM antibodies are found in almost every immune response. Usually, they are formed early in the immune response and only at low levels. They are usually soon dominated by IgG antibodies. (**REF.** 2—p. 349)

134. B. Interferons are not virus-specific, but cell-specific in production and in their effects. Also, a given interferon inhibits viral multiplication most effectively in cells of the species in which it was produced. (**REF.** 2—p. 1003)

135. D. The delayed skin test may sometimes simulate the Arthus reaction. However, the Arthus reaction usually appears about 2 hours after antigen is injected into the skin, is maximal at 4 or 5 hours, and subsides by 24 hours. The delayed-type reaction is later in onset and more persistent. The confusion may arise if a severe Arthus reaction remains conspicuous for 24 hours or more (**REF.** 2—pp. 494–495)

136. C. HAV infection appears to be spread by the fecal–oral route. However, occasionally it is transmitted by parenteral injection, especially in drug addicts. (**REF.** 1—pp. 989–990)

137. D. The respiratory tract is the main portal of entry of *C. psittaci* infection, and the usual source is inhalation of organisms from infected birds and their droppings. (**REF.** 3—p. 791)

138. B. Two to 10 weeks after the appearance of the primary lesion, a generalized skin rash involving the mucous membranes usually appears. All the secondary lesions, particularly those in mucous membranes, contain many spirochetes and are highly infectious if they are located on exposed surfaces. (**REF.** 3—p. 725)

139. B. Autografts are transplants from one region to another of the same individual. (**REF.** 2—p. 533)

140. C. Typical arthrospore formation is characteristic of *C. immitis* when grown in Sabouraud's glucose agar at room temperature. The arthrospores alternate with empty spaces in the hyphae. (**REF.** 2—p. 839)

141. B. *Cryptococcus neoformans* appears in tissue and culture as a thin-walled, oval-to-spherical budding cell. The cells are surrounded by a wide, gelatinous capsule that may equal or exceed the diameter of the cell, which measures 5–15 μm. The presence of the large capsule differentiates this fungus from all other yeast-like organisms. (**REF.** 3—p. 1151)

142. B. In humans and in other mammals, IgA is the principal immunoglobulin in exocrine secretions (colostrum, respiratory and intestinal mucin, saliva, tears, genitourinary tract mucin, etc.). (**REF.** 2—p. 350)

143. B. The young larvae of *T. spiralis* enter circulation and are distributed throughout the body. However, only those entering striated muscles are capable of further development. Within 3 weeks after infection, encapsulation begins. (**REF.** 3—p. 1247)

144. B. The eggs of *S. mansoni* can be recovered from the stools of patients during the acute stage, although it may be necessary to repeat examinations, since they are released in clutches. The eggs are rounded at both ends, measure 115–175 μm × 45–70 μm, and have a conspicuous lateral spine near one pole. (**REF.** 3—p. 1261)

145. A. *Campylobacter* organisms are gram-negative and curved. They are characteristically comma-shaped when seen in infected tissue, but are filamentous or coccoid following laboratory isolation (**REF.** 4—p. 742)

146. B. The V factor released from erythrocytes by mild heat and the heat-stable X factor also derived from erythrocytes are essential for the growth of *H. influenzae* (**REF.** 3—p. 510)

147. C. *Proteus vulgaris* is actively motile at 37°C, producing a thin, translucent sheet of growth on nonselective agars, which is referred to as "swarming." (**REF.** 3—p. 609)

148. A. *Clostridium tetani* produces a spore terminally located and of greater diameter than the vegetative cell, which gives the characteristic "drumstick" appearance. (**REF.** 3—p. 708)

149. E. *Bacillus anthracis* produces the so-called string-of-pearls reaction on the surface of a solid medium containing 0.05–0.5 unit of penicillin G/ml. The cells become large and spherical and occur in chains. This separates the virulent and avirulent *B. anthracis* from *B. cereus* and other aerobic spore-formers (**REF.** 3—p. 675)

150. D. *Pseudomonas aeruginosa* produces the chloroform-soluble pigment pyocyanin, which can be detected in tissue of burn patients as well as in culture. (**REF.** 3—p. 632)

151. A. Profound cellular immunodeficiency in AIDS includes an absence of delayed hypersensitivity and an absolute lymphopenia due to an absence of phenotypic T helper cells due to the reversal of the usual ratio of T helper to T suppressor cells, whereby T helper cells are severely reduced in number. (**REF.** 3—p. 334)

152. E. *Cryptosporidium* is a coccidian protozoan, which causes self-limiting gastrointestinal infection in normal individuals, but in immunocompromised patients a severe illness with chronic, profuse, and watery diarrhea. Oocysts can be identified in the stool; they appear as red bodies when stained with modified Ziehl-Neelsen method. (**REF.** 1—pp. 931, 933)

153. B. The retrovirus genome consists of two identical plus-stranded RNA molecules that are 5000–10,000 nucleotides long. Retrovirus particles are comprised of seven structural proteins; two are glycoproteins that make up the envelope spikes, the larger forming the knobs, the smaller the stalks. (**REF.** 3—p. 938)

154. B. Animal studies have suggested that the usual mode of acquisition of *Pneumocystis carinii* is the airborne route. Sporadic *Pneumocystis* pneumonia is five times more common in the first year of life than at any other age, and over 25% of sporadic illness occurs before the age of 5 years. (**REF.** 1—p. 884)

155. E. HSV–1 and HSV–2 are morphologically indistinguishable. However, they can be distinguished on the basis of certain antigenic, biologic, and biochemical differences. HSV-2 infections do not generally occur before puberty. Thereafter, the acquisition of HSV-2 infections is a function of sexual activity (**REF.** 1—pp. 1114–1115, 1125)

156. B. The incubation period of Legionnaires disease is from 2 to 10 days with a mean of 5.5 days. Cough, dyspnea, and chest pain are common early manifestations. (**REF.** 1—pp. 836–837)

157. C. Every 10–30 years, one or both of the surface antigens of influenza A changes subtype, rendering a previously immune population completely susceptible. Influenza A strains circulating in animals may provide a source of new antigenic subtypes for human influenza A viruses, accounting for antigenic shift. (**REF.** 1—p. 513)

158. C. Herpes zoster (shingles, zoster) occurs most frequently in elderly and immunocompromised individuals. It is caused by varicella-zoster virus (VZV), the same virus that causes varicella. (**REF.** 1—p. 1406)

159. C. *Klebsiella pneumoniae* is found in the respiratory tract and the feces of 5–10% of healthy subjects. It has been determined that approximately 3% of all acute bacterial pneumonias are caused by this organism. (**REF.** 2—p. 659)

160. B. Cytomegalovirus (CMV) is now known to be the most common cause of congenital viral infection and a feared pathogen in post-bone marrow-transplant patients. (**REF.** 3—p. 1005)

7. Pathology

161. D. Instead of the previous classification of amyloidosis, in which primary and secondary forms were recognized, current views support the concept of classifying this disorder into the following categories: immunocyte-derived, reactive systemic, and heredo-familial forms. (**REF.** 1—pp. 198–200)

162. D. Derived from arachidonic acid, prostaglandins (PGG_2, PG_1, PGD_2, and PGF_2) are known to cause vasodilatation, thus potentiating edema formation. Leukotrienes, a group of compounds resulting from the metabolism of arachidonic acid, are known to cause aggregation of leukocytes, vasoconstriction, bronchospasm, and increased vascular permeability. (**REF.** 1—pp. 54–58)

163. D. Patients with Klinefelter's syndrome often have only slightly below normal intelligence; indeed, some have normal I.Q. Pathologic changes in the testis include atrophy and hyalinization of seminiferous tubules; in some patients tubules may appear embryonic. Leydig cell hyperplasia is common. (**REF.** 1—p. 131)

164. D. The association between HLA-B27 and ankylosing spondylitis is well known. Individuals with HLA-B27 have a 90-fold greater chance of developing this disease than do those without it. Less frequently observed is the association between other histocompatibility antigens and Hashimoto's disease, Addison's disease, hemochromatosis, and 21-hydroxylase deficiency. (**REF.** 1—p. 162)

165. B. The pathogenicity of *Vibrio cholerae* is due to the production of a potent enterotoxin, which causes secretion of massive amounts of isotonic solution into the gut, producing the dilute "rice-water" diarrheal stools of cholera. Microscopic changes in the small intestine include congestion and inflammation of the lamina propria, hyperplasia of Peyer's patches, and, less commonly, of mesenteric lymph nodes and spleen. (**REF.** 1—pp. 318–324)

166. D. Two patterns of tissue reaction may be seen with infection with *Coccidioides immitis* (coccidiomycosis): suppuration or granuloma formation. The fungal sperules that are usually found in histiocytes or giant cells are nonbudding and measure 20–60 μm in diameter. The lung is the principal organ involved; however, the disease may involve the bones, adrenal, meninges, liver, spleen, and lymph nodes. (**REF.** 1—p. 357)

167. B. Renal involvement in lead poisoning takes the form of proximal renal tubular acidosis (Fanconi syndrome). Microscopically, the proximal tubules of the kidneys show acid-fast intranuclear inclusion bodies. (**REF.** 1—p. 453)

168. B. Three important features distinguish chronic myelogenous leukemia (CML) from leukemoid reaction: the former shows an increased number of basophils, the presence of Philadelphia chromosomes in about 95% of the cases, and decreased or absent leukocyte alkaline phosphatase in the white blood cells. The circulating white cells are also predominantly neutrophils and metamyelocytes, with a smaller number of immature cells. (**REF.** 1—pp. 676–685)

169. E. Alpha-methyl dopa belongs to the group of hepatotoxins that produce predictable liver reactions. Characteristics of such agents include dose dependence, relatively short interval between ingestion of drug and the onset of reaction, ability to induce a similar disease in experimental animals, and the causation of injury in more than 1% of the population exposed to the drug. (**REF.** 1—p. 914)

170. A. Although the histologic appearance of nephrotoxic acute tubular necrosis usually is nonspecific, some agents may produce distinctive lesions. Mercuric chloride may produce acidophilic inclusions in affected tubular cells, carbon tetrachloride may show accumulation of neutral lipids, and ethylene glycol may produce ballooning and hydropic degeneration with or without deposition of calcium oxalate in tubular lumen. (**REF.** 1—p. 1027)

171. D. People exposed to irradiation in childhood have an increased incidence of papillary thyroid carcinoma. Eighty percent of children who develop thyroid carcinoma have received previous radiation. Papillary carcinoma of the thyroid is a slowly growing tumor usually manifesting as a solitary nodule. Cervical lymph node metastasis is present in about half of the cases at the time of diagnosis. (**REFS.** 1—p. 1219; 2—p. 1411)

172. B. Negri bodies are eosinophilic intracytoplasmic inclusion bodies found in the neurons of Ammon's horn in the temporal lobe and in the Purkinje cells of the cerebellum. (**REF.** 1—p. 1384)

173. D. The features mentioned here aptly describe the typical colonic hyperplastic polyp, the most common type of polyp in this location; they represent about 90% of polyps found incidentally at autopsies. (**REF.** 1—p. 864)

174. A. In familial multiple polyposis the polyps are usually small, measuring about 1 cm in diameter. Less commonly, they may be of the villous type. There is a high incidence of malignant transformation of these polyps. (**REF.** 1—p. 867)

175. B. Found most commonly in the sixth decade or in older individuals, these polyps are sessile and nonpedunculated and present papillary fronds on gross inspection. (**REF.** 1—p. 865)

176. C. Although both types of neoplastic polyps are found more commonly in the rectosigmoid, more of villous adenomas occur in these locations than do adenomatous polyps. (**REF.** 1—pp. 864, 865)

177. D. Usually pedunculated, these polyps are large and histologically show a fibrovascular core containing dilated colonic glands. They are presumed to originate from congenitally malformed glands. These glands pose no danger of malignant transformation. (**REF.** 1—p. 869)

178. C. Tuberculosis is the typical example of cell-mediated (type IV hypersensitivity) tissue reaction, initiated by sensitized T lymphocytes. Bronchial asthma is the most common example of type I hypersensitivity reaction, mediated by IgE antibodies. Other examples of immune complex disease includes membranous glomerulonephritis and systemic lupus erythematosus. (**REF.** 1—p. 166)

179. A. Clinically, Takayashu's arteritis is characterized by ocular manifestations and diminished or absent pulses in the upper extremities (pulseless disease). The disease, which involves the aortic arch or/and its branches, has a predilection for women and patients in the age range 10–50 years. Histologic examination shows adventitial chronic inflammation, perivascular inflammatory cuffing of vasa vasorum, granulomatous inflammation of the media, and fibrosis of the media and collagenosis of the intima. (**REF.** 1—pp. 520–526)

180. D. Follicular center cell lymphomas show four histologic types: cleaved and noncleaved, small- and large-cell types. In general, the cleaved cell types tend to form a nodular pattern much more frequently than do the noncleaved cell types. T-cell lymphomas are much less frequent than B (follicular)-cell tumors. Four types of T-cell lymphomas are recognized: small T-cell lymphoma, convoluted T-cell lymphoma, mycosis fungoides, and Sezary syndrome. (**REF.** 1—p. 664)

181. A. The lesions of familial multiple polyposis are small, pedunculated polyps about 1 cm or less in diameter. The histologic appearance is that of a tubular adenoma (adenomatous polyp). Occasional villous adenoma may be present. Malignant transformation is more likely to recur in diseases of longer duration. Other varieties of familial polyposis include the Peutz-Jegher, Gardner, and Turcot syndromes. (**REF.** 1—p. 867)

182. B. The e antigen is associated with the core particle, but is a distinctive entity. HBeAg appears in the blood usually during acute infection, in the presence of HBsAg, and its presence denotes infectivity. There is controversy as to whether a persistent level of e antigen is a harbinger of chronic hepatitis. (**REF.** 1—p. 901)

183. A. Nodular glomerulosclerosis is the typical glomerular lesion in diabetic mellitus. Also known as intercapillary glomerulosclerosis or Kimmelstiel–Wilson disease, the lesions consist of PAS-positive hyaline masses at the peripheral portions of the glomerular tuft. (**REF.** 1—p. 1021)

184. B. Clear cell adenocarcinoma of the vagina is a rare neoplasm associated with offspring of mothers treated with DES during pregnancy. The tumor, usually located at the anterior wall of the vagina, may be small or large. A tumor of similar morphology may also be found, albeit less commonly, in the cervix. A probable precursor lesion is vaginal adenosis. (**REF.** 1—p. 1120)

185. E. Most commonly encountered in the colon, pseudomembranous enterocolitis is a serious inflammation of the bowel characterized by discrete and later coalescent elevated yellow-green plaques composed of fibrin, mucin, inflammatory cells, and necrotic epithelial cells. The underlying mucosa may be partially or completely necrotic. The disease has also been associated with *Shigella*, staphylococcal, and *Candida* infections. (**REFS.** 1—p. 862; 2—p. 1067)

8. Pharmacology

186. B. Aromatic hydroxylation, deamination of amines, sulfoxide formation, and *N*-oxidation are all oxidative reactions carried out by the hepatic microsomal mixed-function oxidase system. In contrast, *N*-methylation is a conjugation reaction carried out by a number of methyltransferase enzymes, such as phenylethanolamine N-methyltransferase (PNMT). (**REFS.** 1—pp. 36–43; 2—pp. 13–18)

187. B. The safety margin or therapeutic index (TI) is always calculated as the toxic dose over the therapeutic dose, e.g., $\dfrac{TD_{50}}{ED_{50}} = TI$. In each case in the examples given TI comes out to be 10. (**REF.** 1—pp. 8–9)

188. B. Nausea and vomiting, gastrointestinal bleeding, hyperventilation, and tinnitus and deafness are all common symptoms of salicylate poisoning. Hepatic injury manifested by altered liver function tests and in extreme cases by jaundice is more common as a result of acetaminophen poisoning. (**REF.** 1—pp. 159–160, 163–164)

189. C. Muscarinic antagonists (such as atropine) cause both mydriasis and cycloplegia when administered to the eye. Parasympathomimetics (methacholine) and cholinesterase inhibitors (neostigmine) cause miosis and spasm of accommodation. Epinephrine can cause mydriasis, but does not block accommodation. Acetazolamide is a carbonic-hydrase inhibitor that can reduce intraocular pressure. It does not cause mydriasis or block accommodation. (**REF.** 2—pp. 92–95, 107, 123–125, 134, 157)

190. D. Coma, respiratory depression, cyanosis, cold and clammy skin, and pinpoint pupils (miosis) all are typical symptoms of opioid poisoning. Hypertension does not occur. In fact, the patient has a low blood pressure and may be in circulatory failure. Naloxone is a morphine antagonist, which antagonizes morphine at the receptor site. (**REF.** 2—pp. 509, 523)

191. C. The administration of 100% oxygen is the preferred treatment of CO poisoning. The administration of 100% oxygen at 1 atm pressure will hasten the dissociation of carboxyhemoglobin and will decrease the half-life by three-fourths or more. (**REF.** 2—pp. 333, 1633–1634)

192. D. This is obviously a case of anticholinergic poisoning. The indicated therapy is a cholinergic agent that effectively crosses the blood-brain barrier. Only trihexyphenidyl and physostigmine are capable of crossing this barrier on intravenous injection. However, trihexyphenidyl is a relatively weak agent used to treat Parkinson's disease so only physostigmine has had extensive use in anticholinergic poisoning. (**REF.** 1—p. 217)

193. D. Of the agents listed, only cyclophosphamide is an alkyl-
194. B. ating agent, and only methotrexate is a folic acid antagonist. 6-Mercaptopurine is a purine antimetabolite; 5-fluorouracil is a pyrimidine antimetabolite; and leucovorin (folinic acid) is a specific antidote for methotrexate overdosage, since it enters the cellular metabolic scheme past the site of block induced by methotrexate. (**REF.** 1—pp. 404–408, 411, 679–682, 685–687)

195. A. Clonidine has a central action on alpha-receptors in the
196. D. brain, which in turn causes peripheral vasodilation me-
197. E. diated by the autonomic nervous system. Prazosin's main action is on alpha$_1$ receptors (vascular) with relatively little action in alpha$_2$ receptors (neuronal). This results in peripheral vasodilation without feedback inhibition by norepinephrine. Captopril's ability to block the converting enzyme of angiotensin I to angiotensin II inhibits one of the main hypertension-producing mechanisms in the body. Hydralazine and minodoxidil are both direct vascular smooth muscle relaxants. (**REFS.** 1—pp. 205, 302, 306, 307; 3—pp. 118–120, 123)

198. C. Trihexyphenidyl is a cholinergic agent, which easily
199. B. crosses the blood-brain barrier and is suitable especially for the therapy of Parkinson's disease. Bromocriptine is a lysergic acid derivative, which mimics the action of dopamine in the central nervous system, especially in the extrapyramidal tracts. (**REFS.** 1—pp. 142–143; 3—pp. 312, 314)

200. C. Hydrochlorothiazide is a thiazide type diuretic, which is
201. C. commonly used as a first step in the therapy of hyperten-
202. A. sion. Unfortunately, it also wastes potassium, and often
potassium supplementation must be given to patients receiving this
drug. Metoprolol is a beta-blocker with relative beta$_1$ selectivity.
It thus is safer to use in patients who also have asthma as compared
to other beta-blockers, such as propranolol. Of course, there is no
contraindication to the use of thiazides in patients with asthma.
(**REFS.** 1—pp. 290, 302, 305, 308; 3—pp. 110, 118)

203. C. In this experiment the large amount of drug saturated and
overwhelmed the ability of the enzyme to biotransform the drug.
Consequently, the clearance of the drug from the blood depended
only on the rate constant of the reaction. In such cases one obtains
a linear plot of blood concentration versus time. This is known as
zero-order kinetics. A common drug example that follows such
kinetics is ethanol. (**REF.** 1—pp. 30–31)

204. E. All the choices are typical of digitalis toxicity. In modern
digitalis therapy the digitalizing dose will be guided more by elec-
trophysiologic changes than by symptoms that affect the gastrointestinal tract or the visual systems. This is the result of therapy
with relatively pure digitalis glycosides. (**REFS.** 1—pp. 254–255;
2—p. 742; 3—p. 152)

205. B. Nitrous oxide is a weak anesthetic agent, but is useful
because of its rapid induction. It is nonflammable. Halothane is a
commonly used effective volatile anesthetic. (**REFS.** 1—p. 67; 2—
p. 289)

206. B. Isoniazid is one of the most effective drugs for the treatment of tuberculosis. One of the primary pathways by which it is
inactivated is by acetylation in the liver, a process that is genetically
controlled. Slow acetylators can maintain higher plasma levels of
isoniazid and are thus more prone to developing toxic effects, such
as polyneuritis. Fast acetylators, on the other hand, are more prone
to developing hepatotoxicity from a reactive intermediate of isoniazid metabolism. Experience has shown that pyridoxine antagonizes isoniazid's neurotoxic effects without preventing its
antibacterial action. Isoniazid is only one of many examples of

drugs the use of which demands understanding of the interaction between genetic makeup and drug effects. (**REFS.** 1—p. 159; 2—pp. 1200–1202; 3—pp. 546–547)

207. B. Cortisol is an anti-inflammatory glucocorticoid that increases glycogen deposition in the liver and inhibits the utilization of glucose by peripheral tissues. Prolonged treatment with cortisol can cause hyperglycemia and glycosuria, gastric ulcers, and osteoporosis. Other glucocorticoids, such as triamicinolone and betamethasone, will also have these effects. Mineralocorticoids, such as aldosterone, do not. (**REFS.** 1—p. 398; 2—pp. 1471–1475)

208. C. Quinidine and procainamide decrease membrane responsiveness and conduction velocity in ventricular muscle and lengthen the action potential duration. They also reduce ectopic automaticity, thereby inhibiting ectopic premature beats. These actions seem to be important to the antiarrhythmic efficacy of these compounds. (**REFS.** 1—pp. 265–269; 2—pp. 767–769)

209. E. A variety of agents are useful in glaucoma. They may lower intraocular fluid pressure by decreasing secretion or increasing the excretion of intraocular fluid, such as epinephrine and timolol. Agents such as physostigmine and pilocarpine lower pressure by causing miosis and thus increasing the chances for excretion of intraocular fluid by opening the angle of the trabeculae. (**REFS.** 2—pp. 123–125, 177, 200; 3—pp. 70–72, 95, 104)

210. E. Carbamazepine differs chemically from the classical antiepileptic drugs. It also is unique in that it is effective in practically all types of seizures as well as tic douloureux. (**REFS.** 1—pp. 138–139; 2—pp. 457–459; pp. 270–271)

9. Physiology

211. E. Any form of artificial respiration is a must because in each situation listed, except E, the respiratory center fails before the vasomoter center and heart. Any situation involving cessation of respiration requires the need for maintaining oxygenation by artificial methods. (**REF.** 1—pp. 627–628)

212. A. The menstrual cycle may be considered as follows: beginning with regression of the corpus (luteolysis), the estrogen and progesterone levels fall. This causes FSH and LH secretion from the pituitary and starts the development of a new follicle. From there, estrogen secretions rapidly increase and trigger LH secretion via a positive feedback mechanism. At about day 14, ovulation occurs, with formation of a corpus luteum. At this point, both estrogen and progesterone levels rise, and, when high enough, inhibit FSH and LH secretion, which results in luteolysis and a new cycle. Both FSH and LH secretions are controlled by hypothalamic releasing factors. (**REF.** 1—pp. 925–933)

213. C. Parathyroid gland secretion increases the plasma calcium level, mobilizes calcium from bone, and increases urinary phosphate excretion. The rate of parathyroid secretion varies inversely with the plasma calcium level, and its main function is to maintain a constant level of ionized calcium in the extracellular fluid. In addition to the parathyroid hormone, control of calcium metabolism is also under the influence of thyrocalcitonin, which is secreted by the thyroid gland. Its role is to lower plasma calcium. Both act to maintain ionized calcium in the plasma. (**REF.** 1—p. 896ff)

214. B. The pacemaker cells of the heart are characterized by a slow, continuous diastolic depolarization that is automatic (spontaneous). They have a very slow rise time (phase 0) and little or no overshoot and are of low amplitude and short duration. They represent the slow-response action potentials mediated by slow inward currents of Ca^{2+} and Na^+ gates. (**REF.** 1—p. 157)

215. C. Purkinje fibers and all cells of the specialized conducting system are characterized by a stable resting potential, very rapid phase 0, and sharp phase 1 repolarization, and are of long duration (phase 2 is longer than any other cardiac cell type). These fast response calls during phase 0 are mediated by a fast inward Na^+ current. Phase 2 is due to activation of a slow inward Ca^{2+} current and a slow inward Na^+ current. These slow channels are voltage dependent and open at about -40 mV. These currents are offset by an outward K^+ current. The rapid repolarization of phase 3 is due to an outward K^+ current, which starts with the inactivation of the slow Ca^{2+} and Na^+ gates. Ventricular muscle cells are of shorter duration than Purkinje fibers and have a lower rate of initial (phase 1) rapid repolarization. (**REF.** 1—p. 151)

216. D. The QRS of the surface ECG represents the total ventricular muscle cell depolarizations. The voltage changes sensed by the ECG leads record the "muscle" cell alteration because of their mass compared with the total mass of the other cardiac cell types. (**REF.** 1—p. 166)

217. B. An impulse is essentially a series of currents flowing in
218. A. and out of the cell membrane. Action potentials leave the
219. D. membrane ahead of the region of depolarization and act as a cathode (current flow into cathodal electrode). The action potential current acts to stimulate and hence depolarize the area of membrane ahead of it. At this time the membrane permeability is such that Na^+ can move inside while the area behind it is repolarizing and K^+ ion flux is outward. As thus defined, the impulse in the figure is propagating from right to left (i.e., arrow D). At rest the voltage gradient is positive outside and negative inside the cell. (**REF.** 1—p. 41)

220. C. Glucose is actively reabsorbed within the proximal tubule and has a T_m of about 373 mg/minute. Since the GFR is about 125 ml/minute, the theoretical renal threshold for glucose should be about 300 mg/minute, or T_m/GFR. The actual kidney threshold, however, is about 200 mg/100 ml of arterial plasma, and this represents a venous level of about 180 mg/100 ml. The difference between the actual and theoretical values is a result of renal "splay" due to the fact that not all nephrons have the same T_m and filtration rate for glucose cells: some glucose may not be reabsorbed when the filtered amount of glucose is below its T_m. (**REF.** 1—p. 473)

221. D. The hydrogen secretion mechanism is extremely important for acid–base regulation. The ion is secreted both in the proximal and distal tubules as well as in the collecting duct. The H^+ is actively moved across the membrane; for each such ion transported there is an equal Na^+ that enters the cell. Hence, the Na^+ that is exchanged for H^+ moves down its chemical and electrical gradients. The Na^+ moving in may be via diffusion or by a carrier system. The net result, however, is that $H^+ - N^+$ exchange yields one HCO_3 and one Na^+ that can enter the interstitial fluid to be made available as a buffer. (**REF.** 1—p. 526)

222. E. Any shift of the O_2 dissolution curve to the right signifies a decrease in O_2 affinity of the Hb and thus aids oxygen delivery to the cells. Any increase in temperature, H^+ concentration or PCO_2 will enhance the release of O_2 from Hb at any particular pressure of O_2 in the tissue. The organic phosphates, especially 2,3-diphosphoglycerate (2,3-DPG) within the RBC, also aid in the O_2 unbinding, and any increase in 2,3-DPG will increase the amount of O_2; this is an important physiologic response in chronic hypoxia. (**REF.** 1—p. 564)

223. E. In a normal adult both ventilation (V) and blood flow (P) are greater at the base of the lung than at the apex. In addition, the blood flow at the base is greater and more marked in relation to ventilation. As a result, the V/P rate is less at the base. The alveolar PO_2 (and PCO_2) will thus be affected whenever nonuniform ventilation and perfusion exist such that inequality will not maintain as high an arterial PO_2 (and as low an arterial PCO_2) as a lung in which ventilation and perfusion are comparable. Thus, in the normal adult the lower V/P at the lung base will result in a low alveolor PO_2 as compared to the apex. (**REF.** 1—pp. 580, 560)

224. E. All of these factors will cause the blood PO_2 to decrease with hypoventilation. There is less inspired oxygen available, so alveolar ventilation is reduced, with a concomitant fall in arterial PO_2 (and a rise in PCO_2). Since the actual transfer of O_2 and Co_2 from alveoli to blood is by simple diffusion, any barrier to the process, as with thickening of the alveolar wall, will prevent the blood PO_2 from reaching the alveolar value of 100 mm Hg. In addition, any blood that cannot or does not pass through ventilated lung areas is added to the systemic arteries, but is blood that is depleted of O_2 and hence adds to a lowering of systemic arterial PO_2. Finally, the fourth cause of hypoxemia is when there is a mismatch between ventilation (V) and blood flow (P) within the lung. This is represented by the V/P ratio. The normal alveolar PO_2 of 100 mm Hg is a balance between the addition of O_2 by ventilation through the inspired air and its removal by blood flow.

Any increases in ventilation relative to its removal by the blood (as in obstruction of blood flow) means a low arterial PO_2 (high V/P ratio). On the other hand, obstruction of ventilation with an unchanging perfusion (low V/P ratio) will cause a fall in alveolar oxygen to equal mixed venous PO_2. So, when the V/P ratio is high, the alveoli contribute little oxygen to blood compared with the decrease caused by alveoli with low V/P ratio. (**REF.** 1—p. 572ff)

225. B. The presence of glucosteroids and insulin is essential for normal skeletal muscle activity. Insulin is necessary for its action enhancing glucose uptake by the muscle fibers. The glucosteroids, especially cortisol, mobilize amino acids from the blood by decreasing protein synthesis, which then go to the liver for gluconeogenesis. This helps maintain blood sugar and glycogen content of the muscle. Thus, in any pathophysiologic or clinical situation where there is an elevation of these steroids there will appear a diabeteslike and a generalized muscle-wasting condition. Although epinephrine regulates glycogen synthesis and glycogenolysis and may increase contractile tension, the amount needed is extremely high. The thyroid hormone in excess will result in muscle weakness and fatigability. (**REF.** 1—p. 100)

226. E. Type I diabetes mellitus denotes juvenile-onset diabetes; type II is adult-onset diabetes. In each, the clinical signs are the three Ps of diabetes, polyuria, polydipsia, and polyphagia, which are the consequences of hyperglycemia. Eventually there is a large loss of glucose through the urine; the renal threshold for glucose is greatly exceeded. This leads to an obligatory loss of water through the collecting tubules, where the glucose acts as an osmotic diuretic. Although types I and II represent insulin deficiency, the problem in type I is a direct result of an absolute inability of the pancreatic beta cells to secrete insulin, while in type II the plasma insulin level may be normal or even elevated. The defect in type II appears to be a loss of tissue response to the circulating insulin, so this condition represents a "relative" rather than an "absolute" insulin deficiency. (**REF.** 1—p. 830)

227. A. The first heart sound occurs at the beginning of ventricular systole and is best heard over the apex of the heart. It consists of irregular vibrations mainly of a frequency between 30 and 45/

second. These vibrations originate from at least three sources: (1) vibrations from the a.v. valves during and after their closure; (2) vibrations of the eddies in the stream of blood ejected through the aortic orifices as the blood flows into the wider sinuses of Valsalva; and (3) vibrations in the cardiac muscle fibers themselves generated as the heart muscles develop tension from a state of relaxation. In all, the main vibrations develop at the termination of the QRS complex and the beginning of ventricular contraction. (**REF.** 1— p. 226)

228. E. The extrinsic control of ventricular function is by means of the neural stimuli and hormonal stimuli to the heart through efferents of the autonomic nervous system, as well as the chemical content of the blood that supplies the heart muscle. The constant arrival of sympathetic and parasympathetic impulses ensures that the heart force of each contraction can be increased or decreased by altering the frequency of the impulses. In addition, the levels of oxygen, carbon dioxide, and catecholamine in the blood constitute a second group of controls that are extrinsic in nature. Thus, myocardial hypoxia and/or hypercapnea depress contractility, and the force of contraction will be increased by secretions of epinephrine and/or norepinephrine. (**REF.** 1—pp. 212–222)

229. E. All of the factors listed affect gastric motility in some fashion. The fibers of the autonomic nervous system are excitatory (parasympathetic) and inhibitory (sympathetic or catecholamine secretion). The hormone gastrin is like ACh in that both increase the frequency, amplitude, and duration of gastric smooth cell action potentials as well as contractility. The catecholamines decrease the spike potential and spontaneous activity, as well as the force of contraction. The liquid content and volume also play a major role in gastric motility, in that hyperosmolar solutions delay or inhibit contraction, while large fluid volume stretches the smooth muscle fibers and enhance contraction. The net result of these "stimuli" is to alter the rate of stomach emptying by affecting motor activity. (**REF.** 1—p. 654)

230. E. All the factors listed play an important role in the type of blood flowing in any large arterial vessel. When laminar or streamline flow breaks down into a turbulent flow, as occurs at high velocities of flow, the Reynolds number increases, and this can be predicted from the Poiseulle equation. In turbulence, the fluid particles move continuously in varying paths and quite irregularly, sometimes forming eddy currents, while at other times the flow gives the appearance of random motion. This transition from laminar to turbulent flow is greatly dependent upon the density and viscosity of the fluid and extremely dependent upon the vessel radius. The average flow velocity also plays a role. The critical point at which turbulence develops can be determined quantitatively and is referred to as the Reynolds number. It is expressed as Reynolds number $= \dfrac{\overline{V}DP}{\eta}$ where P is the blood density (usually about 1.05 gm/cm^2), D is the diameter of the vessel (cm), $\overline{V}$ is the average velocity (cm/second), and η is the blood viscosity (dyne second/cm$_2$). Usually turbulence in flow will develop at a Reynolds number of 3000 and such turbulent flow is enhanced by increasing velocity, increasing vessel diameter, and decreasing blood viscosity. (**REF. 1**—pp. 132–137)

231. E. Gastric acid secretion is affected by all of the factors listed such that secretion can be either increased or decreased. The excitatory influences on acid secretion during the cephalic phase include sight, smell and taste of food mediated by a release of gastrin and vagal stimulation. During the gastric phase the excitatory influences include local distention as well as the chemical action of peptides and ammino acids, with the activity mediated by local gastric and vago-vagal reflexes as well as gastrin release. The intestinal phase of gastric secretion is mediated by a peptide (enterooxyntin) and stimulated by peptones and amino acids. On the other hand, these excitatory influences are counterbalanced by a number of inhibitory processes, particularly those arising from the duodenum and involving a mucosal factor (bulbogastrone) that prevent or slow down acid secretion. Also involved is an enterogastric reflex with H$^+$ acting as the stimulus. In addition, the presence of secretin and fat in the duodenum will inhibit or markedly reduce gastric acid secretion. (**REF. 1**—p. 709)

232. E. The stimuli listed can elicit the sensation of pain if there is damage or destruction of any living tissue that is innervated— with the singular exception of brain tissue. Pain consists of two components: sensation and reaction. Sensation is the feeling of hurt and is reenforced by experience. Reaction to pain is an autonomic and somatic reflex response and represents an attempt to remove the stimulus and is coupled with an emotional response. Pain involves two afferent types and includes nociceptive units and C-fibers. The former respond to high-threshold tissue-damaging stimuli, giving rise to a hurting, pricky pain. Activation of the C-fibers gives rise to a slower onset, "second" pain, which is more intense and longer lasting, exhibiting a burning quality. The feeling is one of intense hurt. Chemical, thermal, mechanical, and electrical excitation yield pain if they damage or destroy innervated tissue. (**REF.** 1—p. 1134)

233. E. The controlling mechanisms of the sleep–wake pattern lie in the tegmentum of the brain stem, especially the pons, mesencephalon, and lateral hypothalmus. Of these, two areas are essential for the cycles; one area (RAS) keeps us awake, while the other portion (Raphe system) induces sleep as well as its depth and stage. These portions are controlled by different neurohumeral transmitters. It appears that dopamine is the transmitter for the waking system, while serotonin is that for the sleep system. Norepinephrine seems to control the sleep stage referred to as the rapid eye movement (REM) stage. (**REF.** 1—p. 1276ff)

234. B. Parasympathetic (vagal) activity to the heart normally decreases cardiac rate and decreases blood pressure. An increase in vagal tone results in a release of greater amounts of acetylcholine, which directly suppresses sinoatrial activity. Sufficient vagal action results in cessation of all heart activity, leading to cardiac standstill. If such vagal activity is maintained, permanent cardiac arrest does not occur, because the Purkinje fiber network can, and does, develop its own spontaneous depolarizations due to their inherent property of latent automaticity, and this results in "ventricular or vagal" escape. The mechanism of the vagal or acetylcholine action is by its ability to alter cardiac cell permeability, primarily increasing the outward movement of potassium. This rapid outward potassium flux creates a larger inside negativity or hyperpolarization. Such a larger negative potential makes the cardiac cell less excitable. On the other hand, the infusion or release of any catecholamine or any greater sympathetic nerve activity will result in overall greater heart activity. The mechanism for sympathetic actions is probably an increased membrane permeability to sodium and calcium, which can account for the increased heart rate as well as the greater force of contraction. (**REF.** 1—pp. 157–160)

235. E. Body heat is lost through each of the factors listed. Of these, only radiation and evaporation of sweat and insensible perspiration are under direct physiologic control. Radiation accounts for 50% of total body heat loss and represents the rate of cooling of an object that has a temperature gradient between it and the surrounding environment. The body alters this gradient by: (1) blood distribution, which can adjust skin temperature from 15° C to body temperature; (2) variation in blood volume, which in severe heat can shift by 10% in 2–4 hours; this is accomplished by drawing fluid from tissues into the general circulation and can be reversed during extreme cold; and (3) by increasing rate of circulation so that the resulting increase in cardiac output coupled with the enhanced blood flow promotes the transport of heat from inside the body to the surface. The loss of heat by convection is through air movement and increases with increased velocity up to about 60 miles/hour, after which there is no additional loss of heat. The loss of heat by evaporation occurs when the outside temperature is 38° C or higher, since at these temperatures radiation is reversed and the body gains heat. Evaporation is a process by which water is changed from a liquid to a vapor state at the body surface and involves sweating as well as insensible perspiration. In addition, some heat (2%) is lost through the urine and feces. Most heat loss is by way of evaporation (30%). (**REF.** 1—p. 1228)

References

1. Anatomy

1. Carpenter M.B. and Sutin J.: *Human Neuroanatomy*, 8th Edition, Williams & Wilkins, Baltimore, MD, 1983

2. Kelly D.E., Wood R.L., and Enders A.C.: *Bailey's Textbook of Microscopic Anatomy*, 18th Edition, Williams & Wilkins, Baltimore, MD, 1984

3. Moore K.L.: *The Developing Human*, 3rd Edition, E. B. Saunders, Philadelphia, PA, 1982

4. Woodburne R.T.: *Essentials of Human Anatomy*, 7th Edition, Oxford University Press, New York, NY, 1983

2. Behavioral Sciences

1. DiMascio A. and Shader R.: *Clinical Handbook of Psychopharmacology*, Aronson, New York, NY, 1970

2. Haynes R.B.: Strategies to improve compliance with referrals, appointments, and prescribed medical regimens. In Haynes R.B., Taylor D.W., and Sackett D.L. (Eds), *Compliance in Health Care*, Johns Hopkins University Press, Baltimore, MD, 1979

3. Hine F.R. and Pfeiffer E.: *Behavioral Science: A Selective View*, Little Brown, Waltham, MA, 1972

4. Kaplan H.I. and Sadock B. J.: *Modern Synopsis of Comprehensive Textbook of Psychiatry*/IV, 4th Edition, Williams & Wilkins, Baltimore, MD, 1985

5. Millon T.: *Medical Behavior Science*, W.B. Saunders, Philadelphia, PA, 1975

6. Munsinger H.: *Fundamentals of Child Development*, 2nd Edition, Holt, Rinehart and Winston, New York, NY, 1975

7. Nathan P.E. and Goldman M.S.: Problem drinking and alcoholism. In Pomerleau O.F. and Brady J.P. (Eds), *Behavioral Medicine: Theory and Practice*, Williams & Wilkins, Baltimore, MD, 1979

8. President's Committee on Mental Retardation: *Mental Retardation: The Known and the Unknown*, DHEW Publications, Washington, D.C., 1975

9. Robertson L.S. and Heagarty M.C.: *Medical Sociology: A General Systems Approach*, Nelson-Hall, Chicago, IL, 1975

3. Biochemistry

1. Lehninger A.L.: *Biochemistry*, 2nd Edition, Worth, New York, NY, 1975

2. Smith E.L., Hill R.L., Lehman I.R., Lefkowitz R.S., Handler P., and White A.L.: *Principles of Biochemistry*, Vol. I—*General Aspects*, Vol. II—*Mammalian Biochemistry*, 7th Edition, McGraw-Hill, New York, NY, 1983

3. Stryer L.: *Biochemistry*, 2nd Edition, Freeman, San Francisco, CA, 1981

4. Zubay G.: *Biochemistry*, Addison-Wesley, Reading, MA, 1983

4. Biostatistics/Epidemiology

1. Andres R., Bierman E.L., and Hazzard, W.R.: *Principles of Geriatric Medicine*, McGraw-Hill, New York, NY, 1985

2. Armitage P.: *Statistical Methods in Medical Research*, Wiley, New York, NY, 1971

3. Atcheley R.C.: *The Social Forces in Later Life: An Introduction to Social Gerontology*, Wadsworth, Belmont, CA, 1977

4. Birren J.E. and Sloan, R.B.: *Handbook of Mental Health and Aging*, Prentice-Hall, Englewood Cliffs, NJ, 1980

5. Butler R.N. and Lewis M.I.: *Aging and Mental Health: Positive Psychosocial and Biomedical Approaches*, C.V. Mosby, St. Louis, MO, 1982

6. Colton T.: *Statistics in Medicine*, Little, Brown, Boston, MA, 1974

7. Eaton W. W.: *The Sociology of Mental Disorders*, Praeger, New York, NY, 1980

8. Fletcher R.H, Fletcher S.W., and Wagner E.H.: *Clinical Epidemiology*, Williams & Wilkins, Baltimore, MD, 1982

9. Friedman G.D.: *Primer of Epidemiology*, 2nd Edition, McGraw-Hill, New York, NY, 1980

10. Glanz S.A.: *Primer of Biostatistics*, McGraw-Hill, New York, 1981

11. Kessler I.I.: Epidemiologic studies of Parkinson's disease, III: A community-based survey. *Am J Epidemiol*. 96(4):242–254, 1972

12. Last J.M.: *Public Health and Preventive Medicine*, 11th Edition, Appleton-Century-Crofts, New York, NY, 1980

13. Lesko S.M., et al.: Cigarette smoking and the risk of endometrial cancer. *N Engl J Med*. 313(10):593, 1985

14. Levy B.S. and Wegbman D.H. *Occupational Health*, Little, Brown, Boston, MA, 1983

15. Luft H.S.: Competition and regulation. *Medical Care*. 23(5): 383, 1985

16. Morton R.F. and Hebel J.R.: *A Study Guide to Epidemiology and Biostatistics*, 2nd Edition, University Park Press, Baltimore, MA, 1984

17. Report of the Surgeon General, The Health Consequences of Smoking, U.S. Department of Health and Human Services, 1982

18. Rom W.: *Environmental and Occupational Medicine*, Little, Brown, Boston, MA, 1983

5. Genetics

1. Emery A.E.H. and Rimoin D.L.: *Principles and Practice of Medical Genetics*, Churchill Livingston, New York, NY, 1983

2. Thompson J.S. and Thompson M.W.: *Genetics in Medicine*, W.B. Saunders, Philadelphia, PA, 1986

6. Microbiology

1. Braude A.I.: *Infectious Diseases and Medical Microbiology*, 2nd Edition, W.B. Saunders, Philadelphia, PA, 1986

2. Davis B.D., Dulbecco R., Eisen H.N., and Ginsberg H.S.: *Microbiology*, 3rd Edition, Harper & Row, Hagerstown, MD, 1980

3. Joklik W.K., Willett H.P., and Amos D.B.: *Zinsser Microbiology*, 18th Edition, Appleton-Century-Crofts, New York, NY, 1984

7. Pathology

1. Anderson W.A.D. and Kissane J.M. (Eds): *Pathology*, 8th Edition, C.V. Mosby, St. Louis, MO, 1984

2. Robbins S.L. and Cotran R.S.: *Pathological Basis of Disease*, 3rd Edition, W.B. Saunders, Philadelphia, PA, 1984

8. Pharmacology

1. DiPalma J.R. (Ed): *Basic Pharmacology in Medicine*, 2nd Edition, McGraw-Hill, New York, NY, 1982

2. Goodman G.A., Goodman L.S., Rall T.W., and Murad F. (Eds): *The Pharmacologic Basis of Therapeutics*, 7th Edition, Macmillan, New York, NY, 1985

3. Katzung B.G.: *Basic and Clinical Pharmacology*, 2nd Edition, Lange, Los Altos, CA, 1984

9. Physiology

1. West J.B. (Ed): *Best and Taylor's Physiological Basis of Medical Practise*, 11th Edition, Williams & Wilkins, Baltimore, MD, 1985

PART II

The material on the following pages is designed to help you prepare for Day II of the Federation Licensing Examination (FLEX). It includes a total of 520 board-type multiple-choice questions, distributed over the 14 required clinical sciences: anesthesiology, emergency medicine, family medicine, internal medicine, medical ethics, neurology, obstetrics and gynecology, ophthalmology, otorhinolaryngology, pediatrics, public health and preventive medicine, psychiatry, radiology, and surgery. The correct answers, with accompanying comments and page references to textbooks and journal articles, begin on page 309. The reference list for Part II appears at the end of the answer section. The questions are a representative sampling of the topics specified in the Federation's content outline for Day II. They are grouped by question type to familiarize you with the variety of question formats you will see on the actual examination.

10

Anesthesiology
Thomas J. DeKornfeld, M.D.

DIRECTIONS: Each of the questions or incomplete statements below is followed by five suggested answers or completions. Select the **one** that is best in each case.

---

1. A thiobarbiturate induction is contraindicated in patients with
    A. essential hypertension
    B. acute intermittent porphyria
    C. erythropoietic uroporphyria
    D. gout
    E. glucosidase enzyme deficiency (Pompe's disease)

2. The primary goal in the anesthetic management of carotid endarterectomy surgery is
    A. the avoidance of hypertension
    B. the avoidance of tachycardia
    C. the maintenance of cerebral perfusion pressure
    D. the provision of complete muscle relaxation
    E. the provision of deliberate hypotension

3. Which of the following is NOT a good measure of cerebral perfusion during carotid endarterectomy surgery?
   A. Jugular venous oxygen saturation
   B. Electroencephalography
   C. Stump pressure measurement
   D. Evoked potentials
   E. Oculoplethysmography

4. Which of the following muscle relaxants should be AVOIDED in patients with severe chronic renal disease?
   A. Succinylcholine
   B. Vecuronium
   C. Atracurium
   D. Gallamine
   E. d-Tubocurarine

5. The most common neurologic complication of spinal anesthesia is
   A. spinal headache
   B. transverse myelitis
   C. anterior spinal artery syndrome
   D. adhesive arachnoiditis
   E. cauda equina syndrome

6. "Halothane hepatitis"
   A. is a gastroenterologic fiction
   B. is a relatively frequent complication after hepatic surgery
   C. is more common in thin males
   D. is an extremely rare form of toxic hepatitis
   E. is probably a genetically linked defect in females

DIRECTIONS: Each group of questions below consists of five lettered headings followed by a list of numbered statements. For **each** numbered statement, select the **one** lettered heading that is most closely associated with it. Each lettered heading may be selected once, more than once, or not at all.

Questions 7–10:

    A. Enflurane
    B. Fentanyl
    C. Halothane
    D. Isoflurane
    E. Ketamine

7. Is considered a dissociative anesthetic agent

8. May cause convulsions in some patients

9. May cause severe hallucinations in the postoperative period

10. May cause severe postoperative respiratory depression

Questions 11–14:

    A. Prostigmine
    B. Physostigmine
    C. Naloxone
    D. Protamine
    E. Atropine

11. Is used to block emergence delirium

12. Blocks the muscarinic effects of prostigmine

13. Should be used with extreme caution in narcotic addicts

14. Should be given slowly and into a peripheral line

DIRECTIONS: Each set of lettered headings below is followed by a list of numbered phrases. For each numbered phrase select

    A   if the item is associated with A *only*
    B   if the item is associated with B *only*
    C   if the item is associated with *both* A and B
    D   if the item is associated with *neither* A nor B

Questions 15–17:

    A. Orotracheal intubation
    B. Nasotracheal intubation
    C. Both
    D. Neither

15. Is practically free of complications

16. May be assisted by fiberoptic visualization of the glottis

17. May cause severe epistaxis

Questions 18–21:

    A. Spinal anesthesia
    B. Epidural anesthesia
    C. Both
    D. Neither

18. May lead to neurologic complications

19. May be used to provide long-range postoperative pain relief

20. May cause significant hypotension

21. May be used in patients on anticoagulant therapy

DIRECTIONS: For each of the questions or incomplete statements below, **one or more** of the answers or completions given is correct. Select

A if only *1, 2, and 3* are correct
B if only *1 and 3* are correct
C if only *2 and 4* are correct
D if only *4* is correct
E if *all* are correct

Questions 22–30:

22. The purpose of the preanesthetic visit is to
    1. establish a good patient–physician relationship
    2. write preoperative orders
    3. do a careful and specific history and physical exam
    4. allay patient apprehension

23. Malignant hyperpyrexia is
    1. more common in adults than in children
    2. a genetically transmitted predisposition
    3. usually accompanies by profound metabolic alkalosis
    4. both preventable and treatable

24. Malignant hyperthermia can be triggered by
    1. succinylcholine
    2. morphine
    3. halothane
    4. ester-type local anesthetics

25. The earliest clinical symptoms of malignant hyperthermia under anesthesia include
    1. fever
    2. tachycardia
    3. metabolic alkalosis
    4. masseter spasm

Directions Summarized

A	B	C	D	E
1, 2, 3 only	1, 3 only	2, 4 only	4 only	All are correct

26. In a patient with a full stomach the danger of regurgitation and aspiration can be minimized by
    1. the Sellick maneuver (cricoesophageal pressure)
    2. rapid sequence induction
    3. awake intubation
    4. gastric aspiration

27. Preanesthetic medication can be used to
    1. decrease apprehension
    2. provide amnesia
    3. decrease salivation
    4. block vagal reflexes

28. Succinylcholine should not be used in patients with
    1. hypertension
    2. penetrating corneal laceration
    3. hypotension
    4. severe burns

29. In patients with high spinal cord transection, which of the following may present serious anesthetic problems?
    1. Autonomic hyperreflexia
    2. Difficult intubation
    3. Hyperkalemia with succinylcholine
    4. Hypotension

30. Intraoperative monitoring in children must include
    1. blood pressure
    2. ECG
    3. temperature
    4. pulse rate

11

Emergency Medicine

James J. Mathews, M.D., and
David Zull, M.D.

DIRECTIONS: Each of the questions or incomplete statements below is followed by five suggested answers or completions. Select the **one** that is best in each case.

---

31. A patient with a recent wrist injury should be treated for a navicular fracture under which circumstance?
    A. Only if the x-ray is diagnostic
    B. If there is tenderness over the anatomic snuff box, regardless of x-ray findings
    C. If there is tenderness over the ulnar aspect of the wrist
    D. If the fifth finger is numb
    E. None of the above

32. The simplest, most readily available, and most effective method for core rewarming in hypothermia is
    A. colonic irrigation
    B. heated IV fluids
    C. peritoneal dialysis with heated fluids
    D. inhalation of warm, humidified air
    E. extracorporeal circulation

33. The most serious toxic effect of tricyclic antidepressant overdose is
    A. severe headache
    B. early respiratory failure
    C. severe vomiting and diarrhea
    D. acute renal failure
    E. lethal cardiac arrhythmias

34. A 41-year-old male is seen in the emergency room complaining of swelling and numbness of both hands. His car had stalled and he had worked on the engine for 45 minutes without gloves. The outside temperature was 5°F with a wind velocity of 15 mph, creating a windchill index of −25°F. Physical examination reveals cold, pale, cyanotic fingers. There is no capillary filling and the tissue has a woody consistency. Early blister formation is seen. What is the most appropriate immediate treatment of this man's hands?
    A. Passive rewarming with protective cradling, elevation, and numerous blankets
    B. Immersion in antiseptic solution at 98°F with gentle massage for 30 minutes
    C. Immersion in well-agitated water bath at 104–108°F for 20–30 minutes
    D. Immersion in cold water followed by gradual rewarming to 104°F, then reduction to 98°F
    E. Immersion in hot water of 140°F with gradual reduction to 98°F

35. A 30-year-old female is brought to the emergency room following a suicide attempt. She is tachypnic, and has vomitted twice in the emergency room. An arterial blood gas reveals pH = 7.28, $PCO_2 = 22$, $PO_2 = 90$. All the following substances in the poisoning or overdose setting can cause this picture EXCEPT
    A. ethylene glycol (antifreeze)
    B. methyl alcohol (wood alcohol)
    C. glutethimide
    D. cyanide
    E. aspirin

36. A 6-month-old boy is brought to the emergency room following a 3-day history of diarrhea, vomitting, and fever. On examination, T = 102.7°F, R = 48, BP = 60/20. He is lethargic and cranky when stimulated. His eyes appear sunken, the axilla are dry, and the skin turgor is poor. What is the most appropriate initial order for fluid management in this child?
   A. Administer one-half of the child's calculated fluid deficit plus maintenance needs over the next 8 hours
   B. Administer the entire calculated fluid deficit over 1 hour, then continue on maintenance fluids
   C. Administer a fluid bolus of 20 ml/kg over 20 minutes
   D. Administer 4 ml/kg per % estimated dehydration over the first 8 hours
   E. Encourage fluids by the oral route, such as Pedialyte, witholding IV fluids unless vomitting ensues

---

DIRECTIONS: Each group of questions below consists of five lettered headings followed by a list of numbered words or statements. For **each** numbered word or statement, select the **one** lettered heading that is most closely associated with it. Each lettered heading may be selected once, more than once, or not at all.

Questions 37–40: Which set of arterial blood gasses would be associated with the condition tested (PO_2 and PCO_2 in mm Hg)?

   A. pH 7.17, PCO_2 18, PO_2 95
   B. pH 7.36, PCO_2 25, PO_2 50
   C. pH 7.60, PCO_2 15, PO_2 95
   D. pH 7.15, PCO_2 55, PO_2 60
   E. pH 7.42, PCO_2 42, PO_2 80

37. Normal arterial blood gasses

38. Uncompensated metabolic acidosis with respiratory alkalosis

39. Hyperventilation secondary to acute anxiety

40. Acute ventilatory failure

Questions 41–44: For each clinical syndrome, choose the most likely insect sting that could cause it:

A. Brown recluse spider
B. Black widow spider
C. Fire ant
D. Ticks
E. Mites

41. Anaphylaxis

42. Ascending flaccid paralysis progressing from extremities to cranial nerves

43. Vesiculation and discoloration progressing to skin necrosis

44. Severe tetanic muscular spasms, especially of the abdomen

---

DIRECTIONS: Each set of lettered headings below is followed by a list of numbered words or phrases. For each numbered word or phrase select

A if the item is associated with A *only*
B if the item is associated with B *only*
C if the item is associated with *both* A and B
D if the item is associated with *neither* A nor B

Questions 45–47:

A. Esophageal reflex with esophagospasm
B. Acute myocardial infarction
C. Both
D. Neither

45. Severe retrosternal chest pain with radiation to jaw and/or arm, and associated diaphoresis and shortness of breath

46. Relief of pain with nitroglycerin

47. Elevation of the MB band of creatine kinase isozymes

Questions 48–50:

    A. Organophosphate insecticides
    B. Carbon tetrachloride
    C. Both
    D. Neither

48. Absorbed readily through the skin

49. Bradyarrhthmias, bronchorrhea, and muscle twitching

50. Hepatotoxic

DIRECTIONS: For each of the questions or incomplete statements below, **one or more** of the answers or completions given is correct. Select
    A if only *1, 2, and 3* are correct
    B if only *1 and 3* are correct
    C if only *2 and 4* are correct
    D if only *4* is correct
    E if *all* are correct

Questions 51–54:

51. Human bites should be treated with
    1. primary closure in most cases
    2. prophylactic antiobiotic therapy
    3. profuse irrigation with sterile saline before suturing
    4. tetracycline or erythromycin if the patient is allergic to penicillin

		Directions Summarized		
A	**B**	**C**	**D**	**E**
1, 2, 3	1, 3	2, 4	4	All are
only	only	only	only	correct

52. Carbon monoxide poisoning is commonly associated with
  1. marked decrease in arterial PO_2 in most cases
  2. chest pain and cardiac arrhythmias in older patients
  3. absence of central nervous system symptoms, except with severe toxicity
  4. long-term neurologic problems, which may present several weeks after the acute episode

53. Sepsis and meningitis in a 9-day-old child are most commonly caused by
  1. *Neisseria* meningitis
  2. Group B *Streptococcus*
  3. *Hemophilus influenzae*, type B
  4. *Escherichia coli*

54. A 50-year-old male developed progressive pain and decreased vision in his right eye while in a dark movie theater. On arrival to the emergency room, the man appears in moderate distress from the pain and he is vomitting repeatedly. Physical examination reveals a diffusely reddened conjunctiva, the cornea is hazy, and the pupil is mid-dilated and fixed. Visual acuity is decreased and the patient describes halos around lights. What would be appropriate immediate therapy?
  1. Topical pilocarpine
  2. Mannitol
  3. Carbonic anhydrase inhibitors (acetazolamide)
  4. Paper bag breathing

DIRECTIONS: This section of the test consists of situations, each followed by a series of questions. Study each situation and select the **one** best answer to each question following it.

Questions 55–57: An unconscious 28-year-old male is brought to the emergency department after sustaining injuries in an automobile accident. His car was struck head on by a car traveling the opposite direction. Both cars were traveling between 35 and 40 mph when the head-on collision occurred. On arrival to the emergency room, the patient is unconscious; BP = 60/40; R = 28 shallow. There are multiple stellate lacerations on the forehead and mid-frontal area. There are multiple palpable rib fractures on the left chest, which expands on expiration and sinks in on inspiration. In addition, there is palpable crepitus over the pubic bones and blood is noted at the urethral meatus.

55. If the patient's respiratory rate rises to 40 and he appears in greater distress, what is the most definitive intervention?
    A. Sandbag the segment of chest wall involved
    B. Tracheal intubation and positive pressure ventilation
    C. Chest tube insertion
    D. Immediate thoracotomy
    E. 100% O_2 by rebreather mask

56. Two large-bore IV lines are placed and saline is given wide open; transiently the BP rises to 110/80, P = 110, but then drops again to 70/30, P = 140. What diagnostic procedure is most likely at this point to find the cause of the shock?
    A. Thoracic aortography
    B. Head CT scan
    C. Peritoneal lavage
    D. IVP
    E. C-spine x-rays

57. The peroneal injuries are best evaluated by which of the following procedures?
    A. Pelvic x-ray
    B. IVP
    C. Passage of a small urinary cather
    D. Cystourethrogram
    E. Percutaneous bladder tap

Questions 58–60: A 45-year-old male presents with chief complaints of severe headache, malaise, blurring of vision, and chest pain. Review of history reveals a history of low-grade hypertension treated with diurectics and sodium restriction for about 10 years. His last blood pressure check was about 4 weeks earlier and was O.K. per the patient. Otherwise history was negative. On exam his blood pressure was 220/140 in both arms. His weight is about 70 kg.

58. The most likely diagnosis is malignant hypertension. The most prevalent physical finding with this condition is
    A. papilledema and retinal hemorrhages
    B. bibasilar rales
    C. cardiomegally
    D. abdominal pain and flank tenderness
    E. focal neurologic deficits

59. Treatment goals and modalities for malignant hypertension should or may include all of the following EXCEPT
    A. careful reduction by 30–40% of blood pressure from pretreatment levels
    B. initiation of a nitroprusside drip of 70 μg/minute with careful monitoring of blood pressure
    C. immediate injection intramuscularly of 25 mg of hydralazine
    D. admission to the hospital in all cases
    E. assessment of renal function to include urine analysis, electrolytes, and serum creatinine

60. The clinical syndrome of malignant hypertension
   A. is always associated with hypertensive encephalopathy
   B. generally occurs without the presence of papilledema
   C. is diagnosed by a fixed diastolic blood pressure greater than 135 mm Hg
   D. may be the initial presentation of hypertension
   E. includes seizures and coma

12

Family Medicine
John E. Verby, M.D.

DIRECTIONS: Each of the questions or incomplete statements below is followed by five suggested answers or completions. Select the **one** that is best in each case.

---

61. An 82-year-old woman comes to your office complaining of discomfort in the right lower quadrant of the abdomen with minimal tenderness. There is no fever and a normal white blood cell count. She has been healthy prior to this time and has never been hospitalized. The most likely diagnosis needing to be ruled out is
   A. regional enteritis
   B. mesenteric adenitis
   C. appendicitis
   D. gastroenteritis
   E. none of the above

62. What percentage of persons with appendicitis are over 60 years of age?
    A. Less than 10% of patients operated upon for appendicitis
    B. Less than 40% of patients operated upon for appendicitis
    C. More than 40% of patients operated upon for appendicitis
    D. Less than 60% of patients operated upon for appendicitis
    E. None of the above

63. The percentage of patients of the age of this 82-year-old woman who would be expected to have a ruptured appendix is
    A. above 60%
    B. 40%
    C. 20%
    D. 10%
    E. none of the above

64. What percentage of the mortality rate in appendicitis is in the over-60 age group?
    A. Over 50 % of all deaths from appendicitis
    B. 5% of all deaths from appendicitis
    C. 25% of all deaths from appendicitis
    D. 45% of all deaths from appendicitis
    E. Over 75% of all deaths from appendicitis

65. As a family physician, you have just delivered a 7 1/2-lb baby boy, full term, vertex, after 15 hours of active, uneventful labor. You note that the child is not breathing. Which of the following is NOT a possible cause for the baby's apnea?
    A. Compression of the inferior vena cava by a heavy gravid uterus
    B. Compression of the aorta by a heavy gravid uterus
    C. Use of depressant drugs that cause hypotension
    D. Overdeveloped placenta
    E. Meconium aspiration

66. Diabetes mellitus may be deleterious to pregnancy in a number of ways. Which of the following will NOT be harmful to mother or baby?
  A. Fourfold increase in pre-eclampysia–eclampsia
  B. Infection occurs less often in mother or baby and is usually less harmful
  C. Tendency of the fetus to succumb before the onset of spontaneous delivery
  D. Hydramnios
  E. Fetus may be much smaller than usual

67. As a family physician, you have a 34-year-old, normal, white adult female for whom you have delivered three normal babies. She has had no history of spontaneous abortions or stillborns and no serious illnesses since the third delivery 1 year ago. She now presents with left lower quadrant abdominal pain. Her history and physical examination suggest a left tubal pregnancy. Which of the following is the LEAST likely possibility in the differential diagnosis of tubal pregnancy?
  A. Gastrointestinal disturbance
  B. Intrauterine device
  C. Twisted cyst
  D. Terminal ileitis
  E. Salpingitis

68. The factors responsible for chronicity in suppurative middle ear disease are varied. Which of the factors listed below is NOT a factor?
  A. Partial or complete perforation of tympanic membrane
  B. Persistent obstruction to aeration of mastoid spaces
  C. Persistent osteomyelitis in the mastoid
  D. Persistent intact tympanic membrane
  E. Constitutional factors, such as allergy or altered defense mechanisms of the host

69. From 1960 to 1978 the overall death rate in the United States dropped 20%, but in one particular age group it rose 11%. From 40 to 60% of traffic fatalities among this age group were alcohol-related, and this was the leading cause of death. The correct age group is

   A. 85 years of age and above
   B. 65–84 years of age
   C. 35–64 years of age
   D. 25–34 years of age
   E. 15–24 years of age

70. You have in your family practice a number of persons who have seen a psychiatrist and been returned to you with a label of having a personality disorder. Which of the following is NOT a cause of this disorder?

   A. Genetic factors
   B. Epidemiologic factors
   C. Environmental factors
   D. Constitutional factors
   E. Cultural factors

DIRECTIONS: Each group of questions below consists of five lettered headings followed by a list of numbered words. For **each** numbered word, select the **one** lettered heading that is most closely associated with it. Each lettered heading may be selected once, more than once, or not at all.

Questions 71–74: Indicate the nutrient element insufficiency of which can lead to each of these clinical signs or symptoms in an adult.

   A. Pigmentation changes of the skin
   B. Perifollicular petechiae of the skin
   C. Night blindness
   D. Goiter
   E. Thoracic rosary

71. Iodine

72. Vitamin A

73. Vitamin C

74. Vitamin D

Questions 75–79: For each type of disorder, match the diagnosis.

    A. Affective disorder
    B. Schizophrenic disorder
    C. Anxiety disorder
    D. Chemical dependency disorder
    E. Personality disorder

75. Manic

76. Panic

77. Alcoholism

78. Antisocial personality

79. Schizotypical features

DIRECTIONS: Each set of lettered headings below is followed by a list of numbered words or phrases. For each numbered word or phrase select:

    A if the item is associated with A *only*
    B if the item is associated with B *only*
    C if the item is associated with *both* A and B
    D if the item is associated with *neither* A nor B

Questions 80–83:

    A. Interstitial parenchymal disease
    B. Pleural disease
    C. Both
    D. Neither

80. Asbestosis

81. Mesothelioma

82. Silicosis

83. Berylliosis

Questions 84–86:

    A. Anthrax
    B. Psittacosis
    C. Both
    D. Neither

84. Pet shop owners

85. Imported hides

86. Taxidermists

DIRECTIONS: For each of the questions or incomplete statements below, **one or more** of the answers or completions given is correct. Select

    A   if only *1, 2, and 3* are correct
    B   if only *1 and 3* are correct
    C   if only *2 and 4* are correct
    D   if only *4* is correct
    E   if *all* are correct

Questions 87–89:

87. Mechanisms responsible for cardiac arrhythmias include
    1. altered normal automaticity
    2. abnormal generation of impulses
    3. altered fast response
    4. slow responses

Directions Summarized				
A	**B**	**C**	**D**	**E**
1, 2, 3 only	1, 3 only	2, 4 only	4 only	All are correct

88. Agents affecting calcification include
    1. parathyroid hormone
    2. vitamin D
    3. calcitonin
    4. morphine

89. The following drugs exert uterine stimulation:
    1. Ergotamine
    2. Methysergide
    3. Ergnovine
    4. Bromocrystine

DIRECTIONS: This section of the test consists of a situation, followed by a series of questions. Study the situation and select the **one** best answer to each question following it.

Questions 90–92: A 74-year-old black male (former postal worker) comes to your office with painless, gradual loss of vision in both eyes. History reveals he has used chlorpromazine as prescribed by his physician on a number of occasions for a resistant pneumonitis. Examination of his eyes reveals a mature cataract in the right eye and an immature cataract in the left eye.

90. You would expect to see the following in the right eye:
    A. An opaque lens
    B. A semiclear lens
    C. A partially cloudy lens
    D. Brown or white dusting on the anterior lens surface
    E. None of the above

91. A further history reveals that he has been on corticosteroids intermittently for a number of years for bronchial asthma with no known etiology. In this situation you would expect the cataracts to be characterized by which of the following?
   A. Eccentric opacity
   B. Diffuse opacity
   C. Copper spots on the anterior capsule
   D. Posterior subcapsular in origin
   E. None of the above

92. Causes of cataracts include all of the following EXCEPT
   A. hypocalcemia
   B. hypoglycemia
   C. galactosemia
   D. diabetes mellitus
   E. multiple sclerosis

13

Internal Medicine
Michael A. Baker, M.D., F.R.C.P.(C), F.A.C.P.

DIRECTIONS: Each of the questions or incomplete statements below is followed by five suggested answers or completions. Select the **one** that is best in each case.

93. The most common early sign of rheumatoid arthritis is
    A. swelling of proximal interphalangeal joints
    B. pleural effusions
    C. a patellar bulge sign
    D. subcutaneous nodules
    E. splenomegaly

94. An immunodeficient patient who develops interstitial lung infection with *Pneumocystic carinii* is best treated with
    A. penicillin
    B. erythromycin
    C. tobramycin and ticarcillin
    D. amphotericin-B
    E. co-trimoxazole

95. Hormonal treatment for carcinoma of the breast is most likely to be helpful in patients with
    A. a six-month disease-free interval
    B. a tumor over 4 cm
    C. metastatic disease in the liver
    D. cytoplasmic estrogen receptors
    E. premenopausal status

96. Which of the following is most likely to be associated with severe microcytosis?
    A. Iron overload
    B. Beta-thalassemia major
    C. Chemotherapy effect
    D. Myelodysplasia
    E. Malabsorption syndrome

97. A young woman with chronic diarrhea has radiologic findings in the bowel of ileal wall thickening, discontinuous areas of involvement, and fistula formation. The most likely diagnosis is
    A. appendicial abscess
    B. ulcerative colitis
    C. Crohn's disease
    D. lymphoma
    E. ischemic colitis

DIRECTIONS: The group of questions below consists of five lettered headings followed by a list of numbered statements. For **each** numbered statement, select the **one** lettered heading that is most closely associated with it. Each lettered heading may be selected once, more than once, or not at all.

Questions 98–102:

    A. Tolbutamide
    B. Chlorpropamide
    C. Phenformin
    D. Regular insulin
    E. Lente insulin

98. Duration of action is 24–36 hours

99. The excretory product in the urine may give a false-positive test for albumin

100. Treatment of choice for diabetic ketoacidosis

101. The midafternoon blood glucose level dictates maximum morning dose

102. Potentiates antidiuretic hormone effect on the kidney

DIRECTIONS: The set of lettered headings below is followed by a list of numbered phrases. For each numbered phrase select

    A if the item is associated with A *only*
    B if the item is associated with B *only*
    C if the item is associated with *both* A and B
    D if the item is associated with *neither* A nor B

Questions 103–107:

    A. Multiple sclerosis
    B. Guillain-Barré syndrome
    C. Both
    D. Neither

103. Sensory symptoms are not seen

104. Abnormal cerebrospinal fluid protein values are found

105. Patients usually improve following initial symptoms

106. Demyelination is a pathologic finding

107. Visual impairment is a common problem

DIRECTIONS: This section of the test consists of situations, each followed by a series of questions. Study each situation and select the **one** best answer to each question following it.

Questions 108–109: An 18-year-old man develops malaise, nausea, headache, and dark, smoky urine of sudden onset. He has periorbital edema and a blood pressure of 160/105.

108. The most likely diagnosis is
   A. polycystic kidneys
   B. acute glomerulonephritis
   C. renal tubular acidosis
   D. idiopathic nephrotic syndrome
   E. diabetic nephropathy

109. The increased blood pressure is most likely secondary to
   A. sodium and water retention
   B. increased plasma renin
   C. increased plasma aldosterone
   D. glomerular scarring
   E. vasculitis

Questions 110–111: A 62-year-old woman has demonstrated increasing loss of recent memory over a 5-year period, now associated with reduced affect and nominal dysphasia. She dresses neatly and social amenities are preserved. There are no localizing motor or sensory findings.

110. The most likely diagnosis is
   A. cerebral vascular disease
   B. hydrocephalus
   C. Huntington's disease
   D. Alzheimer's disease
   E. Creutzfeldt–Jakob disease

111. Histologic examination of the brain would be likely to show prominent
   A. demyelination
   B. gliosis
   C. infarction
   D. neuronal loss
   E. viral inclusions

Questions 112–113: A 47-year-old woman presents with a history of joint pains of 6 months duration. More recently the joints of her fingers became swollen and red. Upon awakening in the morning her fingers, toes, wrists, and knees are stiff and do not improve until she is up for more than an hour. Physical examination reveals redness and swelling of the proximal interphalangeal joints and multiple small nodules over the extensor surfaces of the elbows.

112. The most likely diagnosis is
   A. osteoarthritis
   B. gout
   C. scleroderma
   D. psoriatic arthritis
   E. rheumatoid arthritis

113. All of the following tests would be abnormal EXCEPT
   A. marrow iron stores
   B. erythrocyte sedimentation rate (ESR)
   C. latex agglutination test
   D. immunoglobulin levels
   E. x-ray of hands

Questions 114–115: A 20-year-old woman presents with fever of 3 days duration. On examination there are painful red nodules on the shins bilaterally but no lymphadenopathy and no hepatosplenomegaly. Ophthalmologic examination reveals anterior uveitis. The chest x-ray is shown in Fig. 13.1.

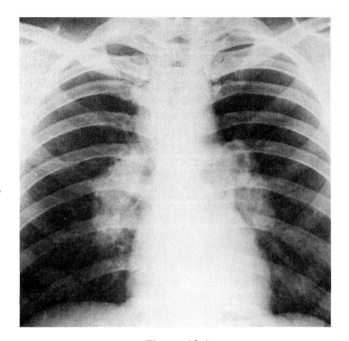

Figure 13.1

114. The most likely diagnosis is
    A. Hodgkin's disease
    B. sarcoidosis
    C. tuberculosis
    D. systemic lupus erythematosus
    E. rheumatic fever

115. The best treatment of this patient includes
    A. corticosteroids
    B. cyclophosphamide
    C. radiotherapy
    D. INH (isoniazid)
    E. salicylates

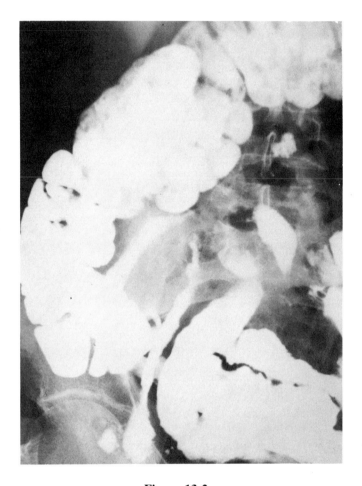

Figure 13.2

Questions 116–117: A 42-year-old American man presents with fever, diarrhea, and a vague ache in the right lower quadrant of the abdomen. Physical examination reveals tenderness on deep palpation. A gastrointestinal x-ray is shown in Fig. 13.2.

116. The most likely diagnosis is
    A. tuberculosis
    B. regional enteritis
    C. appendicitis
    D. ulcerative colitis
    E. lymphoma

117. Treatment may involve all of the following EXCEPT
    A. antidiarrheal agents
    B. Azulfidine
    C. prednisone
    D. parenteral alimentation
    E. high-fiber diet

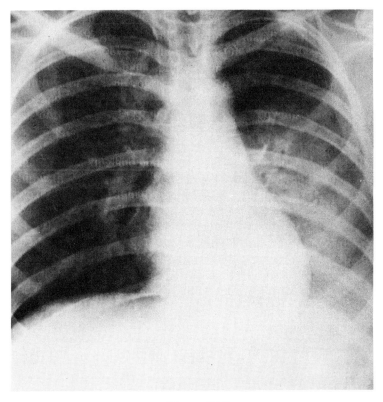

Figure 13.3

Questions 118–119: An 18-year-old man has chills and rigor of sudden onset followed by cough productive of blood-tinged sputum. Initial investigation shows a hemoglobin of 14 gm, white count 18,000 with 80% polymorphs. The chest x-ray is shown in Fig. 13.3.

118. The most likely diagnosis is
    A. pulmonary embolism
    B. lobar pneumonia
    C. leukemic infiltrate
    D. aspergillosis
    E. tuberculosis

119. Specific treatment is most likely to require
   A. heparin
   B. INH
   C. amphotericin B
   D. myleran
   E. penicillin

Questions 120–121: A 70-year-old woman is admitted to hospital with severe weakness and congestive failure of long standing. She had been receiving diuretic therapy and digitalis. The admission ECG shows a ventricular rate of 70/minute and is pictured in Fig. 13.4.

120. The ECG is most suggestive of
   A. first-degree heart block
   B. hypokalemia
   C. hypocalcemia
   D. second-degree heart block
   E. anterior wall infarction

Figure 13.4

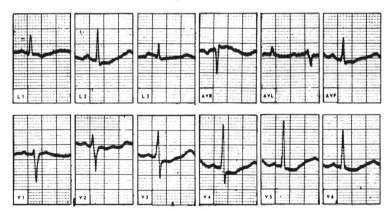

121. The most effective management should include
  A. increased digitalis
  B. increased diuretics
  C. potassium chloride
  D. potassium phosphate
  E. calcium chloride

Questions 122–123: A 60-year-old man presents with a 2-year history of headaches of increasing severity. History further reveals pain in the right hip. An x-ray of the skull is shown in Fig. 13.5.

Figure 13.5

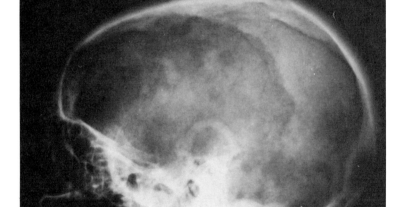

122. What is the most likely diagnosis?
- **A.** Multiple myeloma
- **B.** Metastatic carcinoma to the brain
- **C.** Thalassemia major
- **D.** Paget's disease of bone
- **E.** Hyperparathyroidism

123. Which of the following classes of drugs are potentially helpful in this condition?
- **A.** Folate antagonists
- **B.** Aminoglycosides
- **C.** Diphosphonates
- **D.** Alkylating agents
- **E.** Corticosteroids

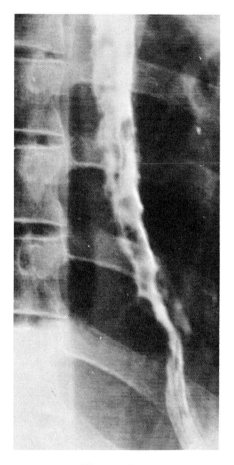

Figure 13.6

Questions 124–125: A 45-year-old man is admitted to the emergency room with hematemesis. A barium swallow shows the esophageal pattern illustrated in Fig. 13.6.

124. The most likely diagnosis is
    A. carcinoma of the esophagus
    B. esophageal varices
    C. foreign body
    D. tertiary waves
    E. Barrett's esophagus

125. The most common cause of the condition shown in this figure is
    A. reflux esophagitis
    B. congenital venous anomaly
    C. coarctation of the aorta
    D. alcoholic cirrhosis
    E. biliary cirrhosis

Question 126: A 30-year-old black woman with a history of recurrent abdominal and skeletal pains has the x-ray of the thoracic vertebrae shown in Fig. 13.7.

Figure 13.7

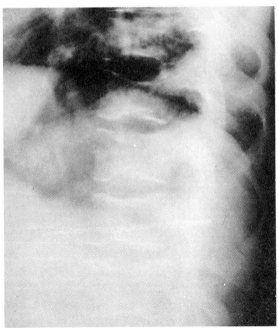

126. What is the most likely diagnosis?
   A. Metastatic carcinoma
   B. Traumatic fracture
   C. Paget's disease of bone
   D. Ankylosing spondylitis
   E. Sickle cell anemia

Questions 127–128: A 60-year-old man presents with a 5-year history of increasing dyspnea. He has diffuse "crackling" rales on auscultation of the lungs. He has been employed in the installation of heat-resistant insulation in a shipyard for 25 years. A lung biopsy is done, and a typical section is shown in Fig. 13.8.

127. The most likely diagnosis is
   A. bronchopneumonia
   B. pulmonary alveolar proteinosis
   C. interstitial fibrosis
   D. pulmonary adenomatosis
   E. asbestosis

Figure 13.8

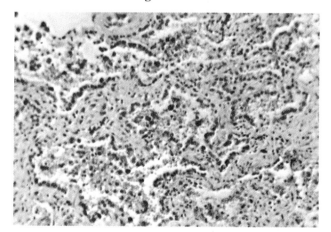

128. The best treatment for the severe dyspnea would include
    A. cyclophosphamide
    B. digitalis
    C. hydrochlorothiazide
    D. corticosteroids
    E. antibiotics

Question 129: A 55-year-old woman presents with renal failure of gradual onset. She has had high blood pressure for several years and diabetes requiring insulin since age 50. She has been taking sulfamethoxasole and trimethoprim for a urinary tract infection. A kidney biopsy is done, and a typical section is shown in Fig. 13.9.

129. The most likely cause of the kidney failure is
    A. nodular glomerulosclerosis
    B. pyelonephritis
    C. precipitated sulfa drugs
    D. malignant hypertension
    E. acute glomerulonephritis

Figure 13.9

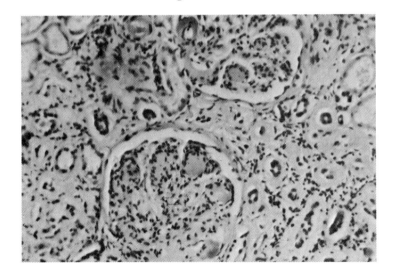

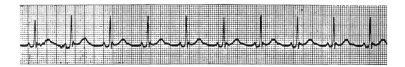

Figure 13.10A

Questions 130–131: A 47-year-old man complains of intermittent chest pain. Although the pain is related to exercise, the characteristics are otherwise "atypical." The resting lead II cardiogram is shown in Fig. 13.10A.

130. What does the ECG in Fig. 13.10A show?
    A. Depressed ST segments
    B. U waves
    C. Normal sinus rhythm
    D. Bradycardia
    E. Wolff–Parkinson–White syndrome

131. After exercise an ECG is taken, and the lead II cardiogram is shown in Fig. 13.10B. The problem most likely affecting this patient is
    A. sinus tachycardia
    B. hyperkalemia
    C. myocardial infarction
    D. myocardial ischemia
    E. Wenckebach phenomenon

Figure 13.10B

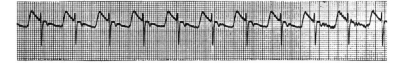

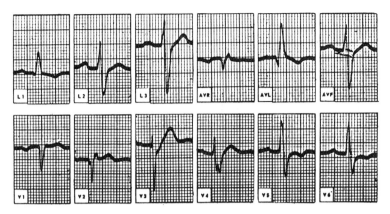

Figure 13.11

Question 132: A 70-year-old man is admitted to hospital with congestive heart failure. He gives a history of angina pectoris of several years duration, with recent exacerbation of symptoms. The ECG is shown in Fig. 13.11.

132. All of the following abnormalities are seen in the ECG EXCEPT
   A. first-degree A-V block
   B. lateral wall infarction
   C. anteroseptal infarction
   D. left axis deviation
   E. left bundle branch block

14

Medical Ethics
Count D. Gibson, Jr., M.D.

DIRECTIONS: The question below is followed by five suggested answers. Select the **one** that is best

---

133. Which of the following statements is NOT correct concerning the 1973 United States Supreme Court decision *Roe versus Wade*?

    A. The decision was based on a fundamental right to privacy
    B. States were forbidden to enact laws regulating abortion in the first trimester
    C. States were forbidden to allow abortions during the third trimester
    D. States were permitted to regulate abortions during the second trimester to ensure that the health of the mother was protected
    E. The Supreme Court decision did not specify when life begins

DIRECTIONS: The question below consists of lettered headings followed by a list of numbered words. For **each** set of numbered words, select the **one** lettered heading that is most closely associated with it. Each lettered heading may be selected once, more than once, or not at all.

Questions 134–135:

    A. Substituted judgment
    B. Basis for a living will
    C. Rights of the mentally ill
    D. Foregoing lifesaving surgery

134. Infant Doe

135. Karen Quinlan

136. Brother Fox

DIRECTIONS: The set of lettered headings below is followed by a list of numbered phrases. For each numbered phrase select

    A if the item is associated with A *only*
    B if the item is associated with B *only*
    C if the item is associated with *both* A and B
    D if the item is associated with *neither* A nor B

Questions 137–141:

    A. Deontology
    B. Consequentialism
    C. Both
    D. Neither

137. Theory of ethics

138. Sanctity of life

139. Law of parsimony

140. Quality of life

141. End justifies the means

DIRECTIONS: For the question below, **one or more** of the answers given is correct. Select

    A if only *1, 2, and 3* are correct
    B if only *1 and 3* are correct
    C if only *2 and 4* are correct
    D if only *4* is correct
    E if *all* are correct

---

142. Which of these terms would be directly relevant to bioethical discussions?
    1. Rawlsian principles
    2. Keynesian principles
    3. Nonmaleficence
    4. Countercurrent distribution

15

Neurology
John Eric Holmes, M.D.

DIRECTIONS: Each of the questions or incomplete statements below is followed by five suggested answers or completions. Select the **one** that is best in each case.

143. In a patient surviving 2 or 3 weeks after subarachnoid hemorrhage, clinical deterioration with failing consciousness may indicate
    A. developing hydrocephalus
    B. metabolic acidosis
    C. hypoventilation
    D. brain stem infarction
    E. subdural hematoma

144. Inability to oppose the thumb to the base of the little finger can be due to a lesion of
    A. C–5 spinal nerve
    B. C–6 spinal nerve
    C. radial nerve
    D. ulnar nerve
    E. median nerve

145. Which of the following anti-Parkinson drugs is a DOPA agonist?
    A. Benztropine (Cogentin)
    B. Trihexyphenidyl (Artane)
    C. Carbidopa-levodopa (Sinemet)
    D. Bromocriptine (Parlodel)
    E. Diphenhydramine (Benadryl)

146. Embolic occlusion of the left common carotid artery can produce
    A. left hemiplegia
    B. blindness in the left eye
    C. ataxia of the left side
    D. left visual field hemianopsia
    E. none of the above

147. Of the symptoms listed, which is most likely to be associated with transient ischemic attacks involving the brainstem circulation?
    A. Aphasia
    B. Hemiplegia
    C. Vertigo
    D. Seizures
    E. Headache

148. A middle-aged man, a known alcoholic, is admitted to a hospital in a confused state. His blood alcohol and drug screen are negative. Physical examination is unremarkable except that he has nystagmus. He quickly lapses into stupor and responds only to pain and loud commands. The most likely diagnosis would be
    A. brain tumor
    B. Klüver-Bucy syndrome
    C. hepatic coma
    D. Wernicke's encephalopathy
    E. Korsakoff's syndrome

DIRECTIONS: Each group of questions below consists of a list of lettered headings followed by a list of numbered words or statements. For **each** numbered word or statement, select the **one** lettered heading that is most closely associated with it. Each lettered heading may be selected once, more than once, or not at all.

Questions 149–152:

    A. Optic nerve
    B. Oculomotor nerve
    C. Facial nerve
    D. Trigeminal nerve
    E. Vagus nerve

149. Loss of taste

150. Dilatation of the pupil

151. Hoarseness of voice

152. Diplopia

Questions 153–156: In the syndrome of central or transtentorial herniation with progressive dysfunction of the brainstem, a progression of signs can be observed in stages which have been given the following designations:

    A. Diencephalic stage
    B. Midbrain–pons stage
    C. Lower pons–upper medulla stage

153. Constricted pupils which react to light

154. Cheyne-Stokes breathing

155. Sustained hyperventilation

156. No response to ice water caloric or to head turning

Questions 157–161:

    A. Frontal lobe cortex
    B. Parietal lobe cortex
    C. Temporal lobe structures
    D. Occipital lobe cortex

157. Amnesia for recent events

158. Inability to name common objects

159. Hemianopsia

160. Denial of blindness (Anton's syndrome)

161. Denial of hemiparesis

Questions 162–164:

    A. Cerebral infarction
    B. Transient ischemic attack (TIA)
    C. Cerebral hemorrhage
    D. Subarachnoid hemorrhage

162. Symptoms last less than 30 minutes

163. Anticoagulant therapy

164. Lumbar puncture is diagnostic

Questions 165–168: Symptoms and signs found in conjunction with lesions of the following:

    A. Femoral nerve
    B. Peroneal nerve
    C. Sciatic nerve
    D. Lateral femoral cutaneous nerve

165. Foot drop

166. Thigh pain with loss of knee jerk reflex

167. Limitation of straight leg raising by pain

168. Numbness and pain over the lateral part of the thigh

DIRECTIONS: Each set of lettered headings below is followed by a list of numbered words or phrases. For each numbered word or phrase select

  A   if the item is associated with A *only*
  B   if the item is associated with B *only*
  C   if the item is associated with *both* A and B
  D   if the item is associated with *neither* A nor B

Questions 169–171:

  A. Alzheimer's disease
  B. Normal aging
  C. Both
  D. Neither

169. CT scan evidence of cerebral atrophy

170. Choreic movements

171. Memory loss

Questions 172–174:

  A. Huntington's disease
  B. Parkinsonism
  C. Both
  D. Neither

172. Dementia

173. Abnormal involuntary movements

174. CT scan reveals enlarged lateral ventricles

Questions 175–178:

    A. Grand mal (tonic-clonic) seizure disorder
    B. Phenytoin (Dilantin) treatment
    C. Both
    D. Neither

175. Nystagmus and ataxia

176. Thickening of facial features: lips, gums, etc.

177. Increased incidence of fetal deformities in the offspring

178. Lymphadenopathy and pseudolymphoma

Questions 179–183:

    A. Petit mal seizure
    B. Complex partial seizure ("psychomotor epilepsy")
    C. Both
    D. Neither

179. Brief spells of loss of consciousness with lip or eyelid movements, blank stare, and amnesia for the attack

180. Loss of consciousness with head turning, body movements, walking, or running

181. Characteristic 3/second EEG waves only during attack

182. Abnormal nonictal EEG only during sleep

183. Carbamazepine (Tegretol) Rx

Questions 184–187:

    A. Trigeminal neuralgia
    B. Bell's palsy
    C. Both
    D. Neither

184. Drooling

185. Facial rash or vesicles

186. Symptoms last only seconds

187. Spontaneous recovery to be expected

Questions 188–191:

    A. Amyotrophic lateral sclerosis (ALS)
    B. Osteoarthritis of the cervical spine with compression of neural structures
    C. Both
    D. Neither

188. Bilateral Babinski signs

189. Atrophy and fasciculation of the hand muscles

190. EMG evidence of denervation in the thigh and calf muscles

191. No specific treatment

DIRECTIONS: For each of the questions or incomplete statements below, **one or more** of the answers or completions given is correct. Select

    A   if only *1, 2, and 3* are correct
    B   if only *1 and 3* are correct
    C   if only *2 and 4* are correct
    D   if only *4* is correct
    E   if *all* are correct

Questions 192–197:

192. A high-pitched systolic bruit heard over the carotid artery indicates
    1. significant stenosis
    2. carotid occlusion
    3. increased risk of embolism
    4. A-V shunt

193. CT scan done 24 hours following a "stroke" due to cerebral infarction with a hemiparesis will reveal
    1. focal lucency in most cases
    2. normal baseline and enhanced scan
    3. evidence of bleeding only on a contrast injection scan
    4. displacement of midline structures in the presence of edema

194. Transient ischemic attack (TIA) in the distribution of the vertebral-basilar circulation may present as
    1. vertigo
    2. loss of portion of visual field
    3. facial paresthesia
    4. "drop attack" with sudden fall

195. A woman with amenorrhea is found to have an elevated blood prolactin.
1. Ovarian dysfunction is the most likely cause
2. Pituitary tumor is the most likely cause
3. Radiation to the gland is the primary treatment
4. Bromocriptine may be adequate treatment

196. In an 18-year-old patient with Guillain-Barré syndrome of 1 week's duration, you would expect to find
1. complete remission 6 months later
2. symmetric flaccid paralysis
3. normal CBC and sed rate
4. elevated CSF protein

197. The syndrome associated with lateral medullary infarction (Wallenberg's syndrome) includes
1. loss of pain sensation on one side of the face and opposite side of the body
2. hemiparesis on the side opposite the presumed infarction
3. arteriographic evidence of thromboembolism of the posterior inferior cerebellar artery
4. loss of consciousness, often only transient

DIRECTIONS: This section of the test consists of situations, each followed by one or more questions. Study each situation and select the **one** best answer to each question following it.

Questions 198–207:

198. A 28-year-old woman complains that when she awoke this morning and looked into the mirror "my face was pulled to one side." Exam reveals inability to close tightly the lips or the eyelids on the left side, and inability to raise the left eyebrow or retract the left corner of the mouth. The rest of the neurologic examination is normal. Her disorder is most likely to be due to
   A. transient ischemic attack (TIA)
   B. right-sided cerebral infarction
   C. herpes simplex encephalitis
   D. glossopharyngeal neuralgia
   E. idiopathic Bell's palsy

199. Although the other cranial nerves are normal on exam, this patient is likely to complain of
   A. diplopia on lateral gaze
   B. loudness of sounds heard in the left ear
   C. numbness of the left side of the tongue
   D. paresthesia in the third division (mandibular n.) of the left trigeminal nerve
   E. sharp shooting pains in the left cheek and left side of the jaw

200. A 22-year-old woman has had seizures for over 10 years. She has a mixture of absence and tonic-clonic attacks. She takes sodium valproate (Depakene) 250 mg t.i.d. Despite this medication, she has two or three "mild attacks" every month. She desires to become pregnant and asks your advice about the effects on her disease on the pregnancy. You advise that she

   A. change to another, less teratogenetic medication
   B. maintain the present Rx, but not increase it
   C. Decrease the valproate until the blood level is just at the lower limit of therapeutic range
   D. Stop the valproate, and not use other anticonvulsants because of their threat to the potential fetus
   E. Increase valproate to control the reported "break-through seizures"

201. An 18-year-old high school student has a history of "spells" in which he loses consciousness but does not fall. His family says he "looks strange," mumbles, walks about the room, and does not answer questions. The spell lasts about 5 minutes, and afterward he has no memory for what occurred. These spells were being controlled by phenytoin (Dilantin) 300 mg/day and carbamazepine (Tegretol) 600 mg/day until 2 months ago. At that time he had three spells in a row, and more recently two more. This patient's "spells" are best characterized as

   A. petit mal seizures
   B. adolescent "acting-out" reaction
   C. complex partial seizures
   D. Jacksonian "march" seizures
   E. pseudoseizures

202. The likeliest cause of the recurrence of attacks in this patient, previously in good control, is

   A. stress of senior year in high school
   B. alteration in drug absorbtion
   C. alteration in rate of drug metabolism
   D. intracranial pathology
   E. noncompliance

203. A 29-year-old female complains of severe headache, and arrives in the emergency room alert. BP 120/60. Neck supple. Over the next 2 hours she lapses into coma. A drug screen is negative. She remains unresponsive except to pain. EKG shows AV dissociation with ST elevation and T-wave inversion in AVL. Most likely diagnosis is
   A. myocardial infarction with cerebral embolism
   B. brain stem infarction
   C. acute hydrocephalus
   D. subarachnoid hemorrhage
   E. migraine

204. A head trauma victim is considered for a kidney transplant donor. He is comatose and on a respirator. To meet the conventional criteria for brain death, this patient would have to fulfill all the conditions below EXCEPT
   A. absent eye movement reflexes
   B. no respiratory effort off the respirator
   C. blood barbiturate level not higher than 30 μg/ml
   D. pupils midposition and fixed to light

205. A number of confirmatory studies on the above victim can be done, but the most important information would be
   A. angiogram showing impaired cerebral vessel filling
   B. isoelectric EEG
   C. firm diagnosis of the cause of the coma
   D. no visually evoked potentials on the averaged EEG
   E. patient is not hypothermic

206. An elderly man had the sudden onset of weakness of the right hand and arm, with less severe weakness of the right leg. There was no aphasia (he has always been right-handed), and no sensory or visual symptoms. BP was 188/120. Blood pressure was treated and recovery was rapid, less than 1 week. Most likely diagnosis is
   A. subdural hematoma
   B. carotid occlusion (thrombosis)
   C. hypertensive encephalopathy
   D. lacunar infarction
   E. cerebral hemorrhage

207. Assume that this hypertensive patient did not respond to antihypertensive treatment and lapsed into coma instead of improving. It is the third hospital day. CT scan shows no hemorrhage and normal ventricles with no shift. The diagnosis to consider first is

A. cerebral infarction
B. hypertensive encephalopathy
C. subdural hematoma
D. cerebral hemorrhage
E. multiple sclerosis

16

Obstetrics and Gynecology
Raymond E. Probst, M.D.

DIRECTIONS: Each of the questions or incomplete statements below is followed by five suggested answers or completions. Select the **one** that is best in each case.

---

208. Those women at highest risk for developing osteoporosis include
    A. black women with a late menopause
    B. white women with larger bone mass
    C. women with a positive family history and who smoke cigarettes
    D. women in their fifth decade of life
    E. white women with a late menopause

209. Which of the following is true concerning the periodic health examination schedule for women?
    A. Women age 20–39 should have a pap smear every 5 years and a mammogram when they reach age 40
    B. Women age 40–49 should have a pap smear every year and a mammogram every 5 years
    C. Women age 50–69 should have a mammogram annually
    D. Women over the age 70 need no longer have a pap smear or mammogram
    E. It is best to do these only when the patient has a complaint

210. The most common reason for antenatal genetic testing is
- **A.** paternal age greater than 50
- **B.** a parent with a balanced translocation
- **C.** Mendelian disorders
- **D.** maternal age 35 or older
- **E.** repeated spontaneous abortions

211. Which of the following drugs, if the patient is not allergic to it, is absolutely safe to use during pregnancy in the treatment of urologic infections?
- **A.** Nitrofurantoins
- **B.** Ampicillin
- **C.** Tetracyclines
- **D.** Sulfonamides
- **E.** Aminoglycosides

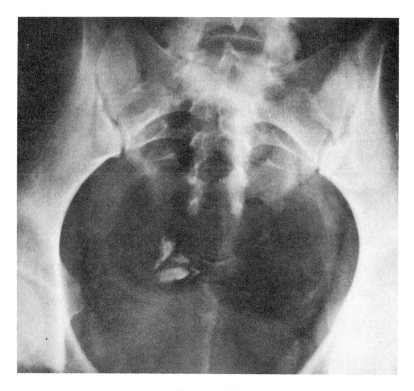

Figure 16.1

Questions 212 and 213 (refer to Fig. 16.1):

212. A 22-year-old white single gravida 0 female is seen by you for a complete physical examination. You feel a mass in the cul de sac. The x-ray is shown in Fig. 16.1. Which of the following is true?
   A. The mass is probably malignant
   B. The lesion is usually made up of one germ cell
   C. It is usually bilateral
   D. Age at peak incidence of this condition is 40 years
   E. The frequency of torsion is great

213. Which of the following is the recommended treatment for this condition?
   A. Posterior vaginal colpotomy and aspiration of the cyst
   B. Laparoscopy and laparotomy
   C. Ovarian cystectomy with incision and inspection of the other ovary
   D. Total abdominal hysterectomy and bilateral salpingo-oophorectomy
   E. Observation

214. Which of the following is usually NOT at issue in the treatment of septic shock?
   A. Restore circulating volume to tissue organ perfusion
   B. Correct alkalosis
   C. Begin empiric antimicrobial therapy
   D. Surgically remove all infected tissue
   E. Monitor vital function to see if therapy is effective

215. Which of the following is a risk factor in developing endometrial cancer?
   A. Obesity
   B. Multiparity
   C. Early menopause
   D. Prolonged oral contraceptive use
   E. Diabetes insipidus

216. In the postmature (after 42 weeks) pregnant female, which is the most definite way to detect fetal distress?
   A. Biomedical profile
   B. Non-stress test
   C. Stress test and decreased amniotic fluid
   D. Estriol determination
   E. Fetal movements

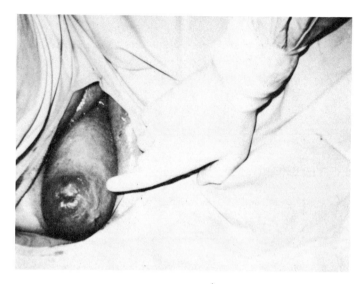

Figure 16.2

217. A 62-year-old white female, gravida 7 para 7, is seen because of a bulging sensation in the perineum. Physical examination reveals the findings as shown in Fig. 16.2. Which of the following is NOT true concerning this condition?
    A. It is due to an attenuation of the cardinal ligaments
    B. A term for this is procidentia
    C. It can cause kinking of the ureters and hydroureters
    D. It is associated with an enterocele and a cystocele
    E. The most common complaint is urinary stress incontinence

218. Which gynecologic neoplasm causes the highest mortality in the United States?
    A. Cervical
    B. Endometrial
    C. Ovarian
    D. Fundal
    E. Tubal

219. A 29-year-old white female, gravida 4 para 4, had a tubal cautery via laparoscopy. Thirty-six hours after surgery she complains of abdominal pain and nausea, has a temperature of 101°F, and has a somewhat distended abdomen. The probable diagnosis is
    A. pelvic inflammatory disease
    B. hemorrhage from the tube
    C. bowel burn
    D. bowel puncture
    E. tubal abortion

220. A 19-year-old single female is seen by you because of severe vulvar pain and swelling and a tender lesion (Fig. 16.3). Which of the following is true?
    A. Exposure time is 14 days
    B. The vagina and cervix are never involved
    C. Inguinal lymphadenopathy is uncommon
    D. Constitutional symptoms of headache may last for 1 week
    E. It is the second most common vulvar viral infection

Figure 16.3

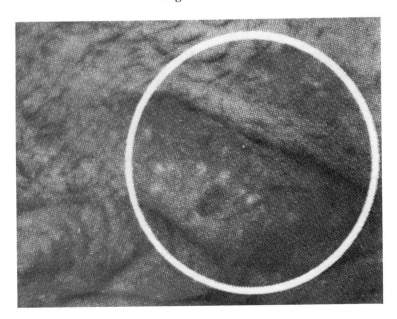

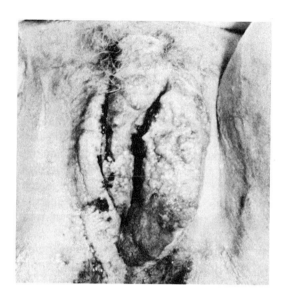

Figure 16.4

221. A 71-year-old white female is seen because of an odorous discharge, bleeding from her genitals, and fatigue. On examination she is found to have lesions as shown in Fig. 16.4. Which of the following is the treatment of choice in this situation?
    A. Biopsy and antibiotics
    B. Radical vulvectomy and inguinal and femoral node dissection
    C. Podophyllin
    D. Simple excision
    E. Radiation therapy

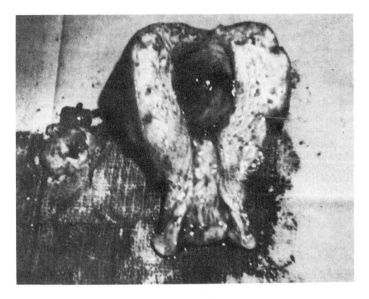

Figure 16.5

222. As shown in Fig. 16.5, which of the following is the most uncommon pathologic change?
    A. Hyalinization
    B. Cystic degeneration
    C. Red degeneration
    D. Fatty degeneration
    E. Sarcomatous degeneration

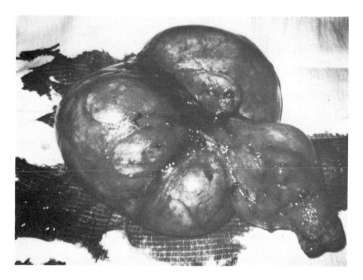

Figure 16.6

223. A 48-year-old black female, gravida 9 para 9, complains of severe lower back pain. She has had heavy menstrual periods for many years. Hemoglobin is 8.5 gm, and a pregnancy test is negative. Which of the following is the most common condition causing misdiagnosis of the problem shown in Fig. 16.6?
   A. Diverticulitis with rupture
   B. Tubo-ovarian abscess
   C. Ovarian neoplasm
   D. Multiple pregnancy
   E. Urachal cyst

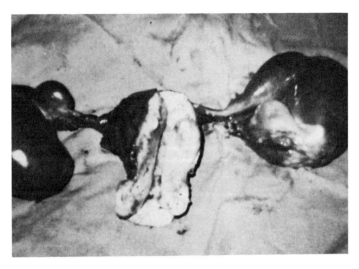

Figure 16.7

224. A 29-year-old single female, gravida 0, is seen because of severe lower abdominal pain of 1 week duration. She had been running a temperature of 102°F and has a purulent discharge, an exquisitely tender abdomen, and a 10-year history of "female infections." Pelvic exam reveals bilateral adnexal masses (Fig. 16.7). The most common cause of this condition is

A. bilateral Brenner tumors
B. acute gonorrheal salpingitis
C. twisted ovarian cysts
D. Krukenberg tumors
E. paraovarian cysts

225. She also complains of severe right upper quadrant abdominal pain. An upper GI and gallbladder series was normal. The most likely cause of this pain is

A. undiagnosed biliary sludge
B. acute pancreatitis
C. stress ulcer of the duodenum
D. Fitz-Hugh and Curtis syndrome
E. Zollinger–Ellison syndrome

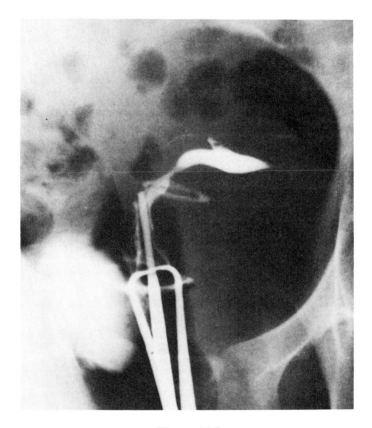

Figure 16.8

226. A patient presents with a complaint of lower abdominal
   pain. Based on the hysterogram shown in Fig. 16.8, what
   is the diagnosis?
   A. Halo sign
   B. Intrauterine pregnancy
   C. Normal intrauterine device
   D. Lost intrauterine device
   E. Calcified fibroid

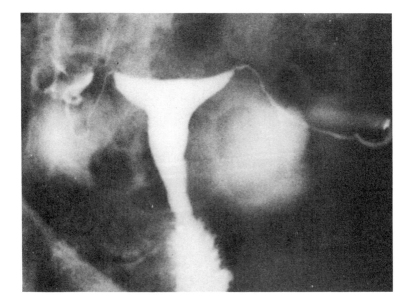

Figure 16.9

227. Which of the following is the usual causative pathologic mechanism in the condition shown in Fig. 16.9?
   A. Oral contraceptives
   B. *Bacteroides* sp.
   C. Diethylstilbestrol
   D. Gram-negative intracellular diplococci
   E. Increased 17-ketosteroids

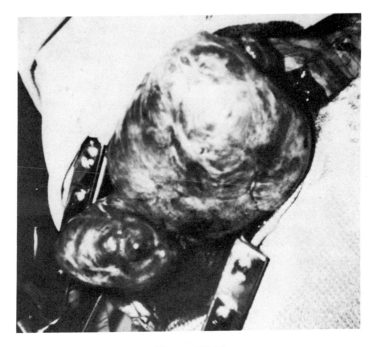

Figure 16.10

228. A 47-year-old female, gravida 6 para 6, complained of a
fullness in the lower abdomen, increasing constipation, fre-
quency of urination, and tightness of the lower abdomen.
A lesion was discovered and on microscopic exam was found
to be benign. Which of the following is true concerning the
condition shown in Fig. 16.10?
A. The treatment of choice is unilateral oophorectomy
B. It can be associated with a mucocele of the colon
C. Treatment of choice is an abdominal hysterectomy and
bilateral salpingo-oophorectomy
D. Such a tumor is often hormone-producing
E. The mass was solid

DIRECTIONS: The group of questions below consists of five lettered headings followed by a list of numbered statements. For **each** numbered statement, select the **one** lettered heading that is most closely associated with it. Each lettered heading may be selected once, more than once, or not at all.

Questions 229–233:

    A. Yeast vaginitis
    B. *Chlamydia trachomatis*
    C. *Gardnerella vaginalis* vaginitis
    D. *Trichomonas* infections
    E. Herpes simplex

229. The simplest method of diagnosis is with a smear

230. Common sites of infection are the pharynx, esophagus, oral cavity, genitals, and skin of the finger (Whitlow)

231. These are Gram-positive and best diagnosed with 10% KOH on a wet mount

232. When 10% KOH is added to the discharge, an aminelike, fishy smell emanates

233. Grouped together in the laboratory with *Lymphogranuloma venereum*

DIRECTIONS: The set of lettered headings below is followed by a list of numbered phrases. For each numbered phrase select

    A if the item is associated with A *only*
    B if the item is associated with B *only*
    C if the item is associated with *both* A and B
    D if the item is associated with *neither* A nor B

Questions 234–238:

    A. Early deceleration
    B. Late deceleration
    C. Both
    D. Neither

234. Can be repetitive in nature

235. Seen in fetal hypoxia

236. Abolished with atropine

237. Usually seen in simple cord compression

238. Positive oxytocin challenge test

DIRECTIONS: For each of the questions or incomplete statements below, **one or more** of the answers or completions given is correct. Select

A if only *1, 2, and 3* are correct
B if only *1 and 3* are correct
C if only *2 and 4* are correct
D if only *4* is correct
E if *all* are correct

Questions 239–247:

239. With regard to the premenstrual syndrome,
   1. 75% of American women experience it
   2. it is usually seen at a younger age
   3. exposure to stress and multiparity are not factors
   4. advancing age and a high intake of carbohydrate are high risk factors

240. Intervention to prevent premature labor may be signaled by the physician inquiring about
   1. low backache
   2. abdominal and pelvic pain
   3. bladder and urinary symptoms
   4. a decreasing fetal motion

241. The highest risk factors in developing breast cancer relate to
   1. women under age 50 from undeveloped countries and of low socioeconomic status
   2. early menarche and late menopause
   3. surgical menopause after ago 40, multiparity, and high-fat diet
   4. fibrocystic disease, cancer in one breast, and a family history of breast cancer

		Directions Summarized		
A	**B**	**C**	**D**	**E**
1, 2, 3	1, 3	2, 4	4	All are
only	only	only	only	correct

242. In caring for the rape patient,
    1. by law the patient cannot refuse examination or forbid release of information to authorities
    2. male as well as female rape must be thoroughly investigated
    3. when obtaining pubic and head hair from the patient, these must be cut so as not to cause discomfort
    4. prophylaxis against gonorrhea is best accomplished with 4.8 million units of procaine penicillin

243. With regard to anatomic considerations of the female pelvis,
    1. the anthropoid pelvis is the most common type
    2. of the midpelvic measurements, the intertuberous is the most important
    3. of greatest importance for a normal vaginal delivery is a convergent pelvic splay
    4. external pelvic measurements are of little value

244. Methods of assessing fetal placental well-being in the pregnant woman include
    1. biomedical profile
    2. non-stress and stress test
    3. estriol determination
    4. ultrasound

245. Absolute contraindications to the use of oral contraceptives include
    1. active liver disease
    2. preexisting undiagnosed amenorrhea
    3. cerebrovascular or coronary artery disease
    4. migraine headaches

246. The maternal ingestion of diethylstilbestrol can produce which of the following in the female offspring?
  1. Vaginal adenosis
  2. Increased risk of breast cancer
  3. Fundal uterine structural changes
  4. Ectopic pregnancy

247. Concerning condyloma acuminata,
  1. the human papilloma virus may be a precursor of squamous cell carcinoma of the genital tract
  2. warts can appear 6 weeks to 6 months after exposure
  3. cryosurgery is a form of treatment
  4. podophyllin is contraindicated in vaginal and cervical condyloma acuminata

17

Ophthalmology
Alfonse A. Cinotti, M.D., F.A.C.S.

DIRECTIONS: Each of the questions or incomplete statements below is followed by five suggested answers or completions. Select the **one** that is best in each case.

248. When faced with a patient with 2-mm pupils that do not react well to light directly or consensually, what is the most appropriate next step?
    A. Order a lab test
    B. Obtain a CT scan of the sella
    C. Look for oculomotor paresis
    D. Examine pupillary reaction to accommodation
    E. Put pilocarpine 1/8% into both eyes

249. In the above patient, what would be the single most important blood test to order?
    A. Chemistry profile (electrolytes)
    B. Erythrocyte sedimentation rate (ESR)
    C. Three-hour glucose tolerance test (GTT)
    D. Anti-nuclear antibody (ANA)
    E. VDRL

250. A 30-year-old female patient presents with bilateral proptosis and difficulty elevating the left eye. The most likely etiology is
    A. rhabdomyosarcoma
    B. euthyroid Grave's disease
    C. shallow orbits
    D. metastatic schirrous carcinoma of the breast
    E. high myopia

251. A 70-year-old woman comes in with sudden monocular loss of vision. She has fevers, unexplained weight loss, lassitude, and depression. Her involved eye has a pale, swollen optic nerve. The most appropriate action is:
    A. Obtain a sedimentation rate; if elevated, arrange a temporal artery biopsy; if positive, start steroids
    B. Obtain a CT scan of the involved optic nerve; if positive, arrange neurosurgical evaluation
    C. Obtain sedimentation rate; schedule rheumotologic evaluation
    D. Obtain a CT scan of the head; if normal, perform lumbar puncture, including measurement of opening pressure
    E. Obtain a sedimentation rate, start steroids, arrange for temporal artery biopsy

252. The most frequently occurring primary intraocular malignancy in childhood is
    A. leiomyoma
    B. melanoma
    C. retinoblastoma
    D. neuroblastoma
    E. rhabdomyosarcoma

253. The most common cause of conjunctivitis in the first 2 days of life is
    A. gonococcus
    B. staphylococcus
    C. chemical irritation
    D. herpes simplex
    E. inclusion conjunctivitis

254. Which of the following is most indicative of severe bilateral visual loss in infants?
A. Exotropia
B. Pendular nystagmus
C. Esotropia
D. Amblyopia
E. Esophoria

255. All of the following may be associated with Horner's syndrome EXCEPT
A. ptosis
B. miosis
C. anhidrosis
D. heterochromia
E. decreased vision

256. Common causes of orbital cellulitis include all of the following EXCEPT
A. sinusitis
B. orbital plane foreign body
C. orbital trauma
D. dental abcess
E. otitis media

257. The most likely organism to cause a "stye" (acute hordeolum) is
A. *Diplococcus pneumoniae*
B. *Staphylococcus aureus*
C. *Pseudomonas aeroginosa*
D. *Escherichia coli*
E. anaerobes

258. Flame-shaped hemorrhages in the retina lie in the
A. layer of rods and cones
B. bipolar cell layer
C. retinal pigment epitheliopathy
D. nerve fiber layer
E. surface of retina

259. Characteristics of damage to the optic nerve head in chronic open angle glaucoma include all of the following EXCEPT
    A. enlargement of the cup
    B. erosion of the neuroretinal rim
    C. angulation of retinal vessels
    D. asymetry between cups of each eye
    E. blurring of disc margin

260. The most commonly used antiglaucoma drug is
    A. atropine
    B. pilocarpine
    C. diamox
    D. timoptic
    E. epinephrine

261. Retinal cotton wool exudates (cystoid bodies) should make you think first of
    A. glaucoma
    B. diabetes
    C. hypertension
    D. chorioretinitis
    E. senile degeneration

262. In hypertensive retinopathy all of the following may occur EXCEPT
    A. arteriovenous crossing defects
    B. copper wire arteries
    C. cotton wool patches
    D. star-shaped figure
    E. dot and blot hemorrhages

263. A patient who has just been examined by an ophthalmologist presents to the ER with blurry vision, a dry mouth, elevated temperature, rubor, mental status changes, and fixed, dilated pupils. The most likely diagnosis and treatment are
    A. metabolic brainstem disorder/admit to ICU and monitor
    B. stroke/admit and observe
    C. atropine toxicity/neostigmine and monitor
    D. atropine toxicity/physostigmine and monitor
    E. none of the above

264. Red–green color blindness is most commonly
   A. autosomal dominant
   B. autosomal recessive
   C. X-linked recessive
   D. a mutation
   E. none of the above

265. Workup and localization of the lesion causing an acquired Horner's syndrome
   A. is important because it may result in blindness
   B. is important because it may result in deafness
   C. is important because there is a significant incidence of associated cerebrovascular accident
   D. is important because there is a significant incidence of associated malignancy
   E. is not important

266. Ocular manifestations of juvenile rheumatoid arthritis
   A. are most often seen in the polyarticular form
   B. are most often seen in the monoarticular form
   C. are seen equally often in the polyarticular and monarticular forms
   D. are not found
   E. are most often seen in males

267. A 42-year-old black female is admitted to the hospital with elevated glucose, tachypnea, serum pH of 6.9, polyuria, unilateral ophthalmoplegia, markedly decreased vision, decreased corneal sensation, ptosis, proptosis, and orbital pain. The most likely etiology is
   A. orbital tumor
   B. mucor mycosis
   C. candida
   D. collagen vascular disease
   E. none of the above

DIRECTIONS: Each group of questions below consists of lettered headings followed by a list of numbered words or phrases. For **each** numbered word or phrase, select the **one** lettered heading that is most closely associated with it. Each lettered heading may be selected once, more than once, or not at all.

Questions 268–272: Match the appropriate visual field in Fig. 17.1 to the most likely location of the lesion that would produce it.

    A. Lesion a–a
    B. Lesion b–b
    C. Lesion c–c
    D. Lesion d–d
    E. Lesion e–e

Figure 17.1

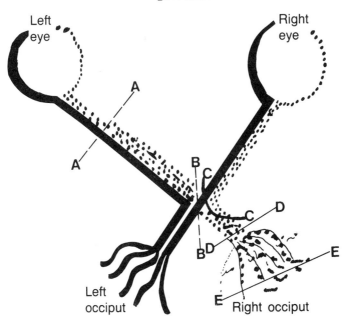

268. Visual field 1

269. Visual field 2

270. Visual field 3

271. Visual field 4

272. Visual field 5

Questions 273–282:

    A. Increased intraocular pressure
    B. Occlusion central retinal artery
    C. Strabismus
    D. Cataracts
    E. Presbyopia
    F. Cholinergic drug
    G. Anticholinergic drug
    H. Sympathetic drug
    I. Anti-inflammatory drug
    J. Antihistamine

273. Sudden loss of vision

274. Glaucoma

275. Gradual loss of vision

276. Blurred vision when reading

277. Cupping of disc

278. Atropine

279. Pilocarpine

280. Neosynephrine

281. Dexamethasone

282. Homatropine

DIRECTIONS: For each of the questions or incomplete statements below, **one or more** of the answers or completions given is correct. Select

    A   if only *1, 2, and 3* are correct
    B   if only *1 and 3* are correct
    C   if only *2 and 4* are correct
    D   if only *4* is correct
    E   if *all* are correct

Questions 283–286:

283. If the eyes are not aligned along the same visual axis,
    1. diplopia may result
    2. etiology may be congenital
    3. amblyopia may result
    4. etiology may be dysthyroid

284. Retinoblastoma
    1. may present with leukocoria (white pupil)
    2. is associated with sarcomas
    3. may be associated with chromosomal abnormalities
    4. is not a cause for concern

285. Retinopathy of prematurity is related to
    1. neonatal administration of oxygen
    2. gestational age
    3. birth weight
    4. use of cephalosporins in pregnant women

286. A cherry red spot in the fovea may be seen in
    1. central retinal artery occlusion (CRAO)
    2. all metabolic storage disorders
    3. Tay–Sachs disease
    4. toxoplasmosis

18

Otorhinolaryngology
Stanley N. Farb, M.D.

DIRECTIONS: Each of the questions or incomplete statements below is followed by five suggested answers or completions. Select the **one** that is best in each case.

287. All of the following drugs are considered ototoxic EXCEPT
    A. quinine
    B. aspirin
    C. aminoglycoside antibiotics
    D. sulfamethoxazole
    E. furosemide (Lasix)

288. Tuning fork tests that reveal bone conduction to be greater than air conduction in one ear (Rinne negative) and a Weber test that lateralizes to that ear suggests
    A. a conductive hearing loss in the ear being tested
    B. a sensorineural hearing loss in the ear being tested
    C. a conductive hearing loss in the opposite ear
    D. a sensorineural hearing loss in the opposite ear
    E. malingering

289. A patient who presents with pain or fullness in the ear aggravated by chewing most likely has
   A. trigeminal neuralgia
   B. a nasopharyngeal neoplasm
   C. eustachian tube dysfunction
   D. temporomandibular joint syndrome
   E. carcinoma of the larynx

290. A large, unilateral nasal polyp which originates from the middle meatus is usually associated with
   A. allergic rhinitis
   B. bronchial asthma
   C. maxillary sinusitis
   D. septal deviation
   E. aspirin sensitivity

291. Sinusitis in children less than 4 years of age
   A. is associated with recurrent ear effusions
   B. does not occur
   C. usually involves the ethmoidal sinus
   D. is associated with nasal polyps
   E. suggests an immune deficiency

292. Patients who snore loudly, have marked restlessness during sleep, and complain of daytime somnolence should be evaluated for
   A. sinopulmonary syndrome
   B. thyroid dysfunction
   C. adenoidectomy
   D. laryngomalacia
   E. sleep apnea

293. A hard, smooth-surfaced, raised swelling in the midline of the roof of the mouth is most likely
   A. torus palatinus
   B. Kaposi's sarcoma
   C. ectopic salivary tissue
   D. midline granuloma
   E. a dermoid

294. A white, plaquelike lesion of oral mucosa that is premalignant is
  A. squamous papilloma
  B. lichen planus
  C. leukoplakia
  D. *Candida albicans*
  E. linea alba

295. A common precursor of oral candidiasis is
  A. antibiotic therapy
  B. blood dyscrasia
  C. contaminated milk
  D. aphthous stomatitis
  E. necrotizing gingivitis

296. In a patient who presents a hard neck mass suspicious for metastitic carcinoma, the first step is
  A. a CT scan of the neck
  B. a thorough search for a primary tumor in the head and neck area
  C. biopsy of the neck mass
  D. wide excision of the neck mass
  E. a CBC and serology

297. The development of left vocal cord paralysis in a long-term cigarette smoker most likely results from
  A. thyroid carcinoma
  B. peripheral neuritis
  C. carcinoma of the esophagus
  D. carcinoma of the lung
  E. metastatic carcinoma of the larynx

298. "Rebound" phenomenon is associated with
  A. excessive noise exposure
  B. histamine-induced headaches
  C. overuse of vasoconstrictor nose drops or sprays
  D. vocal abuse with nodule formation
  E. nasal polyposis

DIRECTIONS: The group of questions below consists of four lettered headings followed by a list of numbered statements. For **each** numbered statement, select the **one** lettered heading that is most clearly associated with it. Each lettered heading may be selected once, more than once, or not at all.

Questions 299–302:

> **A.** Acoustic neurinoma
> **B.** Positional vertigo
> **C.** Meniere's disease
> **D.** Vestibular neuronitis

299. Episodic vertigo, tinnitus, and sensorineural hearing loss

300. Vertigo lasting 1–3 weeks with no change in hearing

301. Unilateral tinnitus with slowly progressive hearing loss

302. Brief dizzy spells related to extension of the neck

DIRECTIONS: Each set of lettered headings below is followed by a list of numbered words or phrases. For each numbered word or phrase select

> **A** if the item is associated with A *only*
> **B** if the item is associated with B *only*
> **C** if the item is associated with *both* A and B
> **D** if the item is associated with *neither* A nor B

Questions 303–306:

> **A.** Acute epiglottitis (supraglottic laryngitis)
> **B.** Acute laryngotracheobronchitis (croup)
> **C.** Both
> **D.** Neither

303. Bacterial etiology in most cases

304. Occurs primarily below the age of 3

305. Dysphagia is an important symptom

306. Endotracheal intubation is often necessary

Questions 307–309:

    A. Intradermal skin testing
    B. Radioallergosorbent (RAST) testing
    C. Both
    D. Neither

307. Measures total circulating IgE in patients suspected of allergy

308. May result in systemic reactions

309. Accurate for testing patients on antihistamines

Questions 310–313:

    A. Acute otitis externa
    B. Acute otitis media
    C. Both
    D. Neither

310. Usually bacterial in origin

311. Associated with cholesteatoma

312. Results in a hearing loss

313. Requires systemic antibiotics

DIRECTIONS: This section of the test consists of a situation, followed by a series of questions. Study the situation and select the **one** best answer to each question following it.

Questions 314–316: A college student presents with severe sore throat, fever, and malaise. After 7 days of penicillin, examination reveals exudative tonsillitis and cervical adenopathy.

314. The most helpful study at this point will be
   A. throat culture and sensitivity
   B. antistreptolysin titer
   C. white blood count with differential
   D. lateral x-ray of the neck
   E. sedimentation rate

315. The causative organism in infectious mononucleosis is thought to be
   A. herpes simplex virus
   B. Epstein–Barr virus
   C. beta-hemolytic streptococcus
   D. cytomegalovirus
   E. *Hemophilus influenzae*

316. If the initial examination had revealed inflammation of one tonsil with marked swelling of the adjacent soft palate, the likely diagnosis would be
   A. diphtheria
   B. pseudomononucleosis
   C. Hodgkin's disease
   D. lateral band pharyngitis
   E. peritonsillar abscess

19

Pediatrics

Daniel L. Coury, M.D., and
Nancy B. Hansen, M.D.

DIRECTIONS: Each of the questions or incomplete statements below is followed by four or five suggested answers or completions. Select the **one** that is best in each case.

317. The infant of a diabetic mother commonly develops all the following problems EXCEPT
    A. hypoglycemia
    B. hyperbilirubinemia
    C. thrombocytopenia
    D. hypocalcemia
    E. polycythemia

318. All of the following events characteristically occur during normal growth in the first 12 months of life EXCEPT
    A. at least a doubling of the initial birth weight
    B. closure of the posterior fontanelle
    C. decrease in subcutaneous tissue
    D. eruption of an average of 6–8 deciduous teeth
    E. increase in length of 25–30 cm

319. A toddler at 24 months of age can do all of the following EXCEPT
    A. link 3–4 words together in simple sentences
    B. assist in undressing self
    C. handle spoon and cup well
    D. climb stairs with alternating feet
    E. build a tower of 5–6 cubes

320. A 10-year-old white male presents to the emergency room with a 24-hour history of painful lower extremities and severe abdominal pain. On physical exam, you note a temperature of 99°F and severe arthritis of both knees along with a purpuric rash located on the lower extremities and buttocks. The stool guaiac is positive, as is a urine dipstick for protein and blood. The most likely diagnosis is
    A. Rocky Mountain spotted fever
    B. juvenile rheumatoid arthritis
    C. Schonlein-Henoch vasculitis
    D. meningococcemia
    E. post-streptococcal glomerulonephritis

321. All of the following therapies would be indicated in status asthmaticus EXCEPT
    A. aminophylline 6 mg/kg loading dose followed by 1 mg/kg/hour
    B. oxygen by nasal cannula
    C. metaproterenol by aerosol
    D. warm humidified air and 30% oxygen by mist tent
    E. intravenous fluids

322. *Hemophilus influenzae* type B is a frequent etiologic agent in all of the following infections EXCEPT
    A. septic arthritis in a 4-month-old infant
    B. osteomyelitis in a 12-year-old child
    C. meningitis in a 3-year-old child
    D. epiglottitis in a 6-year-old child
    E. buccal cellulitis in a 15-month-old infant

323. Pneumococcal sepsis is a distinct possibility in patients with the following underlying diseases EXCEPT
    A. 10-year-old with sickle cell anemia
    B. 5-year-old with Bruton's disease
    C. 30-year-old survivor of Hodgkin's disease following splenectomy
    D. 6-year-old with chronic ascites secondary to the nephrotic syndrome
    E. 8-year-old with chronic granulomatous disease

324. Esophageal atresia might present with all of the following symptoms EXCEPT
    A. excessive secretions noted in the newborn nursery
    B. difficulty feeding with cyanotic episode
    C. inability to pass a catheter into the stomach
    D. a history of polyhydramnios
    E. cyanosis at rest, relieved by crying

325. Which of the following statements concerning Hirschsprung's disease is NOT true?
    A. Although Hirschsprung's disease usually presents as chronic constipation, it can present as diarrhea with intestinal obstruction
    B. It is rarely seen in premature infants
    C. A rectal exam in affected infants is characteristically followed by a slow dribble of liquid stool
    D. It can be differentiated from acquired megacolon (secondary to chronic constipation) by a history of encopresis and the finding of feces in the ampulla on rectal exam

326. Which of the following is the most common cause of epistaxis in children?
    A. Nasal polyps
    B. Hemophilia
    C. Thrombocytopenia
    D. Sinusitis
    E. Self-induced trauma ("nose picking")

327. All of the following are complications of otitis media EXCEPT
    A. hearing loss
    B. brain abscess formation
    C. cholesteatoma
    D. facial nerve paralysis
    E. cauliflower ear deformity

328. Which of the following is the most likely diagnosis in an otherwise normal 3-year-old with a history of recurrent right lower lobe pneumonia?
    A. Cystic fibrosis
    B. Foreign body aspiration
    C. Chronic granulomatous disease
    D. Vascular ring

329. Sick premature infants have a higher incidence for all of the following cardiovascular problems than well full-term infants EXCEPT
    A. symptomatic congestive heart failure secondary to a ventricular septal defect
    B. patent ductus arteriosus
    C. persistent pulmonary hypertension of the newborn
    D. acquired renovascular hypertension secondary to umbilical arterial catheters

330. All of the following statements concerning congenital hypothyroidism are true EXCEPT
    A. newborn screening programs have been initiated in most states due to the difficulty in identifying the affected infant
    B. defective biosynthesis of thryoid hormone accounts for 70% of all neonatal cases
    C. premature infants frequently have transiently low levels of thyrotropin-releasing factor
    D. the breast-fed infant with hypothyroidism is partially protected due to the presence of maternal thyroid hormone in the milk
    E. a neonate with congenital hypothyroidism usually has a normal birth weight, length, and head circumference

331. The most common type of seizure seen in the newborn period is
   A. petit mal seizure
   B. myoclonic seizures
   C. subtle seizures (eye deviations, sucking)
   D. grand mal (tonic-clonic seizures)
   E. psychomotor seizure

332. Which of the following is the most common manifestation of acute valvular disease during the initial stages of rheumatic fever?
   A. Mitral regurgitation
   B. Mitral stenosis
   C. Aortic regurgitation
   D. Aortic stenosis
   E. Pulmonic stenosis

333. The normal infant at birth has all of the following hematologic alterations EXCEPT
   A. polycythemia with a normal Hb of 16–18 and Hct of 45–60
   B. lymphocyte predominance
   C. predominance of fetal hemoglobin
   D. normal white blood cell count ranging from 5000 to 30,000 in the first 48 hours after birth
   E. mildly prolonged prothrombin time

334. The combination of anemia, extramedullary hematopoiesis, jaundice, and hemosiderosis is found in which of the following disorders?
   A. Thalassemia major
   B. Thalassemia minor
   C. Sickle cell disease
   D. Hereditary spherocytosis
   E. Lead poisoning

335. Wilms' tumor is associated with all of the following conditions EXCEPT
   A. hemihypertrophy
   B. aniridia
   C. renal dysplasia
   D. neurofibromatosis
   E. Beckwith-Wiedeman syndrome

336. Hematuria is characteristically seen in all of the following disorders EXCEPT
   A. sickle cell disease
   B. minimal lesion nephrotic syndrome
   C. hereditary nephritis with deafness
   D. acute post-streptococcal glomerulonephritis
   E. cystitis associated with adenovirus infections

337. Low complement levels are seen in association with all of the following renal disorders EXCEPT
   A. post-streptococcal glomerulonephritis
   B. membranoproliferative glomerulonephritis
   C. systemic lupus erythematosus
   D. subacute bacterial endocarditis
   E. Henoch-Schonlein purpura

338. All of the following are characteristic of bilateral renal agenesis (Potter's disease) EXCEPT
   A. severe pulmonary insufficiency after birth
   B. maternal history of oligohydramnios, breech position during the pregnancy
   C. amnion nodosum
   D. extrarenal manifestations of low-set ears, prominent occiput, and limb deformations
   E. vertebral anomalies

339. All of the following neonatal disorders have been associated with hyperinsulinemia EXCEPT
   A. erythroblastosis fetalis
   B. nesidioblastosis
   C. infant of a diabetic mother
   D. Beckwith syndrome
   E. galactosemia

DIRECTIONS: Each group of questions below consists of lettered headings followed by a list of numbered words or statements. For **each** numbered word or statement, select the **one** lettered heading that is most closely associated with it. Each lettered heading may be selected once, more than once, or not at all.

Questions 340–344: Match the following fluid and electrolyte disturbance with the basic pathogenic mechanism:

  A. Na 125, K 4.7, HCO_2 10, Gluc 568, BUN 30
  B. Na 120, K 3.6, HCO_2 18, Gluc 92, BUN 3
  C. Na 135, K 2.7, Cl 85, HCO_3 42
  D. Na 125, K 4.2, HCO_2 10, Gluc 103, BUN 45, Ca 7.8
  E. Na 135, K 4.5, HCO_2 12, Gluc 86, BUN 58, Ca 7.8 mg/dl, phosphorus 9 mg/dl

340. Infant with prolonged diarrhea

341. Five-year-old child with chronic renal failure

342. Ten-year-old with diabetic ketoacidosis

343. Child with *Hemophilus influenzae* meningitis

344. Infant with pyloric stenosis

Questions 345–348: Match the following diseases with the most characteristic clinical features:

  A. Painful abdominal cramping in a previously well 15-month-old, associated with rectal bleeding
  B. Painless rectal bleeding in a previously well 15-month-old
  C. Abdominal distension and rectal bleeding in a premature infant
  D. Acute vomiting and bloody diarrhea in a full-term infant

345. Necrotizing enterocolitis

346. Cow's milk protein intolerance

347. Meckel's diverticulum

348. Intussusception

DIRECTIONS: For each of the questions or incomplete statements below, **one or more** of the answers or completions given is correct. Select

    A   if only *1, 2, and 3* are correct
    B   if only *1 and 3* are correct
    C   if only *2 and 4* are correct
    D   if only *4* is correct
    E   if *all* are correct

Questions 349–363:

349. Colic is characterized by which of the following statements?
    1. The hands are clenched and the abdomen is distended and tense
    2. It is unrelated to feeding routines
    3. It usually resolves spontaneously by 3–4 months of age
    4. "Attack" usually begins insidiously, with gradual increase in fussiness and subsequent development of loud crying

350. Which of the following immunizations would be contraindicated in the immunocompromised child?
    1. DPT
    2. OPV
    3. *Hemophilus influenzae* type B (Hib)
    4. MMR

Directions Summarized

A	B	C	D	E
1, 2, 3	1, 3	2, 4	4	All are
only	only	only	only	correct

351. Staphylococcal infections with elaboration of toxins cause which of the following diseases?
   1. Bullous impetigo
   2. Toxic-shock syndrome
   3. Scalded skin syndrome (Ritter's disease)
   4. Erythrasma

352. Conjugated hyperbilirubinemia in the neonate is associated with
   1. galactosemia
   2. cystic fibrosis
   3. urinary tract infection
   4. hypothyroidism

353. With regard to bronchiolitis,
   1. the etiologic agent most frequently responsible is respiratory syncytial virus
   2. the treatment of choice includes intravenous fluids, mist tent, supplemental oxygen if needed
   3. the most common symptoms include tachypnea, low-grade fever, and expiratory wheezing
   4. roentgenographic findings show hyperinflation of lungs with scattered areas of consolidation

354. Common sites of extramedullary relapse in patients with acute lymphocytic leukemia following chemotherapy include
   1. adrenal gland
   2. central nervous system
   3. thymus
   4. testes

355. Patients with insulin-dependent diabetes have an increased incidence of which of the following associated endocrine disorders?
    1. Hypoparathyroidism
    2. Addison's disease
    3. Hyperthyroidism
    4. Hypothyroidism

356. A child with 21-hydroxylase deficiency might be expected to have which of the following disorders?
    1. Hypervalemia
    2. Female pseudohermaphroditism
    3. Hyponatremia
    4. Hypernatremia

357. Primitive reflexes normally present at birth include
    1. Moro reflex
    2. placing reflex
    3. palmar grasp
    4. parachute reflex

358. Hypotonia is a clinical feature of which of the following disorders at 1 month of age?
    1. Cerebral palsy
    2. Werdnig-Hoffman disease (anterior horn cell atrophy)
    3. Down's syndrome
    4. Duchenne muscular dystrophy

359. Febrile seizures
    1. are usually seen in association with severely brain-damaged children
    2. generally occur after 1 year of age, but before 5 years of age
    3. may be prevented by phenobarbital administration at the onset of fever
    4. usually last less than 15 minutes

Directions Summarized				
A	**B**	**C**	**D**	**E**
1, 2, 3	1, 3	2, 4	4	All are
only	only	only	only	correct

360. Normal findings on the cardiovascular exam in a 5-year-old child include
1. a respiratory rate of 25 and a pulse rate of 100
2. a venous hum heard in the subclavical area
3. a split second heart sound
4. a palpable systolic thrill at the mid-left sternal border

361. A 3-year-old presents to the emergency room with a temperature of 39°C, a respiratory rate of 30, and audible stridor. Which of the following statements is (are) correct?
1. Stridor is usually heard best during expiration
2. Included in the differential diagnosis would be croup and *Hemophilus influenzae* infection
3. Intravenous aminophylline will lessen the symptoms
4. Foreign body aspiration might present with similar symptoms

362. Congenital dislocation of the hip
1. is more commonly observed in girls
2. usually requires corrective surgery by 6 months of age
3. may be detected by apparent shortening of one leg
4. is not more commonly observed in infants with other lower extremity abnormalities, such as club feet

363. With regard to scoliosis,
1. it is a frequent transient finding during the prepubertal growth spurt
2. females are more commonly affected than males
3. the best screening procedure is to observe the child hopping on one foot and then the other
4. all members of a family should be examined once a family member has been identified with scoliosis

20

Public Health and Preventive Medicine
Raymond O. West, M.D.

DIRECTIONS: Each of the questions or incomplete statements below is followed by five suggested answers or completions. Select the **one** that is best in each case.

---

364. When comparing populations for health and disease conditions, it is necessary to use rates. Which of the following statements concerning rates is NOT correct?

  A. A rate must have a numerator and a denominator
  B. An incidence rate is an expression of frequency of occurrence of an event in a population
  C. Prevalence rates are useful for measuring the frequency of conditions that are of considerable duration
  D. Infant mortality rate equals liveborn infants who die before 1 year of age, divided by the number of live births in the same year
  E. Incidence and prevalence rates are, for practical use, identical

365. Which of the following statements concerning cancer trends (secular changes) in the United States from 1930 to 1982 is NOT correct?

A. Mortality due to cancer of the stomach has declined rather dramatically in both men and women

B. Deaths due to cancer of the lung continue to rise in both men and women

C. Mortality due to cancer of the uterus has risen sharply in the past 20 years

D. In men, mortality due to cancer of the prostate continues to rise, but not dramatically

E. Cancer of the breast in women has not shown remarkable secular trends, either up or down, over the past 50 years

366. In considering if one event causes another, which of the following is correct?

A. Most statistical associations are causal

B. The stronger the association between two categories of events, the more likely it is that the association is causal

C. The concept of "web of causation" is less appropriate than the concept of "chain of causation"

D. The stronger the association between two categories of events (as revealed by considering groups of individuals), the less likely is the causal association to be correct

E. The distinction between direct and indirect causal relationships is no longer a valid one. For satisfactory study of causation it is necessary to understand causal mechanisms in their entirety to effect the same preventive measures

367. In conducting case-control studies it is necessary to select a series of controls. Which of the following statements is the most appropriate concerning the choice of controls?
   A. There should be no major differences between case and control groups as to the quality and availability of epidemiologic information
   B. Equal access to important information is not necessary, provided the controls are carefully chosen
   C. When data are obtained by interview, and the same interviewers are used for cases and controls, then it is inevitably certain that the quality of information will be the same for both cases and controls
   D. Cases and controls must be similar in all respects, including the presence of disease being studied in both cases and controls
   E. It is now considered improper for an investigator to attempt to match controls to cases

368. Which of the following statements is correct concerning the leading causes of death in the United States?
   A. Heart diseases still lead all others, comprising about 38.2% of the total
   B. Cancer deaths have now exceeded both heart disease and cerebrovascular diseases, comprising a total of 38.2%
   C. Since the use of seat belts has become more prevalent, accidental deaths have declined to 15th place
   D. Chronic obstructive lung diseases have risen to second place, making up a total of 21.9%
   E. Since the advent of effective antibiotics and flu vaccine, the rubric "pneumonia and influenza" has declined to 15th place

369. Which of the following statements concerning AIDS is NOT correct?

    A. The common accepted name for the AIDS virus is HTLV-III/LAV

    B. Preliminary evidence indicates that in rare cases the AIDS agent can be transmitted from a patient to a person providing care to the patient (and through a nonparenteral route)

    C. AIDS can be transmitted from person to person through blood transfusion

    D. It appears from early evidence that there is a statistical association between the prevalence of pulmonary tuberculosis and AIDS

    E. The Centers for Disease Control do not currently recommend the wearing of gloves routinely during direct contact with AIDS patients, items soiled by them with blood, and body secretions

370. Under which division in Table 20.1 would the Centers for Disease Control, Food and Drug Administration, Health Resources Administration, and the National Institutes of Health come?

    A. Office of Human Development

    B. Public Health Service

    C. Health Care Financing Administration

    D. Social Security Administration

    E. Education Division

Table 20.1 Department of Health and Human Services

Secretary→Under Secretary →	→Office of Human Development
	→Public Health Service
	→Health Care Financing Administration
	→Social Security Administration
	→Education Division

371. Which of the following exercises a direct line of authority for the agencies of the Public Health Service?
    A. Assistant Secretary of Health
    B. Commissioner of Health
    C. Assistant Secretary for Human Development
    D. Administrator for Health Service
    E. Assistant Secretary of Education

372. Which federal agency in Table 20.2 is charged with protecting the public health of this country by providing leadership and direction in the prevention and control of disease?
    A. Health Resources Administration
    B. National Institutes of Health
    C. Centers for Disease Control
    D. Alcohol, Drug Abuse, and Mental Health Administration
    E. Food and Drug Administration

373. The National Center for Health Statistics comes under which agency in Table 20.2?
    A. Food and Drug Administration
    B. Centers for Disease Control
    C. Alcohol, Drug Abuse and Mental Health Administration
    D. National Institutes of Health
    E. Health Resources Administration

Table 20.2 Public Health Service

Centers for Disease Control
Food and Drug Administration
Health Resources Administration
National Institutes of Health
Alcohol, Drug Abuse, and Mental Health Administration
President's Council on Physical Fitness and Sports

374. The National Heart, Lung and Blood Institute—which provides leadership for a national program concerning diseases of the heart, blood vessels, and blood and of the lungs, and in the use of blood and the management of blood resources—comes under which agency?

A. President's Council on Physical Fitness and Sports
B. National Institutes of Health
C. Alcohol, Drug Abuse, and Mental Health Administration
D. Centers for Disease Control
E. Health Resources Administration

375. All of the following are functions of a state health department as defined by the American Public Health Association EXCEPT

A. the study of state health problems and planning for their solution
B. coordination and technical supervision of local health activities
C. financial aid to local health departments
D. the enactment of sanitary regulations applicable in local health departments
E. the establishment of maximum standards for local health work

376. The local health department is usually administrated by a local director of health who is responsible to township, city, or county governments. The basic activities of this department are all of the following EXCEPT

A. collection of vital statistics
B. control of sanitary conditions
C. control of communicable diseases
D. maintenance of a blood collection program
E. protection of the health of mothers and infants

377. Of the following health organizations, which one has the fundamental responsibility to determine the health status and the health needs of the people within its jurisdiction, determine to what extent these needs are being met by effective measures currently available, and take steps to see that the unmet needs are satisfied?
A. U.S. Public Health Service
B. State health departments
C. Local health departments
D. American Red Cross
E. American Cancer Society

378. All of the following United Nations organizations emphasize technical assistance for developing countries and the development of international forums on key health issues EXCEPT
A. UNRWA
B. WHO
C. UNICEF
D. UNFPA
E. FAO

379. All of the following chemicals give evidence of carcinogenicity to man EXCEPT
A. vinyl chloride
B. asbestos
C. benzene
D. phenacetin
E. tetracycline

DIRECTIONS: The group of questions below consists of a diagram with lettered components followed by a list of numbered words or statements. For **each** numbered word or statement, select the **one** lettered heading that is most closely associated with it. Each lettered heading may be selected once, more than once, or not at all.

Questions 380–384 (refer to Fig. 20.1):

380. The mean

381. $\bar{x} - s$ to $\bar{x} + s$

382. Many laboratory standards are based on this value

383. Contains 95% of the data

384. Within three standard deviations (3 SD) of the mean

Figure 20.1

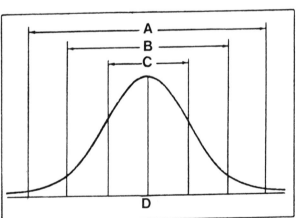

DIRECTIONS: For each of the questions or incomplete statements below, **one or more** of the answers or completions given is correct. Select

A if only *1, 2, and 3* are correct
B if only *1 and 3* are correct
C if only *2 and 4* are correct
D if only *4* is correct
E if *all* are correct

Questions 385–393:

385. The American Red Cross is categorized as a
  1. governmental agency
  2. private, voluntary organization
  3. philanthropic foundation
  4. quasigovernmental agency

386. On July 30, 1965, President Johnson signed into law a major health care bill, of which
  1. Title XVIII is known as Medicare
  2. Title XVIII provides special medical benefits to most everyone 65 or older
  3. Title XIX makes provision for special health benefits to anyone eligible for federally aided public assistance programs
  4. Title XIX is known as Medicaid

387. To reach and understand the health needs of the general public, the social worker has a valuable role. The scope of this role includes
  1. social-work consultation service
  2. program planning, implementation, and policy formulation
  3. social case work for individuals, families, and groups
  4. social research and surveys

Directions Summarized

A	B	C	D	E
1, 2, 3	1, 3	2, 4	4	All are
only	only	only	only	correct

388. Concerning adjusted rates and standardized mortality ratios,
1. the most important variable for which adjustment is required is age
2. adjustment (or standardization) is made for many variables, including sex, race, socioeconomic status, and smoking status
3. there are two basic methods for adjusting
4. the standardized mortality ratio equals observed deaths divided by expected deaths

389. With regard to social determinates of health and disease,
1. studies have shown that higher socioeconomic groups have higher death rates for most causes of death
2. other data indicate that those in top management positions have the lowest blood pressure and that blood pressures rise progressively as one moves down the occupational ladder
3. people who are married have higher mortality rates than people who have never married
4. men generally have higher mortality rates than women

390. Which of the following statements concerning nosocomial infections is/are correct?
1. Urinary tract infections (UTIs) account for about 40% of nosocomial infections nationwide
2. Most nosocomial UTIs are caused by urinary tract manipulation
3. Surgical wound infection is the second most common nosocomial infection, accounting for about 20% of cases
4. Even after effective tuberculosis chemotherapy is administered, the patients remain contagious for many weeks to several months

391. A number of occupations are associated with specific agents that are related to pathologic pulmonary response. Which of the following are correctly matched?
1. Teflon manufacture/polymer fumes (polytetrafluoro-ethylene)
2. Farming (farmer's lung)/*Pseudomonas*
3. Meat wrapping (asthma)/vinyl chloride (phosgene)
4. Airconditioning and humidifer maintenance/*Thermo-actinomyces (vulgarus) sacchari*

392. Concerning world population and public health,
1. the change from high mortality and fertility rates to low mortality and fertility rates is frequently called the demographic transition
2. the rapid population growth rates in most developing countries is due to the fact that mortality rates have dropped considerably while fertility rates have not declined proportionately
3. in recent years in the United States, while the fertility rate for women age 15–19 has been dropping, the number of births has been increasing
4. if a country lowers its fertility rate, the first important effect is on the demand for education

393. Concerning influenza and vaccination for it,
1. we cannot yet identify an absolute level of serum antibody resulting from successful influenza vaccination that can guarantee complete protection against infection
2. titers higher than 1–20 have been associated with significantly decreased rates of infection or illness
3. production of vaccine for a specific flu season must begin in February
4. late outbreaks (March and April) make it impossible to examine influenza isolates in time for vaccine formulation decisions

21

Psychiatry
Edward H. Liston, M.D.

DIRECTIONS: Each of the questions or incomplete statements below is followed by five suggested answers or completions. Select the **one** that is best in each case.

---

394. Electroconvulsive therapy is considered to be absolutely contraindicated in the presence of
    A. multiple myeloma
    B. recent myocardial infarction
    C. third trimester pregnancy
    D. myasthenia gravis
    E. none of the above

395. Diagnostic criteria for schizophrenia include all of the following EXCEPT
    A. thought broadcasting
    B. thought insertion
    C. auditory hallucinations of a voice calling a name
    D. auditory hallucinations of several voices commenting on the patient's actions or thoughts
    E. delusions of being controlled

396. Mania is characterized by all of the following EXCEPT
   A. elated, unstable mood
   B. irritability and impatience
   C. pressured speech
   D. clarity of insight
   E. increased psychomotor activity

397. Which of the following characterizes conversion disorder?
   A. Unconscious conflict is symbolized in some way by the symptoms
   B. Indifference to symptoms is always present
   C. Symptomatology is likely to mimic closely organic physical illness
   D. Patients are always women
   E. The disorder is limited to patients with hysterical character disorder

398. Antisocial personality disorder is characterized by all of the following EXCEPT
   A. onset before age 15 years
   B. alcohol or substance abuse
   C. higher prevalence in females
   D. impulsiveness
   E. repeated lying

399. All of the following are indications for sex therapy EXCEPT
   A. inhibited sexual excitement
   B. delusions about the sexual organs
   C. ejaculatory incompetence
   D. orgasmic dysfunction
   E. functional dyspareunia

400. The most common psychological defense mechanism in reaction to physical illness is
   A. projection
   B. reaction formation
   C. conversion
   D. denial
   E. dissociation

401. The most common etiology of irreversible dementia is
  A. Huntington's disease
  B. multi-infarct dementia
  C. Alzheimer-type dementia
  D. Creutzfeldt-Jakob disease
  E. Pick's disease

DIRECTIONS: Each group of questions below consists of five lettered headings followed by a list of numbered words or statements. For **each** numbered word or statement, select the **one** lettered heading that is most closely associated with it. Each lettered heading may be selected once, more than once, or not at at all.

Questions 402–407:

  A. Behavior therapy
  B. Electroconvulsive therapy
  C. Neuroleptic therapy
  D. Psychotherapy
  E. Lithium therapy

402. Used for maintenance treatment in bipolar disorder

403. Used for maintenance treatment in schizophrenia

404. Phobias are a major indication of this type of therapy

405. Severe depression is the primary indication of this type of therapy

406. Neurotic conflicts are often treated with this type of therapy

407. Useful in treatment of adjustment disorders

Questions 408–410:

    A. Benztropine
    B. Urecholine
    C. Propranolol
    D. Phenoxybenzamine
    E. Physostigmine

408. Treatment of anticholinergic side effects

409. Treatment of anticholinergic toxic effects

410. Treatment of extrapyramidal side effects

DIRECTIONS: Each set of lettered headings below is followed by a list of numbered words or phrases. For each numbered word or phrase select

    A if the item is associated with A *only*
    B if the item is associated with B *only*
    C if the item is associated with *both* A and B
    D if the item is associated with *neither* A nor B

Questions 411–416:

    A. Delirium
    B. Dementia
    C. Both
    D. Neither

411. Always involves clouding of consciousness

412. Is always irreversible

413. Is always reversible

414. May be substance-induced

415. Onset is usually acute

416. Is usually toxic or metabolic

Questions 417–419:

    A. Transference
    B. Countertransference
    C. Both
    D. Neither

417. Involves inappropriate projections and identifications arising from unconscious emotional attitudes

418. A focus of attention in supportive psychotherapy and behavior therapy

419. May be manifested by critical, hostile, or angry feelings or behavior

---

DIRECTIONS: For each of the questions or incomplete statements below, **one or more** of the answers or completions given is correct. Select

    A if only *1, 2, and 3* are correct
    B if only *1 and 3* are correct
    C if only *2 and 4* are correct
    D if only *4* is correct
    E if *all* are correct

Questions 420–429:

420. Toxic delirium has been associated with
    1. anti-inflammatory drugs
    2. anti-infection agents
    3. bromides
    4. anticholinergics

421. Borderline personality disorder is characterized by
1. impulsivity and unpredictability
2. inappropriate, intense anger
3. affective instability
4. desire to be alone

422. Compulsive personality disorder is characterized by
1. perfectionism
2. decisiveness
3. stubborness
4. unconventional behavior

423. Features of histrionic personality disorder include
1. self-dramatization
2. irrational angry outbursts
3. manipulative suicidal threats
4. avoidance of activity and excitement

424. Common side effects of treatment with lithium salts include
1. nausea
2. coarse tremor
3. polyuria
4. nystagmus

425. Signs of lithium toxicity include
1. atrioventricular block
2. poor concentration
3. ataxia
4. epileptiform seizures

426. Characteristics of delirium include which of the following?
1. Psychomotor activity is always increased
2. Disorientation or memory impairment is always present
3. Clinical features tend to be stable over time
4. Clouding of consciousness is always present

427. Characteristics of dementia include
1. impaired abstract thinking
2. impaired judgment
3. aphasia and apraxia
4. personality change

Directions Summarized

A	B	C	D	E
1, 2, 3 only	1, 3 only	2, 4 only	4 only	All are correct

428. Appropriate measures in the diagnostic assessment of organic brain syndrome include
   1. Wechsler Adult Intelligence Scale
   2. Halstead-Reitan Battery
   3. Bender Gestalt Test
   4. Thematic Apperception Test

429. Appropriate modalities in the treatment of chronic alcoholism include
   1. self-help groups
   2. intensive psychotherapy
   3. disulfiram
   4. diazepam

DIRECTIONS: This section of the test consists of a situation, followed by a series of questions. Study the situation and select the **one** best answer to each question following it.

Questions 430–431: A 64-year-old sales clerk presents at an emergency room with disorientation, confusion, visual hallucinations, dry mouth, and tachycardia. Her husband reports that she has always been "moody," but has been worse during recent years, and that she recently was given some medication "for her moods." He thinks that she has taken several of those pills today, but does not know their name. He says that she has been in her present condition for about 4 hours.

430. Of the following, the medication LEAST likely to have produced this picture is
   A. amitryptiline
   B. imipramine
   C. thioridazine
   D. lithium carbonate
   E. chlorpromazine

431. The most appropriate immediate pharmacologic intervention for this patient would be
   A. physostigmine
   B. diphenhydramine
   C. atropine
   D. haloperidol
   E. mannitol

22

Radiology
Alan E. Oestreich, M.D.

DIRECTIONS: Each of the questions or incomplete statements below is followed by five suggested answers or completions. Select the **one** that is best in each case.

---

432. In addition to the ulna fracture on Fig. 22.1, what other injury should be especially suspect?
    A. Dislocation of the ulna at the elbow
    B. Displacement of the distal humeral growth center C
    C. Dislocation of the radius at the wrist
    D. Dislocation of the ulna at the wrist
    E. Dislocation of the radius at the elbow

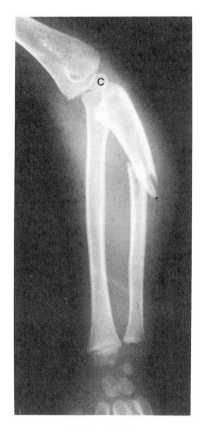

Figure 22.1

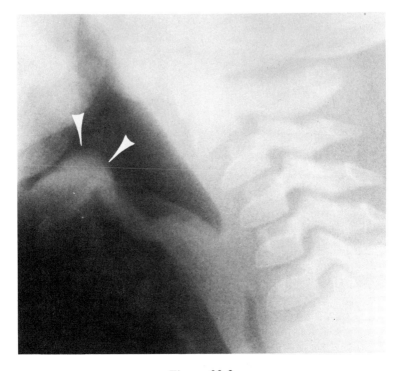

Figure 22.2

433. The young child in Fig. 22.2 has severe respiratory distress. Which of the following statements is LEAST appropriate?

A. If epiglottitis is suspected, the best x-ray view is an overhead lateral with the child recumbent

B. The arrowheads indicate a swollen epiglottis

C. Epiglottitis is a life-threatening condition

D. Subglottic narrowing may be present in epiglottitis

E. Epiglottitis, if clinically evident, does not require radiographic confirmation

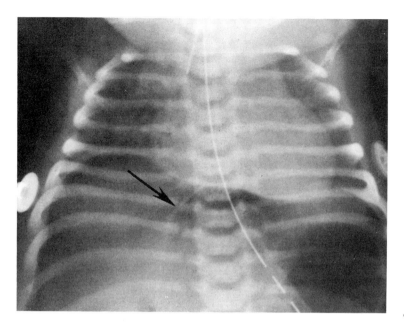

Figure 22.3

434. The child in Fig. 22.3 is supine. Which of the following statements is INCORRECT?
   A. The right lobe of the thymus is seen
   B. The arrow points to bowel loop wall
   C. There are no posterior rib fractures
   D. There is pneumoperitoneum
   E. An endotracheal tube and a nasogastric tube are present

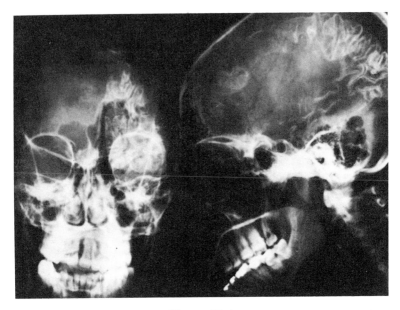

Figure 22.4

435. Figure 22.4 is characteristic of
   A. Sturge-Weber syndrome
   B. Riley-Day syndrome
   C. neurofibromatosis
   D. tuberous sclerosis
   E. multiple sclerosis

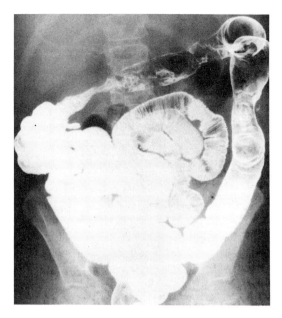

Figure 22.5

436. The pattern on the barium enema in Fig. 22.5 suggests a
most likely diagnosis of
A. ulcerative colitis
B. amyloidosis
C. pancreatitis with spread of enzymes
D. Hirschsprung disease
E. Crohn disease of the colon

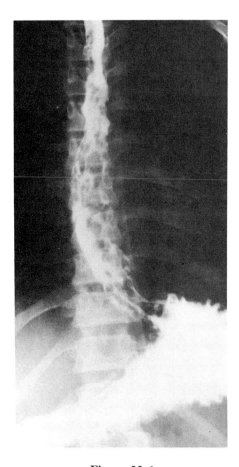

Figure 22.6

437. The esophageal pattern during barium swallow in Fig. 22.6
may be seen in association with
   A. non-beta islet cell tumor of the pancreas
   B. cavitating lesion of the lung apex
   C. portal hypertension
   D. tracheoesophageal fistula
   E. long-term gastroesophageal reflux

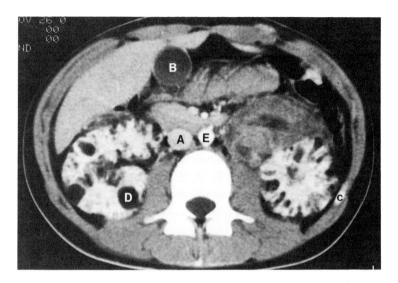

Figure 22.7

438. The CT of Fig. 22.7 was taken immediately following in-
     travenous contrast injection. Which of the following struc-
     tures is correctly identified?
     A. Aorta
     B. Liver cyst
     C. Ureter
     D. Angiomyolipoma of the kidney
     E. Inferior vena cava

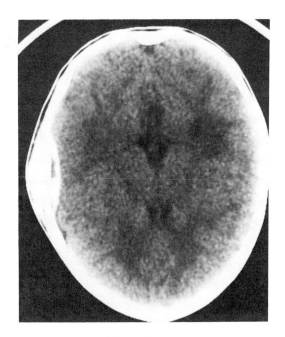

Figure 22.8

439. Which statement about the noncontrast CT on Fig. 22.8 is correct?
   A. There is a several-day-old epidural hematoma
   B. There is hydrocephalus
   C. Gray and white matter cannot be differentiated
   D. Magnetic resonance imaging cannot distinguish hemorrhage from calcification
   E. There is evidence of brain atrophy

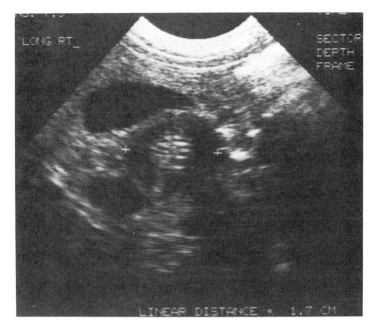

Figure 22.9

440. The 4-week-old boy in Fig. 22.9 has developed vomiting following several weeks of apparently normal feeding. This ultrasound is representative of a real-time study that showed a pyloric region diameter of 16 mm or more (measured between the plus signs on Fig. 22.9). Which statement is correct?

    A. The baby requires a barium study to confirm the diagnosis

    B. The echolucent donut indicated by the plus signs is ascites

    C. If the measured diameter persists, the diagnosis is assured

    D. The normal pylorus has a muscle width of 4–6 mm

    E. There is no physical finding which would make this study superfluous

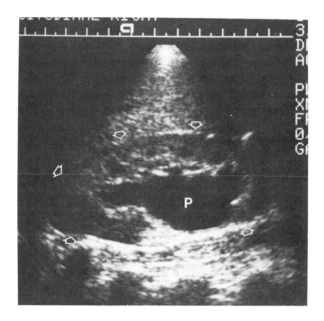

Figure 22.10

441. Figure 22.10 is a longitudinal ultrasound scan through a right
kidney (arrows). The appearance of the renal pelvis (P) may
be due to any but which of the following?
A. Vesicoureteral reflux
B. Page kidney
C. Ureteropelvic junction obstruction
D. Ureterovesical junction obstruction
E. Overdistended bladder

DIRECTIONS: Each group of questions below consists of five lettered headings followed by a list of numbered words or statements. For **each** numbered word or statement, select the **one** lettered heading that is most closely associated with it. Each lettered heading may be selected once, more than once, or not at all.

Questions 442–444:

    A. Ascites
    B. Pneumoperitoneum
    C. Ovarian cyst(s)
    D. Gallstone(s)
    E. Dilated ureter

442. Figure 22.11 (arrows), longitudinal sonogram

Figure 22.11

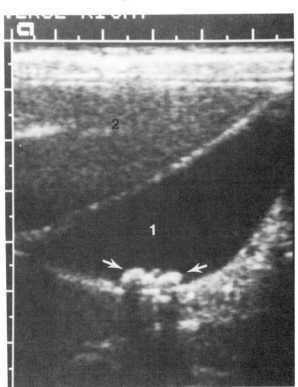

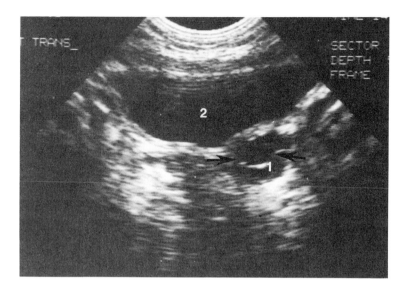

Figure 22.12

443. Figure 22.12 (arrows), transverse sonogram

444. Figure 22.13 (arrows), longitudinal sonogram

Figure 22.13

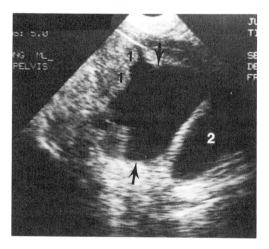

Questions 445–447:

    A. Osteomyelitis
    B. Fracture
    C. Scurvy
    D. Rickets
    E. Osteoporosis

445. Figure 22.14 (horizontal x-ray beam)

Figure 22.14

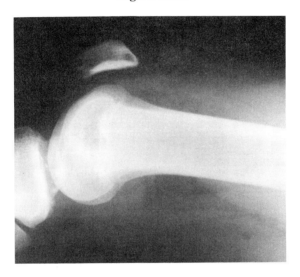

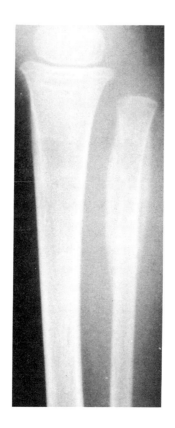

Figure 22.15

446. Figure 22.15 (vertical x-ray beam)

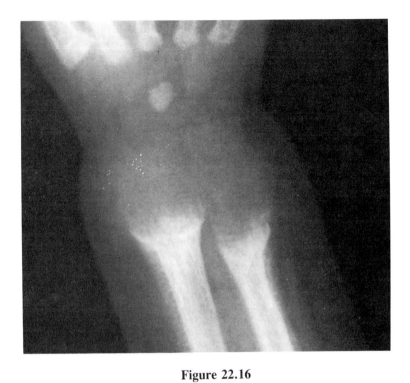

Figure 22.16

447. Figure 22.16 (vertical x-ray beam)

Questions 448–450:

    A. Pneumonia
    B. Left-to-right shunt
    C. Lung metastasis
    D. Check valve hyperaeration from foreign body
    E. Cystic fibrosis

448. Figure 22.17

Figure 22.17

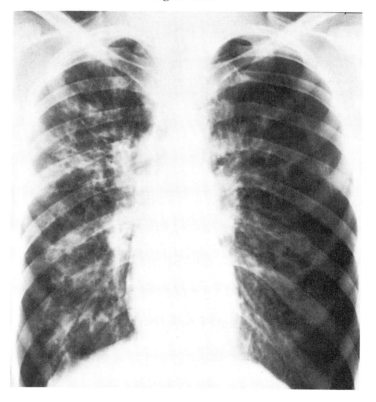

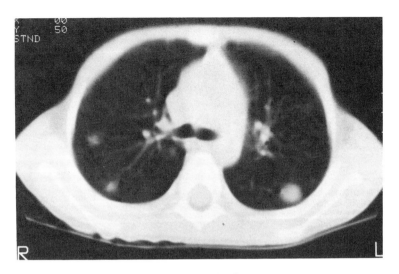

Figure 22.18

449. Figure 22.18

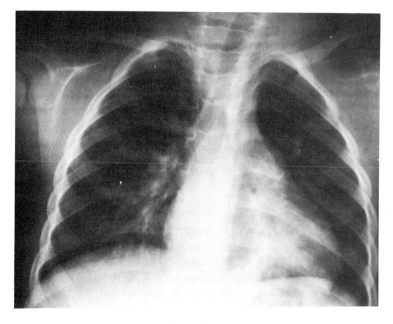

Figure 22.19

450. Figure 22.19

DIRECTIONS: The set of lettered headings below is followed by a list of illustrations. For each numbered illustration select

    A if the diagnosis is associated with A *only*
    B if the diagnosis is associated with B *only*
    C if the diagnosis is associated with *both* A and B
    D if the diagnosis is associated with *neither* A nor B

Questions 451–454:

    A. Ureteral stone
    B. Appendicitis
    C. Both
    D. Neither

451. Figure 22.20

Figure 22.20

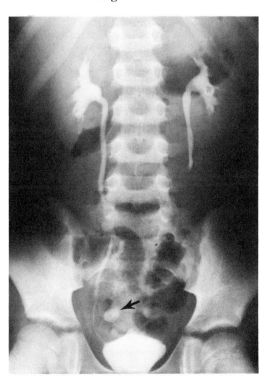

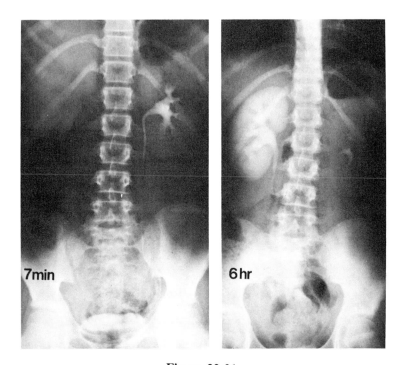

Figure 22.21

452. Figure 22.21

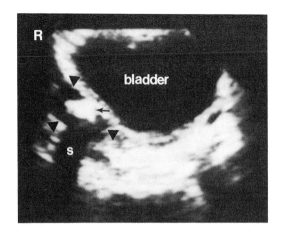

Figure 22.22

453. Figure 22.22

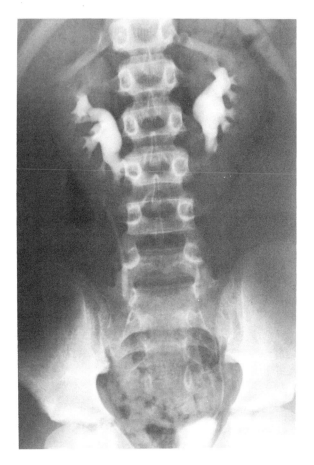

Figure 22.23

454. Figure 22.23

DIRECTIONS: For each of the questions or incomplete statements below, **one or more** of the answers or completions given is correct. Select

    A if only *1, 2, and 3* are correct
    B if only *1 and 3* are correct
    C if only *2 and 4* are correct
    D if only *4* is correct
    E if *all* are correct

455. On Fig. 22.24, the distance between the dens (d) and anterior arch of the C–1 (c) is 7.5 mm.

    1. This distance is always often above normal in Down's syndrome
    2. This distance may vary between flexion and extension
    3. This distance is greater in adults than children
    4. The distance of 7.5 mm in this child is beyond normal limits

Questions 455–459:

Figure 22.24

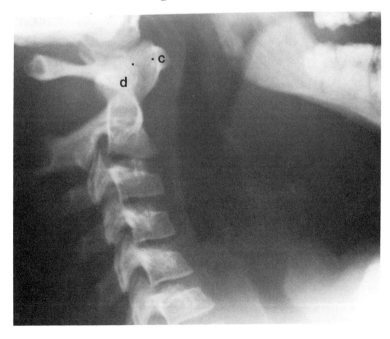

Directions Summarized				
A	**B**	**C**	**D**	**E**
1, 2, 3	1, 3	2, 4	4	All are
only	only	only	only	correct

456. Figure 22.25 is a bone-window axial CT image of a skull following direct trauma. The distance between the two x's is 7 mm.

   1. All children with skull trauma should have plain radiographs as soon as possible
   2. Standard frontal and lateral radiographs usually suffice to demonstrate how depressed a fracture is
   3. The absence of skull fracture after acute trauma is reason for reassurance
   4. This is a depressed skull fracture

Figure 22.25

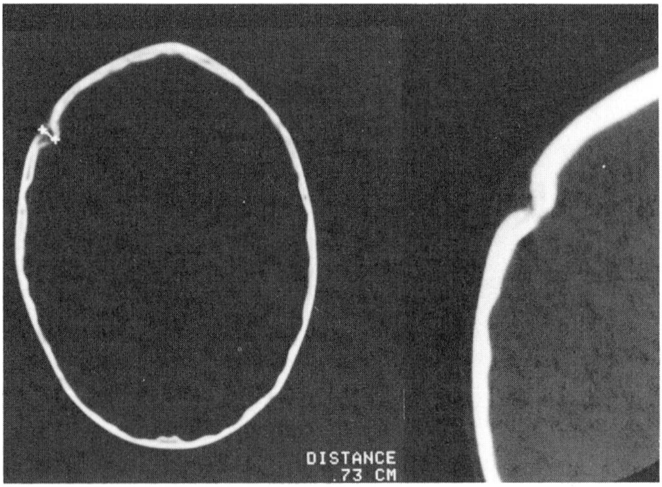

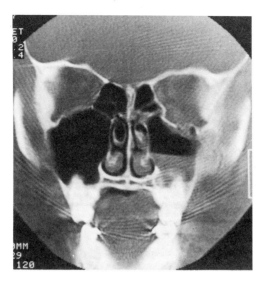

Figure 22.26

457. On Fig. 22.26, a direct coronal CT of the face following facial trauma, the following diagnostic signs are present:

1. Gas-fluid level in the involved maxillary sinus
2. Linear fracture fragment of the floor of the involved orbit
3. Abnormal soft tissue in the roof of the involved sinus
4. Abnormal protrusion of tooth into the involved maxillary sinus

Directions Summarized

A	B	C	D	E
1, 2, 3	1, 3	2, 4	4	All are
only	only	only	only	correct

458. The patient whose wrist radiograph is shown in Fig. 22.27 has wrist pain following trauma the same day.
  1. There is no perilunate dislocation
  2. The pain is likely centered at the medial wrist
  3. The navicular is fractured
  4. There is concern especially for the vascularity of the distal portion of the injured bone

Figure 22.27

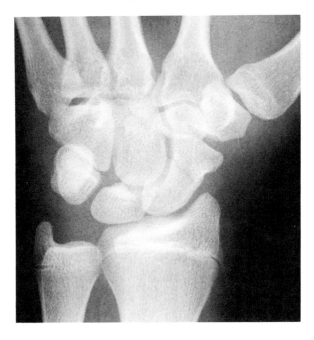

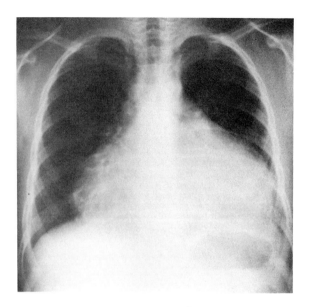

Figure 22.28

459. With regard to the chest shown on Fig. 22.28,
    1. echocardiography can distinguish between pericardial effusion and cardiomyopathy
    2. the patient could have rheumatoid arthritis
    3. there is no azygous fissure
    4. a right pleural effusion is present

DIRECTIONS: This section of the test consists of a situation, followed by a series of questions. Study the situation and select the **one** best answer to each question following it.

Questions 460–461: An apparently healthy 3-year-old boy was discovered incidentally to have a mass in the right side of the abdomen. There was no hepatomegaly, no palpable spleen, and a normal temperature. No hemihypertrophy and no aniridia was noted. Blood pressure was normal. The child was referred for screening abdominal ultrasound (Fig. 22.29). A mass (arrowheads) of mixed echogenicity in the lower right kidney distorts the normal upper kidney (K) on the longitudinal sonogram shown.

Figure 22.29

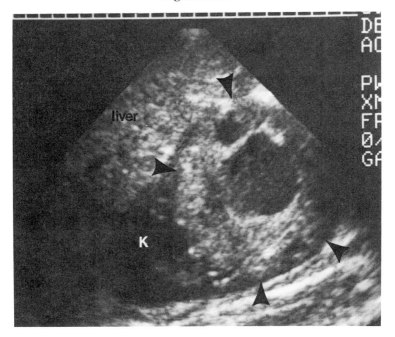

460. The diagnosis most likely is
 A. neuroblastoma
 B. angiomyolipoma
 C. multicystic dysplastic kidney
 D. Wilms' tumor
 E. renal cell carcinoma

461. Further areas important to screen during the ultrasound examination for involvement in this child include especially all of the following structures EXCEPT
 A. right atrium of the heart
 B. inferior vena cava
 C. bladder
 D. left kidney
 E. liver

23

Surgery
Stephen N. Joffe, M.D.

DIRECTIONS: Each of the questions or incomplete statements below is followed by five suggested answers or completions. Select the **one** that is best in each case.

---

462. In a patient suspected to have suffered a pulmonary embolism, immediate primary treatment consists of
    A. pulmonary embolectomy
    B. inferior vena caval clipping
    C. infusion of streptokinase
    D. anticoagulation
    E. endotracheal intubation and positive end expiratory pressure (PEEP)

463. Which of the following types of carcinoma of the breast is most frequently associated with bilateral disease?
    A. Infiltrating ductal cancer
    B. Paget's disease
    C. Mucinous carcinoma
    D. Lobular carcinoma
    E. Medullary carcinoma

464. A 35-year-old female presented with a 3-day history suggestive of bowel obstruction. She had undergone an appendectomy 10 years before this episode. All of the following are consistent with bowel obstruction EXCEPT

A. pain
B. vomiting
C. fever
D. constipation
E. abdominal distension

465. An 8-year-old child had a left supracondylar fracture that was reduced and the arm put in a cast. The same night the mother brought the child back because the child was complaining of pain and could not sleep. Repeat x-ray showed the reduction was still good. The patient should be managed by

A. administration of meperidine and a barbiturate for sleep
B. cutting the cast and extending the elbow from previous flexed position
C. angiography of left arm
D. elevation of arm and active exercises of fingers
E. axillary nerve block to relieve pain

466. A 15-year-old boy presented with complaint of pain in the knee of 6 weeks duration. On examination he had swelling in the lower end of the femur, which was warm. The movement of the knee was limited 20° at extremes of flexion and extension. Radiographs revealed areas of destruction and new bone formation. The most likely diagnosis is

A. giant cell tumor (osteoclastoma)
B. osteosarcoma
C. osteochondroma
D. osteomyelitis
E. osteoid osteoma

467. Antibiotics useful against *Bacteroides fragilis* include all of the following EXCEPT
    A. clindamycin
    B. cephalothin
    C. chloramphenicol
    D. erythromycin
    E. carbenicillin

468. All of the following are indicative of poor prognosis in acute pancreatitis EXCEPT
    A. serum calcium of less than 8.0 mg/100 ml
    B. hyperglycemia
    C. serum amylase of more than five times normal on admission
    D. arterial oxygen tension less than 60 mm Hg
    E. serum lactic dehydrogenase of more than three times normal

---

DIRECTIONS: Each group of questions below consists of five lettered headings followed by a list of numbered words or statements. For **each** numbered word or statement, select the **one** lettered heading that is most closely associated with it. Each lettered heading may be selected once, more than once, or not at all.

Questions 469–472:

    A. Obturator hernia
    B. Umbilical hernia
    C. Ventral hernia
    D. Direct inguinal hernia
    E. Indirect inguinal hernia

469. Romberg-Howship sign

470. Hernia through Hasselbach's triangle

471. Strangulation is rare

472. Common in the young

Questions 473–477:

    A. Alpha-fetoprotein
    B. Carcinoembryonic antigen (CEA)
    C. Chorionic gonadotropin
    D. Vanillylmandelic acid (VMA)
    E. 5-Hydroxyindoleacetic acid (5-HIAA)

473. Hepatoma

474. Carcinoma of colon

475. Testicular tumor

476. Carcinoid

477. Neuroblastoma

Questions 478–481:

    A. Methoxamine
    B. Dopamine
    C. Phenoxybenzamine
    D. Norepinephrine
    E. Isoproterenol

478. Blocks alpha-adrenergic receptors

479. Stimulates beta-adrenergic receptors

480. Alpha-adrenergic stimulator for peripheral circulation and beta-adrenergic stimulator on heart

481. Increases myocardial contractility

DIRECTIONS: The set of lettered headings below is followed by a list of numbered words or phrases. For each numbered word or phrase select

    A if the item is associated with A *only*
    B if the item is associated with B *only*
    C if the item is associated with *both* A and B
    D if the item is associated with *neither* A nor B

Questions 482–485:

    A. Ulcerative colitis
    B. Regional enteritis
    C. Both
    D. Neither

482. Toxic megacolon

483. Massive bleeding

484. Enteroenteric fistula

485. Arthritis

DIRECTIONS: For each of the questions or incomplete statements below, **one or more** of the answers or completions given is correct. Select

A   if only *1, 2, and 3* are correct
B   if only *1 and 3* are correct
C   if only *2 and 4* are correct
D   if only *4* is correct
E   if *all* are correct

Questions 486–488:

486. Regarding salivary gland tumors,
1. they occur most often in the parotid gland
2. the most common tumor is the papillary cystadenoma lymphomatosum
3. most are benign
4. sialography is often valuable in diagnosis and treatment planning

487. In a patient who has a spinal cord injury, indications for laminectomy include
1. debridement for penetrating trauma
2. progressive neurologic deficit
3. bony penetration of the spinal canal
4. complete high cervical cord injury

488. In abdominal aortic aneurysm, frequently there is occlusion of
1. superior mesenteric artery
2. left renal artery
3. right renal artery
4. inferior mesenteric artery

DIRECTIONS: This section of the test consists of situations, each followed by a series of questions. Study each situation and select the **one** best answer to each question following it.

Questions 489–490: A 55-year-old white female was admitted with acute pain in the epigastrium and right upper quadrant. She was a smoker. She had had six children. On admission she had a fever of 103°F, pulse of 120/minute, and marked rigidity and guarding in the upper abdomen, more on the right side. She was initially treated with antibiotics and intravenous fluids, and on ultrasound was found to have gallstones. Four days after admission, she underwent a cholecystectomy. Following this procedure, her temperature decreased, and she made a slow recovery. She had a temporary ileus for 72 hours, but was improving. On the sixth postoperative day, her temperature rose to 99.6°F. On the seventh postoperative day, she suddenly developed severe pain in the right chest associated with cough, shortness of breath, and hemoptysis.

489. The probable cause of this most recent episode is
A. atelectasis, right lower lobe
B. hemolytic crisis
C. subphrenic abscess on the right
D. acute myocardial infarction
E. pulmonary embolism

490. If the cause of her pain is pulmonary embolism, the most likely source of the embolus is the
A. plantar plexus
B. pelvic plexus of veins
C. common femoral vein
D. ovarian veins
E. veins in the upper limbs used for IV infusion

Questions 491–492: A 60-year-old white male was brought to the hospital with sudden onset of pain in his right lower limb. The pain was severe and started after a coughing spell. He had an acute myocardial infarction 3 weeks previously and was discharged 24 hours prior to his present admission.

491. The most likely diagnosis is
A. deep venous thrombosis
B. acute arterial thrombosis
C. acute arterial embolus
D. ruptured disc at L_{4-5} with radiating pain
E. dissecting aneurysm

492. Treatment of this patient's problem is
A. anticoagulation alone
B. bed rest and elevation of leg
C. immediate surgery
D. pelvic traction
E. controlled hypotension

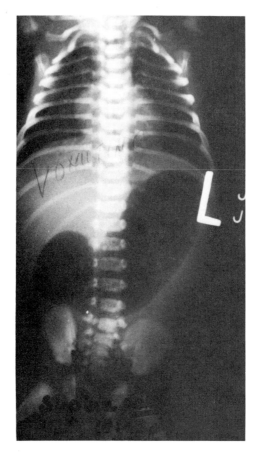

Figure 23.1

Questions 493–494: Forty-eight hours after birth an infant was brought for evaluation because of vomiting that had started 6 hours after birth. The infant was a full-term, normal delivery, and was mildly dehydrated. Physical examination was unremarkable. Plain x-ray of abdomen is as in Fig. 23.1.

493. The diagnostic possibilities include all the following EXCEPT
- **A.** annular pancreas
- **B.** duodenal atresia
- **C.** intestinal malrotation
- **D.** congenital pyloric stenosis
- **E.** peritoneal bands

494. Operation of choice for treatment of this condition is
- **A.** division of annulus of the pancreas
- **B.** pyloromyotomy
- **C.** duodenoduodenostomy
- **D.** gastrojejunostomy
- **E.** Billroth II operation

Questions 495–496: A 65-year-old male was admitted with a history of sudden onset of epigastric pain of 1 hour duration. He had a myocardial infarction twice before and is a chronic smoker. On examination he was pale and sweaty. Temperature of 100°F, pulse, 100/minute; BP, 90/60. The admission x-ray is shown in Fig. 23.2.

495. The most probable diagnosis is
   A. myocardial infarction
   B. acute pancreatitis
   C. acute mesenteric embolism
   D. perforated peptic ulcer
   E. atelectasis of right lower lobe

Figure 23.2

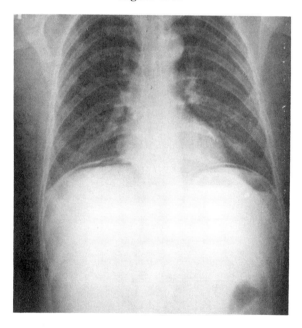

496. Choice of treatment for the above patient is
  A. conservative management with nasogastric suction, intravenous fluids, and antibiotics
  B. laparotomy and drainage
  C. closure of perforated ulcer
  D. partial gastrectomy including the ulcer
  E. resection of necrotic bowel

Questions 497–499: A 65-year-old patient presented with a history of mucous diarrhea, rectal bleeding, and change in bowel habit. Proctosigmoidoscopy revealed a large polypoid lesion 10 cm from the anal margin. Biopsy of the lesion was performed, and the photomicrograph is shown in Figure 23.3.

497. The most likely diagnosis is
  A. hyperplastic adenoma
  B. adenomatous polyp
  C. villous adenoma
  D. carcinoid
  E. carcinoma

Figure 23.3

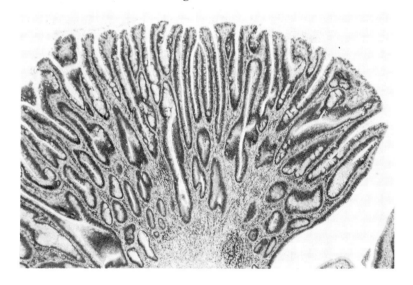

498. Treatment of the lesion is by
  A. excision through a proctoscope
  B. segmental resection of rectum
  C. proctectomy
  D. abdominoperineal resection
  E. fulguration

499. Biochemical abnormalities associated with this tumor include all the following EXCEPT
  A. hypocalcemia
  B. hypokalemia
  C. hyponatremia
  D. hypochloremia
  E. hypovolemia

Questions 500–502: A 45-year-old man presented with a history of swelling in his left scrotum of 3 months duration. On questioning he had no other complaints except that on two occasions during the same period he had painless hematuria, each seen only during one attempt to micturition. On examination the left testis appeared to be normal in size, but the spermatic cord was thickened and bulky. There was an expansile impulse on coughing. Abdominal examination revealed an indistinct lump to the left of the midline in the epigastrium. A routine IVP was obtained (Fig. 23.4).

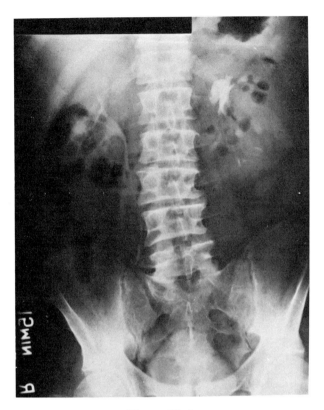

Figure 23.4

500. The most likely diagnosis is
    A. left inguinal hernia and englarged prostate
    B. left inguinal hernia and left renal tumor
    C. left testicular tumor with para-aortic lymph nodal mass
    D. left varicocele and left renal cell carcinoma
    E. left varicocele with a bladder tumor

501. The most useful procedure in further investigation of this patient is
   A. renal scan
   B. ultrasonography of the abdomen
   C. thermography of the scrotum
   D. selective abdominal arteriography
   E. voiding cystourethrography

502. Which of the following may be associated with the lesion?
   A. Elevated chorionic gonadotropin levels
   B. Increased red cell mass
   C. Elevated alpha-fetoprotein levels
   D. Increased vanillylmandelic acid (VMA) levels in urine
   E. Elevated serum acid phosphatase

Questions 503–505: A 45-year-old female presented with a lump in the right lobe of the thyroid. Thryoid function studies were normal. No other masses were palpable. A scintiscan shown in Fig. 23.5 was obtained.

Figure 23.5

503. The next step in the management of this lesion is
  A. suppression therapy with triiodothyronine
  B. fine needle aspiration
  C. open biopsy
  D. enucleation of the lesion
  E. lobectomy

504. If examination of the tissue removed reveals papillary carcinoma, management should be
  A. postoperative irradiation of neck
  B. administration of a large dose of radioactive iodine
  C. total thyroidectomy and standard radical neck dissection on the involved side
  D. near-total thyroidectomy and administration of thyroxin postoperatively
  E. administration of thyroxin alone

505. In the light of the diagnosis made, which of the following is the significant point in the history of this patient?
  A. Childhood iodine deficiency
  B. Treatment with antithyroid drugs
  C. Management of acne by irradiation
  D. Preexisting multinodular goiter
  E. Long-term ingestion of the contraceptive pill

Questions 506–508: A 25-year-old female presents with a history of recurrent abdominal pain, diarrhea, and weight loss of 6 months duration. Physical examination was not remarkable. A barium follow-through of small bowel is shown in Fig. 23.6.

506. Based on the history, findings, and x-ray, the most likely diagnosis is

    A. appendicitis with abscess
    B. Crohn's disease
    C. carcinoid tumor
    D. amoebic disease of intestine
    E. carcinoma of small bowel

Figure 23.6

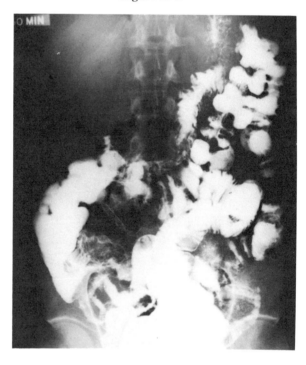

507. Other manifestations of the disease include all the following EXCEPT
A. erythema nodosum
B. gallstones
C. arthritis
D. endocarditis
E. anal lesions

508. Regarding surgical treatment of this disease, all of the following are correct EXCEPT
A. resection is preferable to bypass
B. resection of the diseased bowel will help control systemic manifestations
C. radical surgical treatment prevents recurrence
D. bowel obstruction is the most frequent indication for surgical treatment
E. most patients with the disease require surgery

Questions 509–510: A 25-year-old, otherwise healthy male was admitted with burns of his body surface, including part of the face, upper trunk, and upper arms, sustained in a closed room. His weight was 60 kg, and the burned area was estimated to be 30% of body surface.

509. In the early management of a severely injured patient, the most important initial measure is to
A. control exsanguinating hemorrhage
B. type and cross-match blood
C. establish intravenous access
D. secure an effective airway
E. provide tetanus prophylaxis

510. The best method for achieving temporary control of severe external hemorrhage is by means of
A. arterial tourniquets
B. venous tourniquets
C. direct finger pressure
D. clamping with hemostats
E. application of a gravitational suit

511. A 35-year-old man is brought to an emergency department shortly after being removed from a burning, smoke-filled automobile. The patient is confused, agitated, and tachypneic. His general color is normal, his blood pressure is 80/40 mm Hg, and his pulse is 160 beats/minute. No surface burns are noted. Auscultation of his chest reveals normal air entry bilaterally, with minimal coarse expiratory wheezes. His abdomen is soft, active bowel sounds are present, and the remainder of the physical examination is within normal limits. The neurologic examination is normal except for an acute confusional state. The immediate treatment for the most likely cause of this patient's agitation and confusion is administration of

A. intravenous morphine, 2–3 mg
B. intravenous Ringer's lactate, 1 L over the next hour
C. intramuscular haloperidol, 2 mg, or chlorpromazine, 50 mg
D. 100% oxygen by face mask
E. intravenous methylprednisolone, 2 g, and mannitol, 50 g

Questions 512–514: A middle-aged female presented with right upper quadrant pain radiating to the back. One of the x-rays is shown in Fig. 23.7.

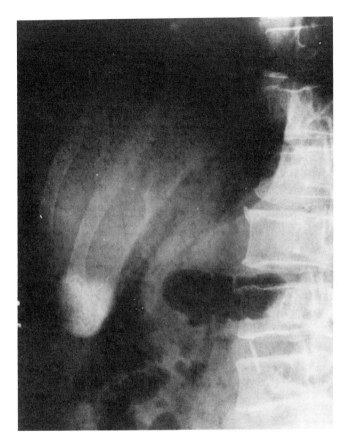

Figure 23.7

512. The most likely cause of pain is
   A. gallstones
   B. renal stones
   C. osteoarthritis
   D. chondrosarcoma of ribs
   E. cholangitis with air in liver

513. All of the following are associated with gallstones EXCEPT
   A. obstructive jaundice
   B. pancreatitis
   C. cancer of the gallbladder
   D. acute cholangitis
   E. sclerosing cholangitis

514. Ideal treatment of cholelithiasis and chronic cholecystitis is by
   A. oral administration of chenodeoxycholic acid
   B. cholecystectomy
   C. cholecystostomy
   D. cholecystectomy and operative cholangiography
   E. cholecystectomy and exploration of common bile duct

Questions 515–517: A 60-year-old white male presented with history of anorexia, weight loss, melena, and occasional vomiting. An upper gastrointestinal series was performed (Fig. 23.8).

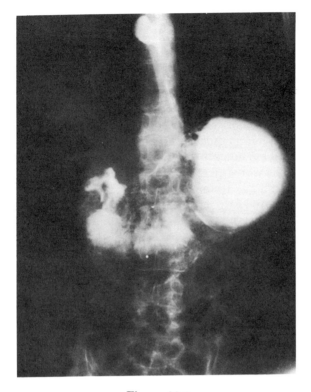

Figure 23.8

515. Probable cause of symptoms in the patient is
    A. chronic duodenal ulcer
    B. chronic gastric ulcer
    C. esophageal diverticulum
    D. gastric cancer
    E. hypertrophic gastritis

516. Etiologic factors associated with gastric cancer include all of the following EXCEPT
   A. sex (males)
   B. atrophic gastritis
   C. high consumption of fish in diet
   D. previous gastric ulcer
   E. gastric polyps

517. At exploration there was a large bulky tumor in the distal half of the stomach. There were a few enlarged lymph nodes at the pylorus and head of pancreas. Operation of choice is
   A. total gastrectomy
   B. partial gastrectomy
   C. radical distal subtotal gastrectomy
   D. gastrojejunostomy
   E. radical pancreaticoduodenectomy

Questions 518–520: An 80-year-old male was seen with an asymptomatic pulsatile mass in the abdomen. An angiogram was performed (Fig. 23.9).

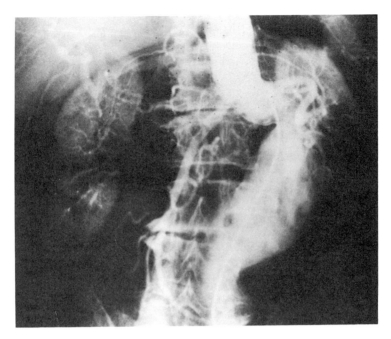

Figure 23.9

518. The angiogram shows
   A. a large vascular tumor in left kidney
   B. an aortocaval fistula
   C. an aortic aneurysm
   D. an aortic occlusion
   E. an aortoduodenal fistula

519. The most common feature in association with an abdominal aortic aneurysm is
   A. involvement of renal arteries
   B. aneurysms of femoral and popliteal arteries
   C. occlusive disease of vessels of the lower extremities
   D. distal emboli
   E. hypertension

520. The patient underwent an abdominal aortic reconstruction with a dacron graft. On the fourth postoperative day the stool was positive for blood. The most likely cause is
  A. aortoduodenal fistula
  B. uremic ulceration of gut
  C. ischemic colitis
  D. operative injury to the bowel
  E. atheromatous emboli in the superior mesenteric artery distribution

Answers and Comments

10. Anesthesiology

1. B. In acute intermittent and variegated porphyria barbiturates must be avoided, since they may trigger acute neurologic injury. (**REF.** 2—pp. 495–498)

2. C. The maintenance of cerebral perfusion pressure is critical. A stump pressure greater than 60 torr is considered adequate. (**REF.** 2—pp. 264–267)

3. A. Jugular venous O_2 saturation will not reflect regional brain ischemia. EEG and evoked potential are becoming increasingly more practical. (**REF.** 2—pp. 266–267)

4. D. Gallamine is excreted almost totally by the kidney. It should not be used in these patients. Atracurium is probably the drug of choice. (**REF.** 1—pp. 898–899)

5. A. Spinal headache occurs in a predictable number of cases. It is more common in young patients. The other complications are exceedingly rare, but devastating when they occur. (**REF.** 1—pp. 1081–1083)

6. D. "Halothane hepatitis" is a toxic hepatitis, seen most often in obese females. The incidence is less than 1 per 30,000. Metabolic products are the presumptive ideologic agents. (**REF.** 2—pp. 343–346)

7. E. Ketamine is classified as a dissociative anesthetic agent. In practice this is difficult to achieve. (**REF.** 1—pp. 815, 1268, 1932)

8. A. Enflurane, similar to other halogenated ethers, may cause convulsions in patients prone to seizures. (**REF.** 1—pp. 815, 1268, 1932)

9. E. Ketamine has an incidence of 10–15% of hallucinations during the recovery period. This incidence can be lowered by the administration of benzodiazepine. (**REF.** 1—pp. 815, 1268, 1932)

10. B. Fentanyl, similar to any other narcotic, can cause severe respiratory depression. Even after reversal, renarcotization can occur in the recovery room.(**REF.** 1— pp. 815, 1268, 1932)

11. B. Physostigmine (1–2 mg) is the agent of choice to treat the central anticholinergic crisis. (**REF.** 1—p. 962)

12. E. Atropine must be given with or prior to prostigmine to avoid the muscarinic effects of this agent. (**REF.** 1—p. 928)

13. C. Naloxone can produce very severe withdrawal symptoms in the narcotic addict. (**REF.** 1—p. 775)

14. D. Protamine when given rapidly or into a central line can cause profound hypotension. (**REF.** 1—p. 1508)

15. D. Both forms of intubation have significant complications. Trauma, esophageal intubation, and airway obstruction are just a few of them. (**REF.** 1—pp. 542–548)

16. C. In difficult oro- or nasotracheal intubation the fiberoptic bronchoscope may literally be a lifesaver. (**REF.** 1—pp. 542–548)

17. B. This is a gift question. (**REF.** 1—pp. 542–548)

18. C. More common after spinal anesthesia, but the anterior spinal artery syndrome occurs most frequently after an epidural anesthetic. (**REF.** 1—pp. 1073ff, 1086ff)

19. B. A catheter epidural is an excellent method to provide postoperative analgesia. (**REF.** 1—pp. 1073ff, 1086ff)

20. C. More dramatic after spinal anesthesia, but common to both techniques. (**REF.** 1—pp. 1073ff, 1086ff)

21. D. Anticoagulant therapy or any serious bleeding disorder is an absolute contraindication. (**REF.** 1—pp. 1073ff, 1086ff)

22. E. All of these are critical factors. In addition, informed consent must be obtained. Absence of adequate preoperative assessment can lead to medical and medicolegal disaster. (**REF.** 1—pp. 226, 227, and 381ff)

23. C. Malignant hyperpyrexia is genetically transmitted. Pretreatment with dantrolene will prevent most cases. Treatment with dantrolene is effective. (**REF.** 2—pp. 785–788)

24. B. Narcotics and esters are reasonably safe. Amid-type local anesthetics and volatile anesthetics must be avoided. (**REF.** 2—pp. 785–788)

25. C. Fever is a later manifestation and may be slight or even absent. Masseter spasm, tachycardia, and metabolic acidosis are the early findings. (**REF.** 2—pp. 785–788)

26. A. Gastric aspiration is practically useless and the nasogastric tube may act as a wick. (**REF.** 1—pp. 2040–2042)

27. A. Belladonna alkaloids are now rarely used in adults. The usual doses of atropine or glycopyrrolate are insufficient to block the vagal reflexes. (**REF.** 1—pp. 382ff)

28. C. Succinylcholine causes increased intraocular pressure and a potentially fatal potassium flux in patients with severe burns or major neurologic injuries. (**REF.** 1—pp. 919–922)

29. A. Hyperkalemia is a major hazard from day 3 of the injury and for several months. Autonomic hyperreflexia is a potentially fatal complication. Intubation may be difficult and dangerous in patients with cervical cord injury. (**REF.** 2—pp. 295–298)

30. E. All are mandatory in modern anesthesiology. (**REF.** 1—pp. 412ff)

11. Emergency Medicine

31. B. Fracture of the navicular bone of the wrist may be difficult to appreciate on x-ray. If tenderness is present in the anatomic snuff box, which is directly over the navicular, these should be treated as a fracture with follow-up and re-x-ray to reduce the complications of nonunion and avascular necrosis. (**REF.** 5—pp. 568–569)

32. D. All of the other methods have been used with success. However, the only method approved for prehospital care is heated aerosol. This method is effective and is available in almost all medical facilities without delay. (**REF.** 5—pp. 483–491)

33. E. Although tricyclics produce many central nervous system effects, the primary problem as a result of an overdose is cardiac toxicity. This presents as both arrhythmias and conduction disturbances. Frequently ventricular fibrillation occurs, which is not responsive to defibrillation in many cases. Treatment is not universally consistent, but alkalinization and physiostigmine are recommended. (**REF.** 5—pp. 1504–1507)

34. C. The patient described has frostbite of both hands. Frostbite to exposed parts, such as the nose, ears, and hands, can occur within several minutes when the windchill index is at or below $-25°F$. The degree of tissue injury in this case is difficult to estimate at initial presentation. Immediate rewarming is critical in order to minimize tissue injury. Water temperatures of 104–108°F have been found to be ideal, whereas higher temperatures may worsen tissue injury; the same is true of more gradual rewarming. There is no advantage of massage or exercise to treat frostbite once it has occurred; in fact, any minor trauma to frozen tissue will cause more damage. (**REFS.** 5—pp. 444–450; 6—pp. 776–780)

35. C. This patient has a metabolic acidosis, which is only partially compensated by hyperventilating. The differential diagnosis of metabolic acidosis is divided into those with an increased anion gap (ketoacidosis, uremia, lactic acidosis, methanol, ethylene glycol, salicylates, and paraldehyde) and those with a normal anion gap (renal tubular dysfunction, diarrhea, and carbonic anhydrase inhibitors). Methanol and ethylene glycol cause acidosis by their metabolism to organic acids, methanol to formic acid and ethylene glycol to glyoxylic acid and oxalic acid. Aspirin causes a metabolic block, with the accumulation of endogenous organic acids. Cyanide poisons the cytochrome system and hence produces lactic acidosis. Glutethimide is a sedative drug that does not cause metabolic blockade or acid metabolites. (**REFS.** 3—pp. 111–117; 7—p. 232)

36. C. This 6-month-old child presents in shock secondary to probable gastroenteritis. Initial management of hypovolemic shock is with a fluid bolus of 20 ml/kg over 20 minutes. If there is no clinical response, one should administer a 10–20 ml/kg repeat bolus of normal saline. Once there is hemodynamic stabilization, a reasonable fluid schedule would be to give one-half of the child's calculated fluid deficit plus maintenance needs over the next 8 hours. (**REFS.** 1—pp. 19–28, 40–50; 2—pp. 236–239)

37. E. Normal arterial blood gasses at sea level. Range: PO_2 80–100 mm Hg, PCO_2 35–45 mm Hg, pH 7.35–7.45. (**REF.** 7—pp. 535–544)

38. A. In this example hyperventilation is present, but the pH is very acidotic, indicating the presence of a severe metabolic acidosis. (**REF.** 7—pp. 535–544)

39. C. In this example the patient is blowing off excessive CO_2, producing a respiratory alkalosis. This is consistent with an anxiety episode, but not diagnostic, since this could occur during extreme exercise. (**REF.** 7—pp. 535–544)

40. D. While one cannot make a diagnosis of cause from this set of gasses, an elevated PCO_2 is diagnostic of ventilatory failure. If acute, the pH will be acidotic, whereas if chronic, the pH should be normal secondary to compensatory metabolic alkalosis. (**REF.** 7—pp. 535–544)

41. C. Insect envenomation causing anaphylaxis is most com-
42. D. monly seen with stings from the Hymenoptera family,
43. A. which includes yellow jackets, honeybees, hornets, wasps,
44. B. bumblebees, and fire ants. An ascending flaccid paralysis is seen in tick paralysis, which is caused by a neurotoxin produced by a very small number of hard tick species, with symptoms occurring after a few days of feeding. The venom of the brown recluse spider produces local tissue destruction, with an area of vesiculation and hemorrhage, leading to progressive tissue necrosis. The venom of the black widow spider is a neurotoxin that causes release of acetylcholine from presynaptic nerve terminals, causing tetanic muscular contractions. Muscular cramping starts in the area of the bite, then spreads diffusely, centering primarily in the abdomen. (**REFS.** 5—pp. 685–690; 6—1626–1633)

45. C. Either of these conditions may produce this set of symptoms. If these are profound, one should consider acute myocardial infarction (AMI) over esophageal reflux, since AMI is a lifethreatening disorder. (**REF.** 7—pp. 672–673)

46. C. Another aspect of esophagospasm that confuses this condition with angina pectoris and AMI. The EKG may be helpful, as is the duration of pain. Often these conditions cannot be differentiated in the Emergency Department. (**REF.** 7—pp. 288–295, 672–673)

47. B. Routine enzymes are not useful in the Emergency Department to rule out or in an AMI, and creatine kinase (CK), LDH, and SGOT are elevated in many conditions. CK-MB isozyme elevation is specific for myocardial muscle, but is not available as a STAT test. (**REF.** 7—pp. 291)

48. C. Both organophosphate insecticides and carbon tetrachlo-
49. A. ride are readily absorbed through the skin and can cause
50. B. severe poisoning by this route. Organophosphates cause inhibition of acetylcholinesterase and hence an accumulation of

acetylcholine with resultant muscarinic effects of sweating, lacrimation, salivation, bronchorrhea, and bradyarrhythmias, and nicotinic effects of fasciculations. Carbon tetrachloride acutely causes CNS depression and gastrointestinal irritation; later hepatic and renal insufficiency may develop. (**REF.** 4—pp. 704–710, 780–783)

51. C. It is safe to say that human bites should not be closed by primary intention. The exceptions are bites on the face less than 24 hours old that are disfiguring lacerations. All human bites should be given antibiotic therapy because of the extremely high rate of infection (>50%). (**REF.** 5—pp. 667–668)

52. C. The earliest signs of carbon monoxide (CO) poisoning are neurologic, beginning with dimming of vision and dizziness, and progressing to seizures and coma as the poisoning becomes more severe. In many patients (up to one-third) there is initial clearing with subsequent development of neurologic problems consistent with a variety of neurologic and psychiatric syndromes. In the older population at risk for coronary artery disease, myocardial ischemia and arrhythmias often occur. Finally, PO_2 levels are not lowered in most patients, although the O_2 carrying capacity of hemoglobin is markedly reduced. (**REF.** 5—pp. 242, 243)

53. C. *Escherichia coli* and group B *Streptococcus* are the most common causes of neonatal sepsis and meningitis. *Staphylococcus aureus*, *Listeria*, and various gram-negative rods are other common organisms. *Neisseria* meningitis is associated with meningitis in adults and older children. *Hemophilus influenzae* can cause bacteremia and meningitis at ages from 6 months to 6 years. (**REFS.** 1—pp. 71–73; 2—pp. 403–405))

54. A. The patient described has acute narrow-angle glaucoma. Entry into a dark room may precipitate an episode by pupillary dilatation. The symptoms and signs described are all very typical of acute glaucoma. Pilocarpine will constrict the pupil and enhance flow of aqueous humor. An osmotic diuretic such as mannitol will reduce intraocular pressure. Acetazolamide inhibits aqueous humor production. Paper bag rebreathing may be useful in central retinal artery occlusion, since it increases cerebrovascular blood flow, but it could aggravate glaucoma. (**REFS.** 5—pp. 702–703; 6—1155–1162)

55. B. The patient described has severe multiple injuries. The respiratory compromise is from a flail chest, in which multiple rib fractures allow a segment of chest wall to move independently from the rest of the rib cage. A flail segment can cause respiratory arrest by increasing the work of breathing, resulting in inefficient gas exchange. Positive pressure ventilation via endotracheal intubation will allow the flail segment to move in unison with the rest of the rib cage. Sandbagging the flail segment will help, but is only a temporizing procedure. Associated hemothorax and pneumothorax is common and chest tube insertion should be done prior to intubation, but it is not definitive treatment for flail chest. There is no reason to do a thoracotomy unless associated cardiac tamponade is highly suspect. (**REFS.** 5—pp. 335–336; 8—pp. 403–408)

56. C. Recurrent shock in blunt trauma is usually from intra-abdominal injury, especially rupture of the spleen or liver. Peritoneal lavage is the best way to evaluate this, short of taking the patient to laparotomy directly. All the other procedures listed should be performed also at some time in the evaluation of this patient, but they are unlikely to reveal the etiology of the shock. (**REFS.** 5—pp. 380–408; 8—pp. 106–108)

57. D. The patient appears to have a pelvic fracture on exam and blood at the meatus is highly suggestive of a urethral tear. Cystourethrogram is the best test to evaluate the integrity of the urethra and bladder in trauma. The IVP is preferred for evaluating the kidney and ureters and will miss bladder injuries and not visualize the urethra at all. Passage of a catheter in this setting is contraindicated. (**REFS.** 5—pp. 409–432; 8—pp. 527–539)

58. A. The diagnosis of malignant hypertension should be questioned if papilledema is absent. Linear retinal hemorrhages are also frequently present. (**REF.** 5—pp. 878, 879)

59. C. Hydralazine is an effective drug in treatment of hypertensive emergencies. However, in the acutely ill, much smoother control can be obtained by other agents. Also, it has been suggested that this agent may exacerbate angina. In any case, a test dose of

5–10 mg should be given first to avoid an unsuspected drop in blood pressure with this agent. (**REF.** 6—pp. 878, 879, 883)

60. D. Hypertensive encephalopathy may occur with or without the presence of malignant hypertension. If seizures and coma occur in the presence of malignant hypertension, one must consider an intracerebral hemorrhage or hypertensive encephalopathy. Malignant hypertension is a clinical syndrome and is not diagnosed simply by the level of blood pressure. It may represent the initial presentation of hypertension, or can occur after a long period of stable, treated high blood pressure. (**REF.** 6—pp. 873–881)

12. Family Medicine

61. C. Appendicitis, because one should be aware of a possible *organic surgical condition* and *not* assume it is a nonsurgical condition. (**REF.** 7—p. 1251)

62. A. Less than 10% of patients operated upon for acute appendicitis are over 60 years of age. (**REF.** 7—p. 1251)

63. A. A total of 67–90% of older patients are found to have a ruptured appendix at the time of operation. (**REF.** 7—p. 1251)

64. A. More than 50% of all deaths from appendicitis correspond to individuals over 60 years of age. (**REF.** 7—p. 1251)

65. D. An "overdeveloped" placenta may prevent apnea, whereas the other items may be primary causes of apnea. (**REF.** 2—p. 180)

66. E. All other elements may jeopardize the mother. (**REF.** 6—p. 600)

67. D. All other elements may simulate a left tubal pregnancy. Terminal ileitis rarely if ever produces symptoms on the left side. (**REF.** 6—p. 430)

68. D. An intact tympanic membrane is not a factor for chronicity in suppurative middle ear disease. All other elements are factors in the disease. (**REF.** 1—p. 1136)

69. E. Much adolescent drinking takes place away from the home, in or around cars and prior to driving. (**REF.** 5—p. 223)

70. B. Epidemiologic factors do not cause personality disorders. (**REF.** 4—pp. 961–962)

71. D. Goiters may be caused by deficiency of iodine. (**REF.** 4—p. 993)

72. C. Night blindness may be relieved by vitamin A. (**REF.** 4—p. 993)

73. B. Perifollicular petechiae of the skin is relieved by vitamin C. (**REF.** 4—p. 993)

74. E. Thoracic rosary may be prevented with vitamin D. (**REF.** 4—p. 993)

75. A. Manic is an affective disorder. (**REF.** 4—p. 993)

76. C. Panic is an anxiety disorder. (**REF.** 4—p. 993)

77. D. Alcoholism is a chemical dependency disorder. (**REF.** 4—p. 993)

78. E. Antisocial personality is a personality disorder. (**REF.** 4—p. 993)

79. E. Schizotypical features are a personality disorder. (**REF.** 4—p. 993)

80. C. Asbestosis is found in both interstitial and pleural disease. (**REF.** 8—p. 227a, Table 559–1)

81. B. Mesothelioma is found in pleural disease. (**REF.** 8—p. 2279, Table 559–1)

82. A. Silicosis is found in interstitial parenchymal disease. (**REF.** 8—p. 2279, Table 559–1)

83. A. Berylliosis is found in interstitial parenchymal disease. (**REF.** 8—p. 2279, Table 559–1)

84. B. Pet shop owners may be seen with psittacosis (**REF.** 8—p. 2279, Table 559–1)

85. A. Imported hides may carry anthrax. (**REF.** 8—p. 2279, Table 559–1)

86. B. Taxidermists may be seen with psittacosis. (**REF.** 8—p. 2279, Table 559–1)

87. E. All elements listed may cause cardiac arrhythmias. (**REF.** 3—pp. 751–754)

88. A. Morphine does not cause calcification in the body. (**REF.** 3—p. 1517)

89. A. Bromocrystine is inactive on the uterus. (**REF.** 3—p. 935)

90. D. Chlorpromazine causes a brown or white dusting on the anterior lens surface. (**REF.** 8—p. 2217)

91. D. Corticosteroids promote formation of posterior subcapsular cataracts. (**REF.** 8—p. 2217)

92. E. Multiple sclerosis is not known to cause cataracts. (**REF.** 8—p. 2217)

13. Internal Medicine

93. A. Swelling of the proximal interphalangeal joints gives a fusiform or spindle-shaped appearance to the fingers. This is generally associated with bilateral and symmetric swelling of the metacarpophalangeal joints. Other joints commonly involved are wrists, knees, and feet. Later involvement may include elbows, shoulders, hips, and ankles. (**REF.** 4—pp. 1913–1914)

94. E. *Pneumocystitis carinii* infects immunodeficient patients and malnourished or premature infants. The pulmonary infection is characterized by dyspnea, tachypnea, and hypoxemia. The initial treatment devised was pentamidine, but this has been supplanted by co-trimoxazole. This drug interferes with the synthesis of folinic acid. Adults are given a 14-day course in four equal oral or intravenous doses. (**REF.** 2—p. 26)

95. D. It is possible to measure cytoplasmic proteins that function as receptors to bind and transfer estrogens to the nuclei of cells. About 60% of primary breast tumors have such receptors. Patients with estrogen receptors are better responders to hormonal therapy. Other criteria favoring response include a disease-free interval over 2 years, a small tumor, metastases confined to bone, skin, lung, and nodes, and the patient's being more than 5 years postmenopausal. (**REF.** 1—p. 858)

96. B. Thalassemias are associated with severe microcytosis, secondary to defective globin chain production. The mean cell volume is usually less than 70fL (normal is over 90fL). Iron deficiency is the commonest cause of microcytosis. Iron overload may be associated with macrocytosis. (**REF.** 3—p. 406)

97. C. Crohn's disease is associated with bowel wall thickening, hyperemia, and adhesions between adjacent loops of bowel. Characteristic x-ray findings include segmental narrowing, obliteration of the normal mucosal pattern, enteroenteric fistula formation, and the classic string sign of contrast medium, especially in distal small bowel. (**REF.** 4—p. 743)

98. B. Daily administration may result in cumulative effect. Chlorpropamide is metabolized by the liver, but is excreted intact by the kidneys. Activity of this drug may extend to 60 hours. It can cause significant water retention by potentiation of ADH. (**REF.** 4—p. 1329)

99. A. Tolbutamide is precipitated by acidifying the urine. Alcohol intolerance has been seen with sulfonylurea administration. The duration of action is 6–12 hours. The drug is metabolized by the liver to inert products. (**REF.** 4—p. 1329)

100. D. Duration of action is 6 hours, with peak onset of action 2–3 hours after injection. Sources of insulin include beef, pork, and human synthetic insulin (made by human DNA cloned in bacteria). (**REF.** 4—p. 1330)

101. E. Lente insulin has zinc as a modifier. It has a peak effect at 8–12 hours and should be used with a midafternoon snack. The duration of action is 18–24 hours. The size of the zinc-insulin crystal is modified by pH in manufacturing; the larger the crystal, the slower the release. (**REF.** 4—p. 1330)

102. B. Chlorpropamide can cause significant water retention and hyponatremia by potentiating ADH effect on the kidney. Hypoglycemia is the major complication of the sulfonylureas and can be particularly severe with chlorpropamide because of its long duration of activity. (**REF.** 4—p. 1329)

103. D. In multiple sclerosis, paresthesias are common and range from vague pins-and-needles discomfort to classic trigeminal neuralgia. Loss of perception of vibration and position at the ankle and toes is common. Sensory symptoms are common in Guillain-Barré syndrome, usually distal paresthesias. (**REF.** 4—pp. 2145, 2191)

104. C. CSF gamma-globulin levels are elevated in 75% of multiple sclerosis patients, particularly after the first year. The gamma-globulin is mostly IgG. CSF total protein is normal for the first 3 days of illness in Guillain-Barré syndrome, then steadily rises and remains elevated for several months. (**REF.** 4—pp. 2144, 2191)

105. C. At least 70% of MS patients improve following initial symptoms, whereas 30% show steady deterioration. Initial recovery may be slight or complete. Guillain-Barré patients usually begin to recover within 2–4 weeks after progression ceases. Within 6 months, 85% of patients are ambulatory. (**REF.** 4—pp. 2145, 2191)

106. C. The lesion of MS consists of scattered areas of dissolution of CNS myelin, within which the axons remain intact. Some areas may show only partial myelin destruction. In Guillain-Barré syndrome, there is inflammatory cell infiltration with lymphocytes and plasma cells followed by segmental demyelineation. Axons are relatively spared and blood vessels are normal. (**REF.** 4—pp. 2144, 2190)

107. A. Visual loss in MS varies in degree from slight blurring with a small central scotoma to no light perception. The patient often has pain on eye movement in the acute phase. Blurring secondary to nystagmus on primary gaze is also noted. Internuclear ophthalmoplegia is common, often unilateral at first, and is due to lesions involving the median longitudinal fasciculus in the pons. (**REF.** 4—p. 2145)

108. B. Acute glomerulonephritis may follow infection with group A streptococcus or a variety of other bacterial and nonbacterial agents, including gram-positive and gram-negative bacteria, viruses, mycoplasma, fungi, protozoa, helminths, and spirochetes. Other primary diseases may present as acute glomerulonephritis, including IgG–IgA nephritis, Goodpasture's syndrome, and idiopathic rapidly progressive glomerulonephritis. (**REF.** 4—pp. 570, 571)

109. A. Hypertension is a common manifestation of the acute nephritic syndrome and may be a presenting sign in older patients. It is largely volume dependent, reflecting impaired renal excretion of sodium and water, with reduced levels of plasma renin and aldosterone. (**REF.** 4—p. 570)

110. D. Patients with Alzheimer's disease have gradual onset of recent memory loss with reduction of affect or increase in anxiety. Social amenities are preserved until very late, so that most patients dress well, maintain neat appearance, and avoid incontinence. Sensory and motor symptoms are rare. (**REF.** 4—p. 2000)

111. D. Pathology includes neuronal loss affecting especially the large pyramidal cells of the parietal and frontal association areas, the hippocampus, and the amygdala. Silver-staining plaques containing degenerating neuronal products are scattered prominently in the cortex and subcortex. (**REF.** 4—p. 1999)

112. E. Rheumatoid arthritis can affect any diarthrodial joint, and those most commonly involved are the small joints of the hands, wrists, knees, and feet. Because of the synovial proliferation and inflammatory destruction of soft tissues, a laxity of ligaments and tendons develops, which, in conjunction with mechanical pressures and regular use, gives rise to typical deformities. (**REF.** 4—p. 1913)

113. A. Serum iron is often low, but TIBC is normal or low, and marrow iron stores are normal. The ESR tends to be elevated, but only roughly parallels the disease activity. The presence of rheumatoid factor by agglutination test is helpful. Hand x-rays show soft-tissue as well as bony deformities. (**REF.** 4—p. 1913)

114. B. There are bilateral hilar enlarged nodes and a paratracheal mass. The clear area between the cardiac silhouette and the enlarged nodes is typical of sarcoidosis. The diagnosis is firmly established when the clinical findings are supported by histologic evidence of widespread epithelioid granulomas in more than one system. (**REF.** 4—p. 432)

115. A. Corticosteroid therapy is the mainstay of treatment. It is particularly indicated for ocular involvement, sever chest disease, hypercalcemia, disfiguring skin lesions, myocardial involvement, and central nervous system involvement. (**REF.** 4—p. 438)

116. B. A long segment of the terminal ileum is involved. A portion is tubular with a wide lumen and without recognizable folds. Skin involvement is helpful in making the diagnosis because of the frequency of fistula formation. Ulcerative colitis more commonly involves the colon and produces thin-walled lesions with discrete ulcers. (**REF.** 4—p. 742)

117. E. In patients with stenotic segments of intestine, a low-residue, low-fiber diet should be recommended. Medical management includes nutritional treatment, if necessary by intravenous total parenteral supplements. Azathioprine may be useful, but studies have been largely uncontrolled. Steroids and drugs to diminish intestinal motility are also useful. (**REF.** 2—p. 395)

118. B. The x-ray shows left lower lobe pneumonia with an air bronchogram effect. Sudden onset of chills and rigor is a typical presentation, as is hemoptysis. The neutrophilia is the expected white cell response. Additional symptoms at presentation are pleuritic chest pain and a racking cough, which raises thick, blood-stained sputum. (**REF.** 4—p. 1498)

119. E. The most common cause of lobar pneumonia is the pneumococcus. This infection responds to intravenous penicillin. If the patient is allergic to penicillin, cephalosporins or erythromycin are used. Other useful agents include tetracycline, clindamycin, or vancomycin. Pneumococci are resistant to aminoglycosides. (**REF.** 2—p. 134)

120. B. Large U waves are visible in the precordial leads. These are characteristic of hypokalemia, and this patient had a potassium of 1.1 mEq/L. The clinical effects of potassium deficiency may be manifest in one or more organ systems, including skeletal muscle, heart, kidneys, and the gastrointestinal tract. (**REF.** 1—p. 1467)

121. C. Potassium chloride is more effective than the phosphate form, since an accompanying hypochloremic alkalosis is inevitable. Oral therapy is preferable, but when gastrointestinal function is impaired, or when neuromuscular manifestations of hypokalemia are present, parenteral therapy with potassium may be advisable. (**REF.** 1—p. 1467)

122. D. There is a rarefied area involving the frontal and parietal bones. Calvarial thickening or foci of radiopacity may appear in the lucent areas with further progression. Headache is a common symptom. After the cranium, the bones most likely to be involved are the clavicles and the long bones, particularly of the lower extremities. (**REF.** 4—p. 1461)

123. C. Potentially useful therapy includes calcitonin, mithramycin, or diphosphonates. Low doses of the disphosphonates are indicated, since high doses paradoxically slow the healing process. Subcutaneous injection of calcitonin given daily or on alternate days is perhaps the most effective single therapy. (**REF.** 2—p. 483)

124. B. The esophageal folds are thick and tortuous, giving rise to a wormy appearance. The radiographic picture would vary with the severity of the varices. The accompanying portal hypertension may be associated with splenomegaly, ascites, and other venous dilatations on the abdominal wall or in the umbilicus. (**REF.** 4—p. 841)

125. D. Alcoholic cirrhosis is the commonest cause of portal hypertension and esophageal varices. Other causes include splenic vein thrombosis, portal vein thrombosis, schistosomiasis, and other causes of cirrhosis of the liver. In alcoholic liver disease, portal hypertension may develop without cirrhosis. (**REF.** 4—p. 842)

126. E. There is a biconcave appearance of the vertebral bodies, giving rise to a "fishmouth" appearance. Sclerotic changes secondary to ischemia are also seen. The major disability is related to painful vaso-occlusive crisis, with secondary end-organ damage as a direct consequence of the sickling phenomenon, and occlusion of the microvasculature. (**REF.** 3—p. 590)

127. C. The histologic picture is one of thickened alveolar septa with fibrous tissue and cuboidal metaplasia of the lining cells. These are characteristic findings of interstitial fibrosis. Inhaled organic or inorganic dust can cause this syndrome. Organic dusts include fungi and animal proteins. Inorganic dusts include silica, silicates (including asbestos), coal dust, and metals. (**REF.** 3—p. 408)

128. D. Steroids improve the feeling of breathlessness and may prevent layering down of new fibrous tissue. Assessment of impairment by lung function tests and assessment of activity by bronchoalveolar lavage and gallium scanning help to follow response to treatment or progression. (**REF.** 3—p. 412)

129. A. This is the most pathognomonic glomerular lesion in diabetes mellitus. The nodules are PAS-positive and contain mucopolysaccharides. Patients with substantial histologic changes can exhibit normal renal function, but with expansion of the mesangium a greater portion of the glomerular volume is occupied and occlusion may occur. (**REF.** 3—p. 1338)

130. C. The rate is 80/minute, the PR interval is normal, and the ST segment is isoelectric. No pathologic diagnosis can be made. Typical anginal pain would have included a clear relation to exercise, effort, and emotion, and relief with rest or nitroglycerin. (**REF.** 1—p. 894)

131. D. There is marked ST depression and T inversion. Patients with angina often have ECG abnormalities occurring during their pain that may be reproduced during exercise. Tests in addition to standard exercise tests include the use of radionuclides in association with exercise. Coronary arteriography is the most reliable diagnostic test. (**REF.** 1—p. 896)

132. E. The patient has an intraventricular conduction defect, which is not left bundle branch block, since there are Q waves in leads I and AVL. First degree heart block is present when the PR interval is greater than 0.2 seconds. (**REF.** 1—p. 457)

14. Medical Ethics

133. C. The decision allowed states to prohibit abortions in the third trimester of pregnancy, except those deemed medically necessary for the life or health of the mother. (**REF.** 3—p. 378)

134. D. Infant Doe had Down's syndrome and was born with a tracheoesophageal fistula. The parents were allowed to refuse corrective surgery and the infant died shortly thereafter. (**REF.** 2—p. 233)

135. A. Karen Quinlan was a comatose patient on a respirator. The court allowed her parents to direct that the respirator be discontinued. (**REF.** 4—pp. 352–361)

136. B. Brother Fox, age 83, suffered a stroke and because permanently comatose, maintained on a respirator. Since Brother Fox had previously expressed the wish while still healthy that he not be kept alive under these circumstances, the judge allowed the respirator to be discontinued. Subsequent legislation for living wills has been based on this reasoning. (**REF.** 4—pp. 371–379)

137. C. Both terms refer to competing and sometimes overlapping theories. Deontology operates from a set of a priori rules, such as "thou shalt not kill." Consequentialism judges interventions by the results they produce. (**REF.** 2—p. 82)

138. A. Sanctity of life is a classic deontologic principle.

139. D. The law of parsimony is a principle in logic, not ethics.

140. B. Quality of life is a typical issue in consequentialist thinking.

141. B. "End justifies the means" is a restatement of consequentialism.

142. B. In *A Theory of Justice*, John Rawls sets forth principles of resource allocation for a just society. The theory is often involved in a discussion of health care resources. Nonmaleficence refers to a primary principle of doing no harm. (**REFS.** 2—pp. 349–354; 3—p. 496)

15. Neurology

143. A. Hydrocephalus. It is thought that the blood components mechanically interfere with outflow and resorbtion of CSF. (**REF.** 8—p. 274)

144. E. A classic symptom of median nerve compression (as in the carpal tunnel syndrome) is weakness of the opponens policis muscle. (**REF.** 7—p. 24)

145. D. Bromocriptine is thought to act directly on the dopamine receptors of the nigrostriatal system. L-DOPA causes an increase in the production of dopamine, but does not mimic dopamine. Benztropine and trihexyphenidyl are anticholinergic drugs, and diphenhydramine, of course, is an antihistamine. All are useful in the treatment of Parkinsonism, although the rationale of their use is not always compelling. (**REF.** 4—pp. 461–472)

146. B. Ischemia of the eye is the result of decreased blood flow in the ophthalmic artery on the same side. When this occurs transiently, it is called amaurosis fugax. Patients are not aware of the possibility of hemianopsia, however, they may describe blindness in symmetric visual fields as "blind in one eye." Hemianopsia may result from involvement of the posterior cerebral artery (supplied by the vertebral–basilar system) or of the blood supply to the optic tract (supplied by the carotid–middle cerebral artery system). (**REF.** 10—p. 67)

147. C. Vertigo is the most common symptom of TIA in the vertebral–basilar circulation. (**REF.** 10—p. 108) Other major symptoms of ischemia in the area supplied by these arteries are visual field loss, facial paresthesia, drop attacks, and paresis (either mono- or hemi-). Incidentally, Toole estimates the prognosis in TIAs by the rule of thirds: One-third of patients will continue to have transient attacks without developing permanent disability, one-third will have a stroke, and in one-third the attacks will cease spontaneously. (**REF.** 10—p. 111)

148. D. The combination of stupor and nystagmus in a known alcoholic raises the diagnostic possibility of Wernicke's encephalopathy. Thiamine treatment is often effective, although the patient may be left with an amnestic syndrome. (**REF.** 8—p. 178)

149. C. Taste sensation from the anterior tongue is conveyed by impulses in the seventh nerve. (**REF.** 6—pp. 12–13)

150. B. Pupillary constriction is mediated by the third nerve. (**REF.** 6—pp. 12–13)

151. E. The tenth nerve (vagus) innervates the vocal cord muscles. (**REF.** 6—pp. 12–13)

152. B. Diplopia can be produced by lesions of the third, sixth, or (rarely) the fourth cranial nerve. (**REF.** 6—pp. 12–13)

153. A. Small reactive pupils are seen early, in the diencephalic stage. (**REF.** 8—pp. 103–108)

154. A. Cheyne-Stokes breathing is also characteristic of the diencephalic stage. (**REF.** 8—pp. 103–108)

155. B. Patients with lesions progressing to the pons, or occurring in the pons, often show persistent hyperventilation (40/minute) for long periods of time. (**REF.** 8—pp. 103–108)

156. C. When the medulla becomes involved in the lesion, respiration is irregular or stops altogether. At this stage, reflex eye turning cannot be induced by turning the head, by ice water calorics, or other maneuvers. (**REF.** 8—pp. 103–108). Plum and Posner's book on coma (**REF.** 8) contains this information in a series of diagrams now considered "classic" by neurologists. The syndrome of progressive brainstem failure also occurs in the "uncal herniation syndrome," where it includes the effects of compression of the third nerve, so that dilatation of one pupil precedes the coma and the other signs.

157. C. Amnesia and the amnestic syndrome are common sequelae of bilateral temporal lobe injury. (**REF.** 6—pp. 325–347)

158. A. Lesion of Broca's area (Brodmann 44) in the left frontal lobe is responsible for these aphasic symptoms. Occasionally a lesion of Broca's area does not cause speech disturbance and in these cases the patient is usually left-handed. (**REF.** 6—pp. 325–347)

159. D. Hemianopsia is the classic symptom of lesions of the visual pathways behind the chiasm: the optic tract, the lateral geniculate nucleus, the optic radiation, and the calcarine cortex. (**REF.** 6—pp. 325–347)

160. D. Denial of the patient's own blindness may occur in bilateral infarction of the occipital lobes. This situation can occur with embolism of the basilar artery at its bifurcation. The patient usually cannot tell light from dark, but stoutly maintains his vision is only slightly impaired. (**REF.** 6—pp. 325–347)

161. D. Denial of the paralysis of a limb or limbs opposite a cerebral infarct occurs when the parietal lobe on the right is lesioned. Sometimes the patient denies that the offending limb belongs to him. This symptom is part of the larger syndrome of the nondominant parietal lobe. (**REF.** 6—pp. 325–347)

162. B. The definition of TIA requires that the symptoms clear in a very short time. (**REF.** 10 —p. 109)

163. B. While the efficacy of anticoagulant therapy in preventing stroke in these patients is not firmly established, all authorities recommend it. (**REF.** 10 —p. 120)

164. D. CSF may be bloody in cerebral hemorrhage, but this is not always the case. CT scan resolves the question of subarachnoid hemorrhage versus other intracranial bleeding. The use of clotting agents, such as the antifibrinolytic agent epsilon-aminocapronic acid, to prevent rebleeding in patients with subarachnoid hemorrhage is advocated by some (**REF.** 3—p. 585) and condemned by others (**REF.** 10 p. 358).

fibula

165. B. Peroneal nerve lesions cause foot drop. Prolonged sitting in one position with the legs crossed (as in an examination) is a common etiologic factor in the transient syndrome of "my foot went to sleep." (**REF.** 3—pp. 701–704)

166. A. Femoral nerve lesions are rarely due to nerve root compression. Disease of the psoas muscle is usually to blame, including hematomas.

167. C. Pain on straight leg raising is a classic sign of sciatica. The usual cause is compression of nerve roots contributing to the sciatic nerve, L4, L5, S1. The pain must be dramatic; most sedentary patients complain of discomfort on stretching the calf muscles. (**REF.** 3—pp. 701–704)

168. D. Meralgia paresthetica is the syndrome produced by compression of the lateral femoral cutaneous nerve. Its symptoms are somewhat bizarre, but not at all uncommon. (**REF.** 3—p. 704)

169. C. Much of the pathology found in Alzheimer's disease is
170. D. also found to a lesser extent in the normal brain of ad-
171. C. vanced age. It includes senile plaques, neurofibrillary tangles, ventricular enlargement, and cortical atrophy. The complaint of memory loss is common to both groups (and many younger normals!). The degree of atrophy on the CT scan correlates poorly with the degree of dementia in those afflicted. At the present time, no specific test for early Alzheimer's disease has been found. (**REF.** 5—pp. 163–170)

172. C. Dementia occurs in as many as half the patients with
173. C. Parkinsonism and is characteristic of Huntington's disease
174. A. at some stage of the illness. Both disorders are also characterized by abnormal involuntary movements (sometimes called AIM), although the character of the movement is different. CT scan often shows enlarged ventricles in Huntington's disease, due in part to the atrophy of the caudate nucleus. This finding may appear years after the initial symptoms, however, and is of little value in establishing the diagnosis. At the present time, the diagnosis of these diseases, like that of Alzheimer's, depends on a cluster of findings, no one of which in isolation is specific. When the diagnosis is in doubt, the best course is still to wait and see how the patient's picture develops. (**REF.** 4—pp. 423, 533–534)

175. B. Although "hypertrophy of the gums" is the side effect of
176. B. phenytoin most of us remember, nystagmus and ataxia
177. E. are by far the most common effects of the drug. Lymph-
178. B. adenopathy and pseudolymphoma as well as a lupuslike picture occur rarely. These more serious effects require that the drug be stopped. Nystagmus is well-tolerated; other effects, such as the ataxia, sedation, and facial changes, may be controlled by lowering the dose. Patients whose seizures are under control should never have their anticonvulsants stopped abruptly for fear of precipitating status epilepticus. The dose should be tapered down, or, in cases where it must be stopped suddenly, the patient should be covered by therapeutic doses of another drug. (**REF.** 3—pp. 361–362)

179. C. Because both of these seizure patterns involve short lapses
180. B. of consciousness without tonic-clonic movements, una-
181. A. wareness of the event, and the "blank stare," they are
182. B. difficult to differentiate. The EEG during an attack of
183. B. petit mal may be diagnostic. Between attacks both types of patients will probably have normal EEGs. Sleep can bring out an abnormality in the complex partial seizure patient, even though there is no clinical convulsion at that time. The abnormality is usually over one or both temporal lobes. The seizure in the complex partial case (psychomotor epilepsy) can include quite a variety of behaviors. Turning, mumbling, chewing, grasping, and walking are all seen. Violence is rare, but does occur, particularly when

the patient is restrained. While ethosuximide is the drug of choice in petit mal, it is ineffective in complex seizures, which respond well to any of the general anticonvulsants used for tonic-clonic seizures. Carbamazepine is recommended as a first choice because of its relative efficacy and low toxicity. (**REF.** 3—pp. 343–358)

184. B. Drooling occurs in Bell's palsy because of the weakness
185. B. of the muscles around the mouth. When Bell's palsy is
186. A. due to herpes zoster of the geniculate ganglion of the
187. B. seventh nerve, the palsy is accompanied by the typical rash in the ear, and is called Ramsey-Hunt syndrome. Herpes of the trigeminal nerve does occur, of course, but it does not produce the pain pattern of trigeminal neuralgia. In trigeminal neuralgia the flashes of pain are very brief, and this may be the only characteristic distinguishing this disorder from some kinds of migraine and from "temporomandibular joint syndrome," where the pains have a similar distribution. Both steroid therapy and surgery have been used for Bell's palsy, but the typical case gets well in several weeks, and only 15% are left with any residual deficit. Both of these disorders are presently idiopathic. The presence of any other cranial nerve abnormality should immediately suggest that the syndrome is not the (relatively) benign idiopathic one, and one should initiate a search for intracranial pathology. (**REF.** 3—pp. 674–679)

188. C. Both of these conditions produce a combination of "long
189. C. tract" signs and lower motor neuron signs. Arthritic cer-
190. A. vical compression, however, produces denervation only
191. A. in the upper extremities, while in ALS there is evidence of lower motor neuron denervation in the legs and feet as well. In ALS the motor neurons in the cord and brain are dying; in cervical osteoarthritis the cord is compressed in the neck and the cervical roots are also trapped as they exit from the spinal foramina. The cervical spine condition can be surgically treated, although the results are only fair. At the present time there is no therapy for ALS. (**REF.** 3—pp. 209–213)

192. B. A systolic bruit over the carotid (and not transmitted from the heart) is an indication of significant stenosis. Occlusion makes no sound. Carotid stenosis is frequently accompanied by ulcerated plaques, which are the major source of cerebral embolism. (**REF.** 10—p. 65)

193. C. After cerebral infarction the infarct fails to show on the CT scan unless there is significant edema. Usually the CT scan is normal for the first 24 hours; then evidence of edema and of altered permeability of the blood–brain barrier begins to appear. The characteristic lucent area does not appear for several weeks. (**REF.** 10—pp. 140–142)

194. E. All these symptoms occur in TIA involving the vertebral and basilar arteries. Vertigo is most common, about 50%, with loss in the visual fields and facial paresthesia in 20% each. Drop attacks, with loss of muscle tone leading to a collapse of posture, occurs less frequently, about 15%. (**REF.** 10—p. 109)

195. C. Prolactin-secreting pituitary tumor can produce this symptom. Dopamine is an inhibitory transmitter in prolactin release, and the dopamine agonist bromocriptine will lower the elevated prolactin levels. Interestingly, many of the tumors regress in size. Only those that continue to grow or that cause other symptoms, such as the classic bitemporal hemianopsia, need to be operated upon. (**REF.** 11—p. 367)

196. A. All of the findings listed occur in Guillain-Barré syndrome, but the elevation of CSF protein does not show up for 10 days. There may be a slight increase in monocytes, usually only to 10–20. (**REF.** 3—p. 689)

197. B. Occlusion of the posterior inferior cerebellar artery is the cause of Wallenberg's syndrome. It produces the startling picture of pain sensation loss on the face (descending tract of 5) and on the opposite side of the body below the neck (ascending spinothalamic tract from the side opposite the lesion). There is no paresis and no loss of consciousness. Other symptoms include vertigo, ataxia, dysarthria, hoarseness, and Horner's syndrome. (**REF.** 3—p. 565)

198. E. Bell's palsy, idiopathic involvement of the seventh nerve only. Cerebellopontine angle tumors, Guillain-Barré syndrome, herpes zoster, and local infection and leukemic deposits can involve the seventh nerve, but rarely fail to involve other structures as well. (**REF.** 3—pp. 677–679)

199. B. Hyperacusis is the only seventh nerve symptom listed. It occurs because of the paralysis of the stapedius muscle. (**REF.** 3— pp. 676–678)

200. A. The relationship between anticonvulsant drugs and fetal abnormalities has probably been overstressed in recent years, but this patient is on valproate, one of the few anticonvulsants most authorities think carries a serious risk to the infant, that of neural tube defects. She should be changed to another medication. The risk of fetal abnormality is slightly higher in epileptic mothers even if they are untreated. The reason for this association is unknown. Incidentally, this young woman, who says she contemplates getting pregnant, should have a pregnancy test done immediately! (**REF.** 2—p. 312)

201. C. Complex partial seizures, also called psychomotor or temporal lobe seizures, are hard to diagnose but are probably the most common seizure disorder. The symptoms are often bizarre. The sleep EEG may be abnormal in doubtful cases, but often the diagnosis must be made on the basis of history alône. (**REF.** 3— pp. 343–358)

202. E. Noncompliance is the commonest cause of failure of anticonvulsant therapy. It can be easily documented, in this case, by getting an immediate blood level. Remember that the laboratory's "therapeutic level" is strictly empirical. Many patients can have their seizures controlled at less than "therapeutic" blood levels. Others are not controlled at levels well above the "therapeutic range." This patient is on a typical dose of two medications; his blood levels should be within the laboratory's standard range or very close to it. Teenage epileptics, like teenage diabetics, have a serious problem adjusting to the disease and the necessity of daily medication. (**REF.** 3—p. 361)

203. D. Subarachnoid hemorrhage. The stiff neck does not develop until hours have passed. EKG changes and other systemic phenomena are not unusual. Plum and Posner (**REF.** 8—p. 273) give a complete case history of a similar case. A history of sudden onset, a bizarre neurologic picture, and obtunded consciousness should always raise a question of SAH. CT scan or LP can confirm the diagnosis. (**REF.** 8—p. 273)

204. C. The blood barbiturate level should be zero. (**REF.** 8— p. 315)

205. C. All the tests listed are appropriate, but knowing the cause of the coma gives the best basis for a hopeless prognosis. The important but ethically difficult diagnosis of brain death should be made by a team that has no connection to the transplant group, and confirmatory studies should be carried out until they feel confident of the prognosis. (**REF.** 8—p. 315)

206. D. A small lacunar infarction in the internal capsule, perhaps only millimeters in size, will produce this picture in a hypertensive patient. The symptom is too localized to be due to encephalopathy or a large infarct, and hemorrhage or hematoma should be evident on the CT scan. (**REF.** 10—pp. 280–282)

207. B. Hypertensive encephalopathy. Another possibility, not listed, is that overenthusiastic treatment of the hypertension in this elderly patient has produced a hypotensive episode and cerebral ischemia. (**REF.** 10—p. 284)

16. Obstetrics and Gynecology

208. C. The disease is usually insidious and asymptomatic. It normally begins during the third decade, and is common among white women with an early menopause and smaller bone mass. Those with inadequate dietary calcium intake are at greatest risk. (**REF.** 11—p. 89)

209. C. Women age 20–29 need a pap smear every 1–3 years, and an initial mammograph between ages 36 and 39. Women age 40–49 need a pap smear every 1–3 years and a mammogram every 2 years. Women age 50 and older need an annual mammogram. (**REF.** 11—p. 89)

210. D. Advanced maternal age, that is, over 35, is the commonest indication for antenatal genetic testing. Several investigators state a paternal age over 55, especially if the mother is over 33 years of age is an indication. In a balanced translocation the actual risk is 10% if the female is a carrier and 2–3% if the father is a carrier. There are over 1200 Mendelian disorders, of which some, such as Tay-Sachs and sickle-cell anemia, can be diagnosed. Most, however, are difficult to detect. (**REF.** 12—pp. 33–35)

211. B. Nitrofurantoins can cause hemolytic anemia, and sulfonamides are related to kernicterus. Tetracyclines can discolor teeth and aminoglycosides can cause ototoxicity and renal toxicity. (**REF.** 2—pp. 496–499)

212. E. Dermoid cysts are usually benign. They are made up of up to three germ cell layers and are bilateral 12% of the time. They usually occur in the 20- to 40-year age group. Teeth can be seen, as in this case, on x-ray and the diagnosis can be made. (**REF.** 2—p. 1129)

213. C. These cysts frequently cause torsion. Treatment is excision of the cyst, leaving the normal ovarian tissue of that ovary, and inspection of the other ovary. Some state that the other ovary should be bisected and inspected in this manner. (**REF.** 2—p. 1130)

214. B. These individuals are in acidosis, not alkalosis. The treatment of septic shock begins with a strong sense of suspicion and prompt recognition of the disease. The infection must be controlled by appropriate antibiotics. The fluid therapy must be appropriate and proper. Steroids are occasionally used. The most important thing is the treatment of the infection with antibiotics, surgery, or both and reversal of the acid–base imbalance. (**REF.** 7—p. 484)

215. A. Obesity, nulliparity, late menopause, diabetes mellitus, hypertension, advanced age, and prolonged use of exogenous estrogens all have an effect producing unopposed estrogen stimulation, which predisposes to endometrial cancer. (**REF.** 12—pp. 646–654)

216. C. The contraction stress test can be of great help in ascertaining if the fetus is at risk. If it is positive, then delivery should be immediate, because of possible ensuing fetal demise. Even if it is negative, there are reported cases of fetal death several days after a normal stress test. Ultrasound of the fetus to see if there is a decreased amniotic fluid is present is of great value. If the amniotic fluid is decreased with a negative stress test, delivery is indicated. (**REF.** 7—p. 763)

217. E. This patient has a third-degree procidentia or complete uterovaginal prolapse with cystocele, urethrocele, rectocele, and enterocele. If a good urethrovesical repair is not done after the vaginal hysterectomy, then these women will complain of some varying degree of urinary stress incontinence; it is thus important to do this. (**REF.** 2—p. 964)

218. C. Nearly 18,500 new cases of ovarian carcinoma are detected each year in the United States. It is the fifth leading cause of cancer death in this country. The annual death rate is 7/100,000 in white women and slightly lower in blacks. At age 70 the incidence is about 70/100,000 women. (**REF.** 2—p. 1133)

219. C. Hemorrhage, puncture of the bowel, and cautery of the bowel occur in about 0.6% of the cases done. Bowel burn leads to peritonitis with ensuing symptoms. (**REF.** 2—p. 255)

220. D. Herpes simplex virus is the most common viral genital infection. It has an exposure time of 3–7 days with inguinal adenopathy and headache due to aseptic meningitis lasting 1 week. (**REF.** 2—p. 980)

221. B. One of the most common problems associated with the treatment of vulvar carcinoma is procrastination on the part of the patient and doctor. After biopsy and staging, at which time it would be ascertained that this patient has a stage III epidermoid carcinoma, she should be treated by radical vulvectomy with inguinal and femoral node dissection by a gynecologic oncologic surgeon familiar with the procedure, and who performs it frequently. (**REF.** 2—p. 1031)

222. E. Sarcomatous degeneration of a fibroid occurs in less than 1% of the cases. This diagnosis is done by the pathologist and is almost never a primary diagnosis. (**REF.** 2—p. 1074)

223. C. Because of the size of this mass, it is frequently misdiagnosed as an ovarian neoplasm, when in reality it is a large, fibroid uterus. With the advent of ultrasound and CT scanning, the diagnosis can be made with relative certainty preoperatively. (**REF.** 2—p. 1073)

224. B. Hydrosalpinx is the result of tardily or untreated gonorrhea with occlusion of the fimbria. (**REF.** 2—pp. 972)

225. D. Fitz-Hugh and Curtis syndrome is gonorrheal perihepatitis, which causes "violin string" adhesions of the liver with severe pain simulating acute cholecystitis. (**REF.** 2—p. 990)

226. D. In this picture the IUD has perforated and is outside the confines of the uterus. Perforation usually takes place when it is being put in. It occurs in about 1 in 1000 insertions. Most can be removed by laparoscopy. (**REF.** 2—p. 250)

227. D. *Neisseria gonorrhea* are gram-negative, intracellular diplococci, which attach to columnar and transitional cells. They attract leukocytes, causing a purulent discharge. (**REF.** 2—p. 972)

228. C. This woman has a large, mucinous cystadenoma of the ovary. These are bilateral about 5–7% of the time. They can cause pseudomyxoma peritoneii if their contents are spilled into the abdominal cavity. At this age the best treatment is abdominal hysterectomy and bilateral salpingo-oophorectomy. (**REF.** 2—p. 1120)

229. D. The protozoan is best diagnosed by a wet smear with saline, taking a specimen from the posterior fornix and examining it immediately to see the flagellated organism. The presence of a single organism can make the diagnosis. Cultures can also be made, but are time-consuming and sometimes are negative. (**REF.** 1—pp. 238–241)

230. E. HSV–1 and HSV–2 are associated with encephalitis, stomatitis, generalized herpes, and genital herpes. The viruses cause syncytial giant cells. They can be cultured and diagnosed in this manner. They are very highly sexually transmissible. (**REF.** 1—pp. 238–241)

231. A. *Candida albicans* and *Tolulopsis globrata* are found in 25–50% of female carrying yeast patients. They can also be isolated from the mouth, throat, and large intestine, as well as the prepuce in the male. There is no uniform accepted serologic test for them. (**REF.** 1—pp. 238–241)

232. C. *Gardnerella vaginalis* vaginitis is a sexually transmitted disease caused by a nonencapsulated gram-variable rod. It can be cultured one-third of the time. It produces Clue cells on wet stain, which is diagnostic of the disease. It can be carried in the male urethra in 90% of male sexual partners of infected women. (**REF.** 1—pp. 238–241)

233. B. These two organisms are closely related, but not identical. They are nonmotile, gram-negative, obligate, intracellular parasites, which replicate within the cytoplasm of the host cells. In women they produce cervicitis followed by acute salpingitis, spread via the lymphatics, and can also cause conjunctivitis in the neonate. They are susceptible to tetracyclines. (**REF.** 1—pp. 238–241)

234. C. Both can be repetitive in nature. Early decelerations represent slowing of the heart rate at the onset of the uterine contractions, but they rapidly return to normal or the baseline by the end of the contractions. These are type I dips. In late decelerations the onset of slowing occurs as the contraction intensifies and recovery is not until the contraction finishes or even later. (**REF.** 7—pp. 281–288)

235. B. There is uteroplacental insufficiency with fetal hypoxia. The fetus undergoes stress and if the stress is not immediately corrected, then delivery is necessary at once. (**REF.** 7—pp. 281–288)

236. A. These are seen in early decelerations due to vagal stimulation from head compression. This is due to increased intracranial pressure. (**REF.** 7—pp. 281–288)

237. D. Variable or nonuniform decelerations are seen in this condition. Often, changing the position of the mother will allow the cord to slip away and not be compressed, relieving the deceleration. (**REF.** 7—pp. 281–288)

238. B. A positive oxytocin challenge test shows late deceleration, which is a sign of uteroplacental insufficiency, and fetal distress, necessitating immediate delivery. (**REF.** 7—pp. 281–288)

239. D. Thirty percent of American women experience PMS, with factors such as advancing age, multiparity, stress, marriage, toxemia in the past, and a high dietary intake of refined carbohydrate increasing their chances of suffering from this affliction. (**REF.** 4—p. 107)

240. A. At each visit the physician should inquire into such complaints as low backache, abdominal and pelvic pain, uterine cramps, contractions, vaginal pain, passage of blood or mucus, and vaginal pressure and bladder and urinary symptoms. (**REF.** 9—pp. 20–32)

241. D. It is seen more in women over 50, from developed countries, with a high socioeconomic status, a surgical menopause under 40, and nulligravity. (**REF.** 10—p. 183)

242. C. By law a patient can refuse any part of the treatment and can forbid release of information to authorities; therefore, informed consent is mandatory to take a history, collect evidence, take pictures, and give treatment. The vulva and head should be combed, and five hairs pulled from each. (**REF.** 8—pp. 84–91)

243. D. Gynecoid is the most common, with bispinous and divergent splay most important. (**REF.** 2—p. 629)

244. E. The use of evaluation of fetal tone, activity, breathing measurements, body movements, and amniotic fluid volume as well as the non stress and if necessary stress test with the others is of importance. (**REF.** 5—p. 103)

245. B. Active liver disease and cerebrovascular or coronary artery disease may be greatly exacerbated by the use of the pill. Other absolute contraindications to the use of the pill are thrombophlebitis and thromboembolic disease, as well as a history of cancer of the breast or endometrium and cigarette smoking over the age of 35. Relative contraindications also include depression. (**REF.** 2—p. 243)

246. E. There is an increased risk of ectopic pregnancy and tubal structural defects in women exposed to DES. (**REF.** 3—pp. 204–222)

247. A. Podophyllin should be used only for vulvar lesions, because absorption from the vagina can lead to severe side effects, such as bone marrow depression, motor sensory neuropathy, and death. (**REF.** 6—p. 31)

17. Ophthalmology

248. D. The first step is always to complete the examination, and the pupillary exam is not complete until the near reflex is checked. If the pupils do not react to near, the next step might be different than if they did react. (**REFS.** 3—p. 514; 4—p. 107)

249. E. Small pupils that exhibit a light-near dissociation are a possible marker for syphilis. (**REFS.** 3—p. 514; 4—p. 107)

250. B. Although shallow orbits and high myopia can mimic proptosis, they are unlikely to cause motility disturbances. Although rhabdomyosarcoma can present this way, bilateral symmetric involvement is unusual. Schirrous carcinoma is often monocular and typically causes enophthalmos. Grave's disease, regardless of thyroid function status, is the most common cause of proptosis in adults. The medial rectus is the most commonly involved muscle, leading to difficulty in elevation. (**REFS.** 3—p. 426; 4—p. 512; 1—pp. 432–434)

251. E. These findings are classical for temporal arteritis. One should, if this disease is suspected, immediately draw a sedimentation rate and start steroids. A biopsy should be scheduled, but the risk of visual loss in the fellow eye is too great to withhold therapy until the biopsy result is available. (**REF.** 3—pp. 503, 434–435)

252. C. Rhabdomyosarcoma is the most frequent primary orbital malignancy in childhood. Melanoma occurs only in adults. Neuroblastoma and leiomyoma do not occur in the eye. (**REFS.** 2—p. 306; 3—p. 328)

253. C. This occurs secondary to silver nitrate prophylaxis. (**REF.** 3—pp. 321–322)

254. B. Unilateral visual loss in infants usually produces esotropia and may be secondary to amblyopia. Nystagmus results from severe bilateral visual impairment in infancy, such as bilateral congenital cataracts. (**REF.** 3—p. 513)

255. E. Horner's syndrome affects the sympathetic nervous system and therefore does not affect vision. Congenital Horner's syndrome affects iris pigmentation and thus may result in heterochromia. (**REF.** 2—p. 250)

256. E. Sinusitis is the most common cause of orbital cellulitis. Otitis media is not a cause of orbital cellulitis. (**REF.** 2—p. 239)

257. B. Acute infections of the glands of Zeis associated with the cilia are most often due to staphlococcus. (**REF.** 2—p. 181)

258. D. Because the orientation of the axons is horizontal, blood that accumulates there tends to assume a horizontal or flame-shaped configuration. (**REF.** 2—p. 280)

259. E. The first four choices are all characteristic of damage to the optic nerve found in glaucoma. Blurring of the disc margin is a finding in papilledema. (**REFS.** 2—p. 346; 3—p. 204)

260. D. Timoptic (timolol maleate) is a beta-blocker, which is the most commonly used glaucoma agent because of its convenience and efficacy. Other recently approved beta blockers are Betoptic (betaxolol HCl) and Betagan (levobunolol HCl). (**REFS.** 1—p. 11; 2—346)

261. C. Cotton wool spots are infarctions of the nerve fiber layer which are common in hypertensive retinopathy. (**REF.** 2—p. 471)

262. E. Dot and blot hemorrhages are common in diabetic retinopathy. All other responses are typical of hypertensive retinopathy. (**REF.** 2—pp. 469–472)

263. D. Atropine or atropine-like drugs are commonly used in ophthalmic diagnosis. Any ocular medication is absorbed systemically. The patient described has typical anticholinergic signs. Physostigmine is the agent of choice because it crosses the blood–brain barrier. (**REF.** 2—p. 103–104)

264. C. Red–green color blindness is most typically X-linked recessive and therefore is more commonly found in males. (**REF.** 2—p. 278)

265. D. Horner's syndrome may be caused by first-, second-, or third-order lesions. Second-order lesions often result from tumors, particularly Pancost tumors and thyroid tumors. (**REF.** 2—pp. 249–250)

266. B. The monoarticular form of juvenile rheumatoid arthritis is associated with uveitis. It is distinctly uncommon in the polyarticular form. (**REF.** 2—pp. 484–485)

267. B. Loss of vision, ophthalmoplegia, loss of corneal sensation, and proptosis are signs of a lesion in the orbital apex. The patient described is in diabetic ketoacidosis. One must think of the possibility of mucormycosis in a ketoacidotic or immunocompromised patient. (**REF.** 2—p. 392)

268. E. The more posterior the defect, the more congruous it is. Lesion d–d is not correct because the more anterior lesion would cause the less congruous defect. (**REF.** 2—p. 448)

269. B. This is a bitemporal hemianopia, the classical field defect for a chiasmal lesion. (**REF.** 2—p. 448)

270. D. Posterior to the chiasm, the lesion gives a homonymous hemianopia. Since this is not far posterior in the visual pathway, the lesion is less congruous than that of lesion e–e. (**REF.** 2—p. 448)

271. A. Central scotomas without involvement of the other eye must be anterior to the chiasm. (**REF.** 2—p. 448)

272. C. This is the classical junctional scotoma. All the fibers from the right eye are affected, as are the nasal fibers (temporal field) from the left eye. (**REF.** 2—p. 448)

273. B. Loss of perfusion to the retina would result in an acute cessation of function and, therefore, sudden loss of vision. (**REF.** 2—p. 287)

274. A. Increased intraocular pressure is a hallmark of glaucoma. (**REF.** 2—p. 343)

275. D. Cataracts or opacification of the crystalline lens typically are slowly progressive and therefore cause a gradual loss of vision. (**REF.** 2—p. 325)

276. E. Loss of accommodative ability occurs with increasing age. This results in decreased ability to read. Presby is a prefix that refers to age. (**REF.** 2—p. 376)

277. A. Cupping of the disc is characteristic of glaucoma; refer to question 274. (**REF.** 2—p. 343)

278. G. Atropine is an anticholinergic agent. (**REFS.** 1—p. 2; 2—p. 103)

279. F. Pilocarpine is a cholinergic agent. (**REFS.** 1—p. 3; 2—p. 102)

280. H. Neosynephrine is a sympathetic agent. (**REFS.** 1—p. 2; 2—p. 107)

281. I. Dexamethasone is a steroid used to reduce inflammation. (**REFS.** 1—p. 9; 2—p. 118)

282. G. Homatropine is an anticholinergic agent. (**REFS.** 1—p. 2; 2—p. 104)

283. E. If the eyes are not aligned, different objects are seen, which is not well-tolerated by the brain. Suppression and amblyopia result. Various etiologies of strabismus include Grave's disease and congenital etiologies. Prompt ophthalmologic evaluation is essential. (**REF.** 2—pp. 356–359, 435)

284. A. Retinoblastoma is the most common intraocular malignancy of childhood. It may present with a white pupil (leukocoria). It is associated with sarcomas of the long bones, and is seen in association with partial deletion of long arm of chromosome 13. (**REF.** 2—pp. 306–307)

285. A. Retinopathy of prematurity is a disorder seen in premature infants of low birth weight. Often there is an associated history of perinatal oxygen administration. (**REF.** 2—pp. 286–287)

286. B. The so-called cherry red spot is the normal blush of the fovea seen in the midst of a whitened, edematous nerve fiber layer. This occurs most commonly in central retinal artery occlusions in some of the metabolic storage diseases and sphingolipidoses, including Tay–Sachs disease. (**REF.** 2—pp. 287–288, 413–418)

18. Otorhinolaryngology

287. D. Quinine, aminoglycosides (gentamicin, tobramycin, kanamycin, neomycin, and streptomycin), and certain diuretics (furosemide, ethacrynic acid) cause permanent sensorineural hearing loss; that following large doses of aspirin is reversible when the drug is withdrawn. (**REF.** 3—p. 82)

288. A. Bone conduction greater than air conduction (Rinne negative) implies a conductive hearing loss. A tuning fork placed on the middle of the forehead or skull (Weber test) lateralizes to the poorer hearing ear when a conductive hearing loss exists. (**REF.** 3—pp. 44–45)

289. D. Patients with temporomandibular joint syndrome often have malocclusion of the teeth, a history of bruxism, and spasm of the muscles of mastication. (**REF.** 3—p. 234)

290. C. A unilateral polyp that extends from the middle meatus into the posterior nasal passage is often associated with infection of the maxillary sinus; allergic polyps are usually bilateral. (**REF.** 3—p. 116)

291. C. The ethmoidal sinus is well developed at birth; the others develop later. (**REF.** 1—p. 215)

292. E. Snoring is a primary symptom of sleep apnea; the diagnosis is confirmed by polysomnographic studies and corrected by surgery on the soft palate and uvula with or without a tracheotomy. (**REF.** 2—p. 57)

293. A. Torus palatinus is the result of embryologic malfusion and requires no treatment. (**REF.** 2—p. 31)

294. C. Leukoplakia is seen in smokers or where there is chronic irritation from a tooth or denture. (**REF.** 2—p. 37)

295. A. Antibiotic therapy may suppress normal oral and gastrointestinal organisms, permitting fungal overgrowth, often *Candida albicans*. (**REF.** 3—p. 151)

296. B. Most malignant neck masses originate from a primary in the head and neck region. Identification and biopsy of the primary lesion is preferable to biopsy of the metastatic mass.

297. D. An enlarging carcinoma in the hilum of the left lung invades the recurrent laryngeal nerve and causes paralysis of the left vocal cord. (**REF.** 2—p. 91)

298. C. The initial vasoconstriction is followed by vasodilatation and nasal congestion, which necessitates further application of the nose drop or spray. (**REF.** 1—p. 199)

299. C. The episodes of vertigo with Meniere's disease last several hours. The patient often notes intra-aural pressure prior to the onset of the acute attack. (**REF.** 1—p. 1259)

300. D. Vestibular neuronitis, presumably of viral etiology, is characterized by vertigo, vomiting, and nystagmus, but with no change in hearing. (**REF.** 1—p. 1249)

301. A. Acoustic neurinoma, a slowly growing benign tumor of the eighth cranial nerve, usually causes unilateral tinnitus followed by a slowly progressive hearing loss, with dizziness a later symptom. (**REF.** 1—p. 1264)

302. C. Paroxysmal positional vertigo is a self-limiting disorder characterized by brief episodes of vertigo and nystagmus when the head is in certain positions; occasional cases are related to a central nervous system disease rather than the more common type, which represents utricular dysfunction. (**REF.** 1—p. 1249)

303. A. Unlike croup, which is usually viral, epiglottitis is bacterial, most commonly *Hemophilus influenzae*. (**REF.** 1—p. 455)

304. B. Acute epiglottitis tends to affect children above 3 years of age, and often occurs in adults. (**REF.** 1—p. 455)

305. A. Sore throat, pain on swallowing, and drooling occur early in the course of epiglottitis. (**REF.** 1—p. 456)

306. C. Both groups of patients are candidates for tracheal intubation or tracheotomy with the development of any significant airway obstruction. (**REF.** 1—p. 456)

307. D. The PRIST (paper radioimmunosorbent) test measures total IgE and identifies patients at risk for development of atopic allergies. (**REF.** 1—p. 148)

308. A. In highly sensitive individuals, intradermal skin tests may result in a systemic reaction. RAST testing, performed on a blood sample, is free from reactions. (**REF.** 1—p. 151)

309. B. RAST testing may be used on patients unable to stop antiallergic medication, whereas antihistamines must be discontinued 3–4 days prior to skin testing. (**REF.** 1—p. 150)

310. C. The commonest cause of otitis externa is *Pseudomonas aeruginosa*, with fungus a less frequent occurrence. While otitis media may be viral initially, bacterial infection is the commonest situation (*Streptococcus pneumoniae, Hemophilus influenzae,* or group A *Streptococcus pyogenes*). (**REF.** 3—pp. 55, 63)

311. D. Cholesteatoma is a sac of infected squamous epithelium which may develop in ears with chronic otitis media where there is a perforation of the uppermost part of the tympanic membrane (pars flaccida). (**REF.** 3—p. 67)

312. B. Although accumulated debris may block the ear canal in external otitis, this infection produces no hearing loss once the external auditory canal has been carefully cleaned out. (**REF.** 3—p. 63)

313. B. Most cases of otitis externa can be treated with topical medication—acidic drops with antibiotics and steroids as needed; systemic antibiotics are reserved for severe cases of otitis externa accompanied by high fever, auricular swelling, and cervical adenopathy. All cases of otitis media require systemic antibiotics. (**REF.** 3—p. 63)

314. C. Tonsillitis with cervical adenopathy in a young adult that fails to improve on penicillin is often indicative of infectious mononucleosis. The white blood count usually exhibits a lymphocytosis with many atypical lymphocytes. (**REF.** 1—p. 272)

315. B. The viral etiology (Epstein–Barr) of infectious mononucleosis explains why antibiotics are of no value unless secondary bacterial invaders can be demonstrated. (**REF.** 1—p. 272)

316. E. Peritonsillar abscess forms deep to one tonsil and requires antibiotics plus surgical drainage. (**REF.** 1—p. 310)

19. Pediatrics

317. C. The infant of a diabetic mother most commonly develops problems with reactive hypoglycemia due to hyperinsulinemia. Other frequently observed problems include hyperbilirubinemia, hypocalcemia, and polycythemia. These infants also have an increased incidence of congenital malformations, including heart and skeletal defects. (**REF.** 2—pp. 854–857)

318. C. Most full-term infants double their birth weight by 6 months and triple their birth weight by 12 months of age. The anterior fontanelle closes at 9–18 months and the posterior fontanelle at 2–4 months. By 12 months of age, most infants have 6–8 deciduous teeth. (**REF.** 1—p. 16–17)

319. D. The normal toddler has achieved all of the listed milestones except the ability to climb stairs with alternating feet, which usually does not occur until the third birthday. (**REF.** 1—p. 37)

320. C. Schonlein–Henoch vasculitis is a childhood disorder of unknown etiology. The most common clinical manifestations include fever, skin lesions (most typically on lower extremities, ranging from wheals to petechiae and frank purpura), arthritis of large joints, gastrointestinal symptoms (colicky pain and GI bleeding), and renal involvement. (**REF.** 1—pp. 577–579)

321. D. An acute episode of bronchospasm is best treated by bronchodilators (theophylline, beta-adrenergic agents), oxygen, and intravenous fluids. A mist tent would be contraindicated because it would obscure vision of the patient and the large humidified air droplets would not reach the bronchospastic airways. (**REF.** 4—pp. 1561–1562)

322. B. *Hemophilus influenzae* type B accounts for 95% of serious infections due to *H. influenzae*. It is the leading etiologic agent in meningitis, septic arthritis, and buccal cellulitis in the under 2-year age group. In the older child, this bacterium is usually associated with acute epiglottitis or pneumonia. *H. influenzae* is an uncommon etiologic agent in osteomyelitis, especially in a 12-year-old, where the more common organism would be staphylococcus. (**REF.** 1—pp. 656–658)

323. E. Pneumococcal sepsis is more common in patients with asplenia (functional, as in sickle cell anemia, or surgical), ascites, and B-cell immune disorders (Bruton's disease). Chronic granulomatous disease with WBC dysfunction more commonly results in serious infection with *staphylococcus aureus* or gram-negative organisms. (**REF.** 1—pp. 520–521, 638–641)

324. E. Esophageal atresia is commonly associated with tracheoesophageal fistula. A common presentation includes a history of polyhydramnios, increased oral secretions followed by choking, and cyanotic episodes, especially following feedings. Cyanosis at rest relieved by crying suggests either choanal atresia or hypoventilation. (**REF.** 2—pp. 496–497, 460–465)

325. C. Hirschsprung's disease is the most common cause of colon obstruction and is due to aganglionic segments of bowel. Clinical manifestations range from acute obstruction to chronic constipation. It is rare in premature infants. On rectal exam one usually finds an empty, nondilated rectum, followed by an explosive discharge of feces and gas. (**REF.** 1—pp. 910–911)

326. E. Nosebleeds are most common during childhood, decreasing in incidence during infancy and after puberty. While all of the listed disorders may be associated with epistaxis, by far the most common etiology is trauma. (**REF.** 1—pp. 1012)

327, E. Otitis media is one of the most prevalent infectious diseases in childhood. Infancy is the period of highest risk due to mechanical or functional obstruction of the eustachian tube. *S. pneumoniae* followed by *H. influenzae* are the most common causative agents. Antibiotic therapy usually resolves an acute episode, although many young children develop recurrent episodes and require either prophylactic antibiotic therapy or pressure-equalizing tubes. Complications include, most commonly, acute hearing loss and perforation of the tympanic membrane, and rarely seen complications include cholesteatoma (a saclike structure lined with squamous epithelium), facial nerve paralysis, and intracranial infection (brain abscess, meningitis, and focal encephalitis). Cauliflower ear deformity is seen in association with trauma to the external ear cartilage. (**REF.** 1—pp. 1025–1028)

328. B. Although foreign body aspiration causes initial symptoms of choking, cough, and dyspnea, if not recognized immediately a relatively symptom-free period occurs followed by recurrent episodes of wheezing and atelectasis, pneumonia, or localized air trapping. Cystic fibrosis and chronic granulomatous disease usually cause symptoms during infancy, as do most vascular rings. Although atelectasis and pneumonia do occur in patients with asthma, the recurrent nature of this patient's pneumonia make this diagnosis less likely. (**REF.** 4—pp. 1517–1518)

329. C. Premature infants have less smooth muscle throughout their pulmonary vascular bed, and thus characteristically develop the symptoms of left to right shunting through a ventricular septal defect or patent ductus arteriosus at a younger postnatal age than term infants. Similarly, the incidence of persistent fetal circulation is decreased in premature infants. Since premature infants are more likely to require umbilical arterial catheters, they are at increased risk for acquired hypertension secondary to thromboembolic disease. (**REF.** 2—pp. 522, 567–570)

330. B. Congenital hypothyroidism must be diagnosed promptly, since delay in therapy can lead to brain damage, yet overt symptoms are rarely present in the neonatal period (infants usually have normal weight and length and rarely have poor feeding and prolonged jaundice). Defective embryogenesis (agenesis/dysgenesis) accounts for 70–80% of all cretinism. Breast milk contains low levels of T4 and may partially treat an infant with congenital hypothyroidism. Premature infants are often identified by screening programs due to transiently low T4 levels in association with low-normal TSH levels of thyrotropin-releasing factor. (**REF.** 2—pp. 890–893)

331. C. The most common type of neonatal seizures are subtle seizures, consisting of eye deviation, sucking movements of the mouth, and posturing with the extremities. It may be difficult to differentiate between jitteriness and subtle seizures. (**REF.** 4— pp. 1848–1849)

332. A. Acute rheumatic fever with myocardial involvement is primarily manifested by tachycardia, cardiomegaly, pericardial effusions, and mitral regurgitation. Valvular stenosis is a later developing complication. (**REF.** 4—pp. 384–387)

333. B. Normal hematologic values in the full-term infant include polycythemia, predominance of fetal hemoglobin, a wide range in total leukocyte count, and granulocyte predominance. In later infancy, lymphocyte predominance develops. Both premature and full-term infants have moderate prolongation of partial thromboplastin (PTT) and prothrombin (PT) time. Since there is no transplacental transmission of clotting factors, vitamin K should be administered after birth. (**REF.** 2—pp. 708–710, 715–717)

334. A. All of the disorders except thalassemia minor may cause anemia and some degree of extramedullary hematopoiesis. However, only patients with thalassemia major are severely anemic, transfusion dependent, and thus develop the complication of hemosiderosis. (**REF.** 4—pp. 798–806, 1149–1167)

335. D. Wilms' tumor, which accounts for virtually all renal neoplasms in childhood, occurs before 5 years of age in 80% of patients. An important feature of Wilms' tumor is its association with other congenital anomalies, including genitourinary disorders, hemihypertrophy, aniridia, and Beckwith-Wiedeman syndrome (macroglossia, hypoglycemia, gigantism, and umbilical hernia). The most frequent presentation for this tumor is an abdominal mass. (**REF.** 1—pp. 1277–1279)

336. B. Hematuria is detected relatively commonly in pediatric practice. Although hematuria is usually associated with glomerular disease, it is also seen with genitourinary tract disease and hematologic disorders. Renal causes of hematuria include glomerulonephritis, interstitial nephritis, cystic diseases, hereditary nephritis, infection, neoplasm, renal vein thrombosis, and trauma. GU causes of hematuria include urolithiasis, infection (classically, hemorrhagic cystitis associated with adenovirus), polyps, trauma, and tumors. Nonrenal causes include hemoglobinopathies (sickle cell disease), disorders of coagulation, strenous exercise, and congestive heart failure. (**REF.** 4—pp. 312–313)

337. E. Low C3 levels are characteristic of all the renal disorders listed except Henoch–Schonlein purpura. All of these diseases may present in childhood as hematuria, proteinuria, hypertension, and renal failure. (**REF.** 1—pp. 1331–1340)

338. E. Potter's anomaly consists of oligohydramnios with resultant pulmonary hypoplasia, typical facial appearance (low-set ears, skin crease under eyes, and prominent occiput), the positional deformation of club feet, and vernix nodules (amnion nodosum) on the placenta. Most infants have bilateral renal agenesis, but any condition that results in early and severe oligohydramnios may cause this syndrome. Most infants die within a few hours after birth from pulmonary insufficiency. (**REF.** 2—p. 793)

339. E. Hyperinsulinemia in the fetus and newborn results in neonatal hypoglycemia. The majority of affected infants have mothers with glucose intolerance, but other etiologies include erythroblastosis, Beckwith-Wiedemann syndrome, and B-cell nesidioblastosis. Galactosemia is another cause of neonatal hypoglycemia, but is not associated with hyperinsulinemia. (**REF.** 2—p. 850)

340. D. An infant with diarrhea has hyponatremia, dehydration, and acidosis, but does not have severe hyperphosphatemia. (**REF.** 1—pp. 239–240)

341. E. Chronic renal failure is associated with increased BUN, acidosis, hypocalcemia, and hyperphosphatemia. (**REF.** 1—p. 1363)

342. A. Diabetic ketoacidosis is associated with hyperglycemia and acidosis. (**REF.** 1—p. 1408)

343. B. Inappropriate ADH secretion with meningitis results in hyponatremia. (**REF.** 1—p. 1440)

344. C. An infant with pyloric stenosis has hypochloremic alkalosis. (**REF.** 1—p. 242)

345. C. Colic is a disorder of unknown etiology occurring in young
346. D. infants (under 3 months of age). Attacks begin suddenly
347. B. with loud cries and apparent distress in the infant. (It may
348. A. sometimes be due to overfeeding, formula intolerance, or
349. B. air swallowing, but most often the cause is not identified.)
Relief occurs with maturation of the child, and generally offering
a supportive, sympathetic attitude is more effective than formula
changes or sedation. (**REF.** 1—p. 163, 912–913, 915, 925, 926–927)

350. C. The immunocompromised child should not receive live
attenuated viral vaccination. (**REF.** 3—p. 36)

351. A. Staphylococcal infections with elaboration of exotoxins
may cause all of the listed disorders except erythrasma, a chronic
superficial infection associated with the diphtheroid corynebacte-
rium. (**REF.** 1—pp. 650–653, 1712–1715)

352. A. Neonatal conjugated hyperbilirubinemia is seen in association with galactosemia, cystic fibrosis, and urinary tract infection
(especially in male infants). Hypothyroidism results in prolonged
*un*conjugated hyperbilirubinemia. (**REF.** 2—pp. 760–766, 774–
777)

353. E. Acute bronchiolitis is caused most commonly by respiratory syncytial virus, although other etiologic agents include para-
influenza, mycoplasma, and adenovirus. The peak incidence is at
6 months of age and the clinical manifestations include tachypnea,
low-grade fever, and expiratory wheezing, secondary to inflammation of the lower airways. Roentgenographic findings of hyperinflation are characteristic. Treatment includes close
observation and supportive care. Intravenous fluids and humidified
air decrease insensible water loss and supplemental oxygen may
be needed. (**REF.** 1—pp. 1044–1045)

354. C. Acute lymphocytic leukemia is the most common form
of childhood cancer, and has a peak incidence at 3–4 years of age.
Initial symptoms are usually nonspecific, but progress to pallor,
fatigue, bleeding, or fever. Initial remission can be expected in
virtually all patients with combination chemotherapy. The most

common sites of extramedullary relapse include the central nervous system and the testes. (**REF.** 1—pp. 1262–1266)

355. C. Diabetes mellitus in childhood is associated with an increased incidence of autoimmune thyroiditis (Hashimoto's thyroiditis) and adrenal insufficiency. (**REF.** 1—p. 1418)

356. A. Congenital adrenal hyperplasia encompasses several enzymatic defects in the pathway of cortisol synthesis. 21–Hydroxylase deficiency accounts for 90–95% of cases. Female infants are virilized (female pseudohermaphroditism) due to overproduction of cortisol precursors, which lead to increased androgen production. One-third of patients are salt-losers and may develop hyponatremia, hyperkalemia, and volume depletion shock. (**REF.** 2—p. 916)

357. A. A neonate has many reflexes at birth, including the Moro, placing, and palmar grasp reflexes. The parachute reflex does not appear until approximately 9 months of age. (**REF.** 4—pp. 161–162)

358. A. Hypotonia is a prominent feature of both Down's syndrome and anterior horn cell atrophy. Infants with cerebral palsy are also initially hypotonic and later become hypertonic. Duchenne muscular dystrophy is the one disorder that would not present as neonatal hypotonia. (**REF.** 4—pp. 1880–1881)

359. C. Uncomplicated febrile seizures typically occur in otherwise normal children from 6 months to 3 years of age. It has been demonstrated that phenobarbital given at the onset of the fever is not efficacious in preventing subsequent febrile seizures. Most children do not develop later epilepsy. (**REF.** 4—pp. 1853–1854)

360. C. All of the physical findings are normal, with the exception of the palpable thrill. (**REF.** 1—pp. 1100–1104)

361. C. Stridor is heard predominantly during inspiration and is never a normal finding. Common etiologies include croup, epiglottitis, and foreign body aspiration. Intravenous aminophylline would not be expected to lessen the symptoms, since it primarily relaxes the smooth muscle of more peripheral airways. (**REF.** 4— p. 1548)

362. A. Congenital dislocation of the hip occurs more frequently in females and is easily detected in infancy by apparent shortening of one leg, or asymmetric skin folds, or by passively dislocating the femoral head from the acetabulum. However, x-rays of the pelvis are particularly difficult to interpret during infancy. (**REF.** 1—1617–1620)

363. C. Scoliosis is a common orthopedic problem in childhood, and always requires orthopedic evaluation and intervention. The best screening device is to observe the symmetry of the child's back while the child is bending from the waist. Scoliosis is more frequent in females, and all members should be examined in affected families. Late complications in untreated cases include pulmonary insufficiency and cardiac decompensation. (**REF.** 1—1624)

20. Public Health and Preventive Medicine

364. E. It is important for health workers to understand the difference between incidence and prevalence rates, because incorrect labeling of incidence and prevalence is common among those inexperienced in their use and results in erroneous conclusions and errors in logic. The denominator for rates is commonly called "the population at risk." Many commonly used rates use as their denominator information derived from the 10-year census. The incidence rate is essentially an expression of average frequency of an event in a population. Numerators of rates are the events.

Prevalence rates are especially useful in chronic diseases. The relationship between incidence, prevalence, and duration of disease is simply expressed by the formula Prevalence = Incidence × Duration (equilibrium is assumed). Infant mortality rate as given in statement D is correct. There is also a neonatal mortality rate, whose numerator is liveborn infants who die before 1 month of age. (**REF.** 6—pp. 13–15)

365. C. It is not correct that mortality due to cancer of the uterus has risen. Indeed, it has shown steady and gratifying decline over the past 50 years. Each of the other statements is true. It may come as a surprise to some readers that mortality due to cancer of the breast has not shown remarkable trends. This indeed is true and appears to be so in spite of advances in both early diagnosis and treatment. Cancer of the colon and rectum continues to be a major source of death in both men and women. In recent decades, there has been a gratifying decline in women, but the same decline is not seen in men. Cancer of the colon and rectum in men continues to be a leading cause of death and surpasses death due to prostate cancer. (**REF.** 9—pp. 14–15)

366. B. Only a minority of statistical associations are causal. The concept of "chain of causation," although useful, is an oversimplification. Causation is multiple and is more likely to form a "web" of causation than a "chain." The stronger an association between two categories of events as revealed by grouping rather than by individuals, the more likely is the assumption that the association is correct. The distinction between direct and indirect causal relationship is a valid one and depends upon the interpretation of *current* knowledge. In order to effect appropriate preventive measures, it is not necessary that we understand causal mechanisms in their entirety, for sometimes breaking the single strand of a "web" is sufficient to make the entire causation mechanism collapse. (A good example of this is cigarette smoking and bronchogenic carcinoma of the lung. Ed.) (**REF.** 7—pp. 20–25)

367. A. There should be no major differences between case and control groups as to the quality of available information. Availability of information implies tabulating both (1) how much information is obtained concerning each case and control, and (2) what proportions of the case and control groups will or can supply it. Equal access to important information previously recorded in a similar fashion for both cases and controls may strongly favor the use of a particular control group.

When data must be obtained by interview, the quality of available information may differ due to differences between cases and controls. Differences could be in relation to, for example, emotional state, knowledge of the disease studied, educational or socioeconomic status, and location of the interview—whether in home, hospital, or elsewhere.

Biases may be known or unknown. Thus, the investigator attempts to find controls that are similar in a general way to the cases (except for the essential difference of whether the disease under investigation is present or absent).

An investigator will often attempt to match the controls to the cases with regard to some important characteristic, such as age or sex. (**REF.** 3—pp. 105–107)

368. A. Heart diseases still lead among the causes of death, with a total of 38.2%. Including the third place cerebrovascular diseases adds another 7.7%, making the total for heart and stroke 45.9%. Cancer is in second place, with a total of 21.9%. Accidents are in fourth place, with 4.6% of total deaths. Pneumonia and influenza hold fifth place at 2.8% of the total, and chronic obstructive lung diseases (COLD) is in sixth place, with a total of 2.3%. (**REF.** 2—p. 10)

369. E. CDC guidelines have emphasized that in hospital and home care settings, health care workers should wear gloves routinely during direct contact with mucous membranes or nonintact skin of such patients. Also, they should wear gloves in handling items soiled with blood and other body secretions or excretions. Gowns, masks, and eye coverings may be appropriate if procedures involving more extensive contact with blood and secretions are performed. Each of the other statements is true. Evidence supports the hypothesis that human T-lymphotrophic virus type III/lymph-adenopathy-associated virus (HTLV-III/LAV) infection of persons with the tubercle bacillus has caused an increase in tuberculosis in some areas. (**REF.** 9—pp. 74–78)

370. B. The other agencies that are included under the Public Health Service are the Alcohol and Drug Abuse and Mental Health Administration, and the President's Council on Physical Fitness and Sports. (**REF.** 11—pp. 284–292)

371. A. The Assistant Secretary of Health exercises direct line authority over the Public Health Service. This individual also has a staff office known as the Office of International Health, which is responsible for international health policy and program coordination. (**REF.** 12—pp. 344–346)

372. C. The Centers for Disease Control is comprised of eight major operation components: Bureau of Epidemiology; National Institute of Occupational Safety and Health; Bureau of Laboratories; Bureau of Health Education; Bureau of State Services; Bureau of Smallpox Eradication; Bureau of Tropical Diseases; and Bureau of Training. (**REF.** 11—pp. 284–292)

373. E. The Health Resources Administration provides leadership relating to the requirements for and distribution of health resources, including manpower training. Other components of the HRA include the Bureau of Health Manpower (deals with question of foreign medical graduates); Bureau of Health Planning and Resources Development; and National Center for Health Services Research. (The Health Resources Administration has been merged with the Health Services Administration to form HRSA. Ed.) (**REF.** 11—pp. 284–292)

374. B. The mission of the National Institutes of Health is to improve the health of the American public. Among the other major components of NIH are National Cancer Institute; National Eye Institute; National Institute of Allergy and Infectious Diseases; National Institute of Arthritis, Metabolism, and Digestive Disease; and National Library of Medicine. (**REF.** 11—pp. 284–292)

375. E. The state health department is required to establish minimal standards for local health work. Its other functions are the maintenance of central and branch laboratory services, including diagnostic, sanitary, chemical, biologic, and research activities; the collection, tabulation, and analysis of vital statistics; the collection and distribution of information concerning preventable disease; the maintenance of safe quality of water and the control of waste disposal; establishment and maintenance of minimal standards of milk sanitation; provision of service to aid industry in the control of occupational hazards; the establishment of qualifications for health personnel; and formulation of plans in cooperation with other organizations for meeting all health needs. (**REF.** 1—p. 52)

376. D. The blood program is usually considered to be a responsibility of the American Red Cross. Some other basic responsibilities of the local health department are provision of laboratory services and education of the public on health matters. (**REF.** 1—pp. 54–55, 58)

377. C. Although the federal and state health organizations can fulfill these criteria, it is the local health department that has the fundamental responsibility to implement these goals. (**REF.** 1—p. 54)

378. A. The United Nations Relief and Work Agency mainly aids Palestinian refugees in education and vocational training, housing, health services, and food. WHO (World Health Organization), UNICEF (United Nations Children's Fund), UNFPA (United Nations Fund for Population Activities), and FAO (Food and Agriculture Organization) meet the criteria set forth in the question. (**REF.** 11—pp. 42–64, 181)

379. E. Authoritative sources do not implicate tetracyline as carcinogenic. All of the others are more than suspect. Many more could be added, such as arsenic, benzidine, and diethylstibesterol, to name only a few. (**REF.** 6—p. 516)

380. D. The mean (the average of the set of numbers) is always located in the middle of a normal distribution. (**REF.** 5—pp. 74–77)

381. C. Plus or minus one standard deviation from the mean would contain 68% of the data. (**REF.** 5—pp. 74–77)

382. B. Most "normal" laboratory tests are based on evaluation of a "normal" population. The standards are then based on 95% of this "normal" population. This would be within two standard deviations of the mean. (**REF.** 5—pp. 74–77)

383. B. The area containing 95% of the data is $\bar{x} - 2s$ to $\bar{x} + 2s$. (**REF.** 5—pp. 74–77)

384. A. The area within three standard deviations ($\bar{x} - 3s$ to $\bar{x} + 3s$) contains 99.7% of the population. (**REF.** 5—pp. 74–77)

385. D. The American Red Cross is a quasigovernmental agency because it has been appointed by the Congress to act as the medium of communication and voluntary relief between the American people and their armed forces, and to carry on a system of national and international relief to prevent and mitigate suffering caused by disasters. This organization has developed its own programs, such as water safety and first aid. (**REF.** 1—pp. 57–59)

386. E. Medicare (Title XVIII) provides medical assistance to anyone 65 or older for hospitalization, nursing home care, home visits by nurses or other health specialists after hospitalization, and hospital diagnostic tests. The Medicaid (Title XIX) portion allows eligible individuals (the aged, the blind, the disabled, and families receiving Aid to Dependent Children) similar assistance to Medicare. (There are some individuals over 65 who have never been eligible for Social Security and thus are not eligible for Medicare. This number is rapidly dwindling. Ed.) (**REF.** 4—pp. 626–627)

387. E. The role of the social worker must be varied in order to meet the needs of the community. They are consultants to individuals, families, and agencies regarding the needs and services of their community. They can plan, implement, and formulate programs because of their understanding of their community. Social case work for the individual, family, or group allows the social worker to integrate services within the community; and the social worker must develop adequate methods of research, study, and survey in order to maintain an awareness of the needs and services within their community. (**REF.** 4—pp. 335–343)

388. E. Standardizing removes the effect of differences in composition of populations being compared and age is most often removed because of its effect on morbidity and mortality.

In the direct method of adjustment, age-specific rates observed in two or more study populations are applied to an arbitrarily chosen population of known age structure referred to as the "standard" population. The indirect method is used if in one of the comparison populations the age-specific rates are not known. In this method, the more stable rates of the larger population are applied to the population of the smaller study group.

Comparison of the number of expected deaths in the smaller population with the number actually observed yields a measure known as the standardized mortality ratio (SMR). The SMR equals observed deaths divided by expected deaths. (**REF.** 8—pp. 136–137)

389. C. Men (but not women) in lower socioeconomic groups have the highest death rates for most causes of death (except motor vehicle accidents). It has been known for years that people who are not married (whether single, separated, widowed, or divorced) have higher mortality rates than married people. In 1980, in the United States, men had an age-adjusted death rate 80% higher than women and men live about 7.5 years less than women. (**REF.** 6—pp. 956–958)

390. A. Most nosocomial UTIs are caused by urinary tract manipulation, such as an indwelling urinary catheter. The prime determinate of infection risk seems to be the surgeon's skill. The third most common source of nosocomial infection is lower respiratory infection (pneumonia, lung abscess, empyema, and bronchitis) and these make up 16% of the total. Patients with pulmonary tuberculosis become noncontagious rapidly, sometimes within a week or so following the administration of appropriate chemotherapy. (**REF.** 6—pp. 298–301)

391. B. Those involved in the manufacture of Teflon are exposed to polymer fumes and meat wrappers are exposed to the fumes of vinyl chloride. Farmer's lung, however, does not come from *Pseudomonas*, but rather from *Aspergillus*, a fungus, and those involved with airconditioning and humidifiers do not react to *Thermoactinomyces*, but rather to amoeba such as *Acathamoeba* or *Naegleria*. Sugar cane workers may be affected by bagassosis in connection with exposure to *Thermoactinomyces sacchari*. (**REF.** 6—pp. 563–565)

392. E. All of these statements are correct. Over the last 200 years mortality rates have declined almost everywhere in the world. In developing countries, mortality declines are recent and often more dramatic. The factors responsible for these declines are (1) increases in the level of education and related socioeconomic changes, and (2) the application of public health measures, such as immunization and malaria control programs. (**REF.** 6—pp. 83–96)

393. E. All of the statements are true. If each season's vaccine is to be available for use by fall, strain selection and production must begin early in the year—by February. In past epidemics (for example, influenza B outbreaks), outbreaks often occurred toward the end of the influenza season rather than during the earlier January–February peak months. Thus, it was not always possible to examine the influenza isolates from these late outbreaks in time to decide on vaccination formulation and get into production. (**REF.** 10—pp. 92–94)

21. Psychiatry

394. E. The listed conditions are relative rather than absolute contraindications for ECT. Some authorities consider intracranial space-occupying lesion as an absolute contraindication to ECT. (**REF.** 2—p. 1562)

395. C. Auditory hallucination of a voice calling a name is a nonspecific finding seen in several conditions other than schizophrenia. (**REF.** 1—pp. 188–190)

396. D. Manic patients typically lack significant insight into the nature of their difficulty. The other characteristics are included in the diagnostic criteria set for mania. (**REF.** 1—pp. 208–210)

397. A. Indifference to symptoms (la belle indifférence) may or may not be present. Symptoms do not usually closely mimic organic illness—hysterical conversion is seen in men as well as women and in patients with many different character types or psychotic diagnoses. (**REF.** 3—pp. 453–460)

398. C. Antisocial personality disorder is approximately three times as prevalent in men as in women. (**REF.** 1—pp. 320–321)

399. B. Delusions about sexual organs are indicative of a psychotic process and should be treated accordingly. (**REF.** 3—p. 459)

400. D. Denial is the most common reaction. (**REF.** 6—pp. 53–55)

401. C. Alzheimer-type dementia accounts for more than 50% of all causes of irreversible dementia. (**REF.** 2—p. 861)

402. E. Lithium salts are used for prophylaxis against recurrence of manic episodes. (**REF.** 2—p. 832)

403. C. For patients with schizophrenia requiring maintenance medication neuroleptic drugs are the treatment of choice. (**REF.** 2—p. 719)

404. A. Phobias are a major indication for behavior therapy. (**REF.** 5—pp. 357–481)

405. B. Severe depression is the primary indication for ECT. (**REF.** 5—pp. 357–481)

406. D. Neurotic conflicts are a primary indication for psychotherapy. (**REF.** 5—pp. 357–481)

407. D. Adjustment disorders are usually successfully dealt with by psychotherapy. Behavior therapy is not indicated and the other choices are contraindicated for adjustment disorders. (**REF.** 2—p. 1099)

408. B. The anticholinergic side effect of urinary retention may be successfully treated with urecholine. (**REF.** 2—p. 1526)

409. E. Physostigmine is an appropriate intervention for toxic anticholinergic effects such as may be seen with overdose of tricyclic antidepressants. (**REF.** 2—p. 1527)

410. A. Benztropine, among other anti-Parkinsonian agents, is useful in the treatment of extrapyramidal side effects of neuroleptic medications. (**REF.** 2—p. 1507)

411. A. This is the hallmark of delirium. (**REF.** 1—p. 104)

412. D. Dementia may be reversible. (**REF.** 1—p. 108)

413. D. Delirium may be irreversible. (**REF.** 1—pp. 104–107)

414. C. Both may be substance-induced. (**REF.** 1—pp. 104–108)

415. A. Dementia usually has an insidious onset. (**REF.** 1—p. 108)

416. A. Dementia is most often idiopathic. (**REF.** 1—p. 108)

417. C. Both transference and countertransference stem from unconscious sources and are by definition inappropriate to the situation. (**REF.** 4—pp. 745–786)

418. D. Transference and countertransference tend to be focused upon in psychoanalysis or other insight-oriented psychotherapies, but not in supportive or directive psychotherapy or in behavior therapy. (**REF.** 4—pp. 745–786)

419. C. Although often having a positive emotional valence, both transference and countertransference may involve negative feelings or behavior. (**REF.** 4—pp. 745–786)

420. E. High doses of phenylbutazone, indomethacin, and salicylates produce delirium, as do sulfonamides, penicillin, and many antituberculosis agents. Anticholinergics are notorious delirium producers. Although the chronic syndrome is more common, acute bromine-induced toxic psychosis has been described. (**REF.** 3—pp. 404–411)

421. A. Patients with borderline personality disorder are intolerant of being alone. (**REF.** 1—pp. 322–323)

422. B. Patients with compulsive personality disorder tend to be indecisive and conventional in their behavior.(**REF.** 1—pp. 327–328)

423. A. Persons with histrionic personality disorder crave activity and excitement. (**REF.** 1—p. 315)

424. B. A fine rather than a coarse tremor is seen as a side effect of lithium. Nystagmus indicates lithium toxicity. (**REF.** 2—p. 831)

425. E. Cardiac conduction defects, impaired mentation, cerebellar dysfunction, and seizures are all signs of lithium toxicity. (**REF.** 2—p. 831)

426. C. In delirium, psychomotor activity may be increased or decreased and clinical features tend to fluctuate over time. (**REF.** 1—p. 107)

427. E. All are included in the diagnostic criteria for dementia. (**REF.** 1—pp. 111–112)

428. A. The Thematic Apperception Test (TAT) is a projective personality test. The others are used for assessment of organic brain dysfunction. (**REF.** 2—pp. 526, 535–543)

429. B. Neither intensive psychotherapy nor minor tranquilizers have been shown to be effective in chronic alcoholism. Self-help groups, such as Alcoholics Anonymous, and treatment with disulfiram are useful modalities in some cases. (**REF.** 2—pp. 1025–1026)

430. D. The clinical picture is strongly suggestive of anticholinergic toxicity. Lithium carbonate has no significant anticholinergic effects. (**REF.** 2—pp. 721, 827, 831)

431. A. Physostigmine is useful in effecting the immediate reversal of anticholinergic toxicity. The use of atropine in such a circumstance would be absolutely contraindicated. (**REF.** 2—p. 827)

22. Radiology

432. E. This patient has the setup for a Monteggia fracture; that is, whenever there is a fracture of the proximal shaft of the ulna, a proximal radius dislocation may be associated if no radius fracture is evident. Although the radius shaft appears to point normally to the distal humeral capitellum center (C) on one view, a film at right angles is needed to rule out dislocation. It was indeed dislocated in this case. (**REF.** 7—pp. 125, 153) (Fig. 22.1 is reprinted from **REF.** 7, with permission.)

433. A. All of the answers are true, except that it is dangerous for a patient suspected of epiglottitis to be recumbent—breathing may become impossible. The arrowheads point to the diagnostic short, wide, swollen epiglottis. Subglottic narrowing, typical of croup, may also be seen in up to 25% of patients with epiglottitis. (**REF.** 6—pp. 68–69)

434. B. The arrow points to the *falciform ligament* anterior to the liver. It is seen in supine patients (children or adults) only when there is air on either side of it. Thus, it is a strong sign of pneumoperitoneum. The normal space between posterior ribs and vertebral transverse processes should not be confused with fracture. (**REF.** 6—pp. 283–288)

435. A. Sturge–Weber syndrome characteristically has serpiginous cerebral calcification unilaterally as illustrated, along with ipsilateral brain hypoplasia (note shift of midline cranial structures to the side of the calcification, and the larger frontal and ethmoid sinuses on that side). (**REF.** 3—pp. 367–368)

436. E. The discontinuous areas of narrowing and irregularity, incomplete involvement around the colon circumference, as well as the deep ulceration of the proximal lateral descending colon are characteristic of Crohn disease rather than ulcerative colitis or the other entities. (**REF.** 6—pp. 265–269)

437. C. The large varices of the distal two-thirds of the esophagus, which appear as wormlike filling defects, are often associated with portal hypertension, as in this patient. (**REF.** 6—pp. 219–220)

438. D. The intrarenal abnormality (D) has a negative CT number (i.e., blackness), less than, for example, the bile in gallbladder (B). Thus, it likely contains fat, as do many of the angiomyolipomas in this patient with tuberous sclerosis. The aorta (E) is strongly opacified by the contrast injection, while the inferior vena cava (A) is somewhat less dense. The rib (C) just enters the CT slice. (**REF.** 9)

439. A. There is a nonuniform lenticular abnormality of the lateral periphery of the brain typical in form for epidural hematoma. There is little associated midline shift. (**REF.** 6—pp. 25, 28)

440. C. A *persistent* pyloric diameter of over 13 mm during real-time ultrasound study of infants is diagnostic of hypertrophic pyloric stenosis, as is a muscle diameter of 4 mm or a pylorus length of over 20 mm. The echolucent donut represents the hypertrophic muscle. If a typical olive had been felt on physical examination, no imaging would have been required. (**REF.** 8)

441. B. The kidney shows a dilated pelvis, but this image does not disclose whether or not the ureter is dilated. If no dilated ureter is present, ureteropelvic junction obstruction may be present; if the ureter is dilated, vesicoureteral reflux of at least grade 2 (of 5), ureterovesical junction obstruction, or a sufficiently distended bladder may be the cause. In a Page kidney, there is a subcapsular hematoma. (**REF.** 6—pp. 306–317)

442. D. Gallstones. Three small echogenic gallstones (with shadowing) are indicated by the arrows. They lie in the anechoic gallbladder (1) behind the smoothly marginated liver (2). Ultrasound is the screening imaging method of choice for gallstones. (**REF.** 2—pp. 137–146)

443. C. An ovarian cyst. The anechoic (echo-free) physiologic follicular cyst is a common, normal finding on ultrasound examination of the ovary (1). It lies behind the fluid-filled, and thus anechoic, bladder (2). Ultrasound is the screening imaging method of choice for ovary visualization. (**REF.** 4—p. 212)

444. A. Ascites. The anechoic (echo-free) fluid in the peritoneum outlines bowel loops (1) and lies above the bladder (2). Pneumoperitoneum, containing air, would have reflected echoes rather than transmitting them. Ultrasound, CT, and MR imaging are excellent for demonstrating ascites, ultrasound being the readiest available and least expensive; plain abdominal radiographs can suggest ascites as well, but in less detail. (**REF.** 2—pp. 270–281)

445. B. The finding of a fat-fluid level on a horizontal beam (cross-table) view makes the diagnosis of associated knee fracture highly likely. The fat-fluid level lies in the suprapatellar bursa of the knee joint, behind and superior to the patella and anterior to the distal femur. The proximal tibia spine fracture is not well shown on this film. (**REF.** 7—pp. 177, 225)

446. A. The periosteal reaction along the proximal fibula could be due to osteomyelitis, fracture, or metastasis. No fracture is present and metastasis is not offered as a choice. (**REF.** 7—pp. 7–8, 66–74)

447. D. The child shows the cupped, frayed, widened distal radius and ulna metaphyses typical for rickets. There is also secondary hyperparathyroidism, which yields an unsharp, washed-out cortex, unlike osteoporosis, which would manifest a thinned, but well-defined cortex. (**REF.** 7—pp. 9–10, 97–98)

448. E. Cystic fibrosis is present in this 19-year-old, who has acute chest pain from left pneumothorax, a not infrequent complication. Small heart and lung fibrosis and bronchiectasis (with nodules of density in some dilated bronchi) are other characteristic radiographic changes which are present. (**REF.** 3—pp. 856–859)

449. C. Round densities of varying sizes, without calcification, are seen in the lungs of this child with rhabdomyosarcoma. Such metastases are often seen on CT sooner than on plain radiographs or conventional whole-lung tomograms. (**REF.** 1)

450. A. Localized density in the left lower lobe *behind the heart* represents pneumonia. Always look behind the heart. (**REF.** 6—pp. 100–103)

451. B. The stone indicated by an arrow is clearly not in the ureter, but may well be an appendicolith in this patient with burning on urination. His rectal exam was strongly tender to the right. The appendiceal abscess is shown in Fig. 22.22. The presence of a calcified appendicolith in a patient with right lower quadrant pain strongly suggests appendicitis. (**REF.** 6—pp. 270–273)

452. A. This excretory urogram (IVP) pattern is typical for a stone acutely in the distal right ureter. There is delayed visualization of the calyces, pelvis, and ureter on the right (at 7 minutes), and prolonged density of the right kidney, collecting structures, and ureter at 6 hours. (**REF.** 3—pp. 718–721)

453. B. Just behind the filled bladder to the right lies a shadowing (s) appendicolith (arrow) within a low echogenicity abscess (arrowheads) on this transverse sonogram. Whenever an appendicial abscess is near the bladder, ultrasound is an effective method of diagnostic imaging. (**REF.** 6—pp. 270–273)

454. D. The bladder in this patient with typical horseshoe kidneys is merely indented on the right by gas and stool in bowel. The horseshoe kidneys are connected inferiorly in front of the vertebral column, resulting in their unusual position. (**REF.** 6—p. 310)

455. C. The normal dens–anterior arch of C–1 distance should not exceed 3 mm in adults or 5 mm in children. Atlantoaxial subluxation is frequently seen in Down's syndrome, and, as in this child, is often found on screening of the asymptomatic trisomy 21 child. Especially when there is ligamentous laxity or other abnormality, the dens–anterior arch distance does vary between flexion and extension. (**REFS.** 5—pp. 113–114, 7—p. 269)

456. D. This is a depressed skull fracture in a child, which at 7 mm was sufficiently deep for the neurosurgeon to operate. The absence of skull fracture should not reassure—the level of consciousness, state of pupil reaction, and neurologic signs are far more important. CT is the current imaging technique if intracranial hemorrhage is suspected; hemorrhage may be present without fracture. Tangential views or CT are usually necessary to show how depressed a fracture is. Skull radiographs do not rule out intracranial injury and may delay proper treatment. (**REF.** 6—pp. 23–28)

457. A. This patient with a blowout fracture of the orbit shows the three classic imaging findings: (1) gas-blood level in the maxillary sinus; (2) fracture fragment of the orbital floor; and (3) hematoma and/or extraocular muscle protrusion into the roof of the sinus. Both sides show normal slight protrusion of tooth roots at the floor of the sinus. (**REF.** 3—pp. 1173–1174)

458. B. There is a transverse fracture of the navicular, which is on the lateral side of the wrist. The lunate (medial to the navicular) is normally aligned with radius and capitate. It is the *proximal* navicular that may develop avascularity problems following such a fracture. (**REF.** 3—pp. 154–155)

459. E. This patient has an enlarged central silhouette from pericardial effusion, as well as a thin right lateral stripe of pleural effusion. Ultrasound easily distinguishes pericardial effusion from cardiomegaly. The azygous fissure variant shows a curvilinear line of the medial right upper lobe, which is indeed not present in this patient. (**REF.** 6—pp. 415–417)

460. D. Wilms' tumor is an intrarenal tumor, often found incidentally in children this age. Neuroblastoma, the other common intraabdominal tumor of young children, is extrarenal, most often in the adrenal. Renal cell carcinoma is uncommon below the age of 10. This lesion has neither anechoic cysts nor the heavy echoes of fat as might be seen in angiomyolipoma. (**REF.** 4—pp. 190–196)

461. C. Except for the bladder, each site is important to search for extension of Wilms' tumor or metastases. (**REF.** 6—pp. 44–45)

23. Surgery

462. D. Anticoagulation using heparin is the primary therapy for pulmonary embolism. Recurrent embolism might require inferior vena caval clipping and/or pulmonary embolectomy. Streptokinase has been of some value in experimental studies. (**REF.** 1—p. 1740)

463. D. Lobular carcinoma has been reported to be bilateral in up to 20% of patients. The exact significance of this is not fully appreciated. Simultaneous breast cancer occurs in 1–2% of women, and a further 8–10% develop a secondary primary in the remaining breast. (**REF.** 2—p. 539)

464. C. The history of this patient and the fact that the most common cause of bowel obstruction is adhesions would indicate that this is mechanical bowel obstruction. Fever is not an accompaniment of early mechanical obstruction. It is seen in paralytic and strangulated obstruction. (**REFS.** 1—pp. 802–806; 2—pp. 1034–1045)

465. B. The history is characteristic of the patient who has compromise of arterial flow. Immediate treatment is to cut the cast and extend the elbow. At this stage one should check for return of radial pulse at the wrist. Delay in performing this might lead to Volkmann's ischemic contracture of the hand. (**REF.** 2—p. 1970)

466. B. Osteosarcoma is the most common malignant tumor in young adults. The most frequent site is on either side of the knee joint. The tumor may be associated with fluid in the joint and mechanical limitation of range of function. Classically it is associated with destruction of old bone and neoplastic new bone formation. (**REF.** 2—pp. 1935–1936)

467. B. Cephalothin is not effective against *Bacteroides fragilis*. All the other antibiotics listed are effective. Some of the newer cephalosporins, such as cefoxitin, are effective against *Bacteroides*. (**REF.** 2—p. 156)

468. C. Serum amylase value is of no significance in the prognosis of patients with acute pancreatic disease. All others are well-documented features that indicate poor prognosis. (**REFS.** 1—p. 1180; 2—p. 1352)

469. A. The Romberg-Howship sign is seen in obturator hernia. This sign is the association of pain in the knee joint with increased pressure in an obturator hernia and is due to stretching of the obturator nerve that passes through the same opening as the hernia. (**REF.** 1—p. 1248)

470. D. A direct inguinal hernia usually occurs through Hasselbach's triangle, which is bounded laterally by the inferior epigastric vessels, medially by the lateral border of the rectus sheath, and inferiorly by the inguinal ligament. (**REF.** 1—p. 1235)

471. C. Ventral hernias usually occur through scars of previous operations and have a wide neck. Consequently, strangulation is rare, although incarceration is seen frequently. (**REF.** 1—p. 1249)

472. E. Indirect inguinal hernia is seen commonly in young individuals and is caused by a congenital sac. (**REF.** 1—p. 1240)

473. A. Alpha-fetoprotein is normally formed in the fetus and also in the serum of patients with malignant hepatic tumors. It is found in about 50% of liver tumor patients in the African population, but only in 30% of those in the Western countries. Following complete removal of the tumor, this protein disappears from the serum, but may reappear with recurrence. (**REF.** 1—p. 1086)

474. B. CEA is another fetal antigen that appears in the serum of patients with carcinoma of the colon. It is also found in patients with cancer of the pancreas and has a similar prognostic value as in the previous situation. (**REF.** 2—p. 1206)

475. C. Testicular tumors, particularly the undifferentiated chorionic varieties, cause elevated levels of serum chorionic gonadotropin. (**REF.** 1—p. 1676)

476. E. Functioning carcinoid tumors secrete 5-hydroxytryptamine (5-HT). The end product of 5-HT is 5-hydroxyindoleacetic acid (5-HIAA), and this is found in urine. Elevated levels of 5-HIAA in urine are helpful in the diagnosis and followup of patients with carcinoid tumors. (**REF.** 2—p. 1157)

477. D. Neuroblastomas are histologically related to pheochromocytomas and usually arise from adrenal medulla. These tumors also may secrete epinephrine or norepinephrine and the end products of breakdown of these can be found in the urine as VMA. (**REF.** 2—p. 1533)

478. C. Phenoxybenzamine is an alpha-adrenergic receptor blocking agent. Its use in shock is to improve tissue perfusion, but it is essential to make sure that there is adequate volume and adequate right-sided filling pressure. (**REF.** 1—p. 685)

479. E. Isoproterenol is a pure stimulant of beta-adrenergic receptors. It produces a tachycardia and thereby increases cardiac output. By reducing peripheral resistance, it improves blood flow to all organs except the brain. (**REF.** 1—p. 2452)

480. D. Norepinephrine is a primary alpha-adrenergic receptor stimulator on the peripheral circulation and has a beta-adrenergic stimulating activity on the heart and metabolism. Its use results in an increase in arterial blood pressure due to an increase in peripheral resistance. (**REF.** 1—p. 679)

481. B. Dopamine is an intermediate product in the synthesis of epinephrine and norepinephrine and is effective in increasing myocardial contractility without the peripheral vasoactive effects on the other amines. (**REF.** 1—p. 2451)

482. A. Toxic megacolon is associated with ulcerative colitis and not with Crohn's enteritis. (**REF.** 2—p. 1178)

483. A. Massive bleeding is a feature of ulcerative colitis. There may be a minor bleed with regional enteritis, but massive bleeding is very uncommon. (**REF.** 2—pp. 1178, 1180)

484. B. Crohn's disease is associated with fistula formation and this fistula may be enteroenteric, enterocolic, or enterovesical. On the other hand, ulcerative colitis is not often associated with fistula formation. (**REF.** 2—p. 1180)

485. C. Both diseases are associated with a number of extraintestinal manifestations and arthritis is seen in both diseases. (**REF.** 2—pp. 1178, 1180)

486. B. Salivary gland tumors are the most common in the parotid gland, which is the largest of the salivary glands, and most are benign. The most common tumor is a mixed tumor, also called a pleomorphic adenoma. Sialography is not helpful in the diagnosis or management of these tumors. (**REF.** 1—pp. 1359–1361)

487. A. Although indications for laminectomy are somewhat controversial, most neurosurgeons feel that compression or bony penetration of the spinal canal, injury of the cauda equina, or progressive neurologic deficit in any patient who has a partial spinal cord lesion justifies surgical exploration. The most difficult decision in the early treatment of spinal cord injury is whether or not to decompress the spinal cord; while some surgeons perform a laminectomy in any severe injury in the belief that the procedure is of some general value in reducing edema and swelling, others perform laminectomy only when there is a later progression of neurologic deficit. Penetrating wounds that result in total cord injury are rarely improved, however, by exploration, although some benefit may be gained from exploration of incomplete lumbar or cervical injuries. A high, complete cervical spinal cord lesion accompanied by respiratory paralysis contraindicates surgical intervention. (**REF.** 2—p. 1796)

488. D. The inferior mesenteric artery is usually occluded by thrombus or clot formation within the aneurysm. Collateral circulation is usually through the marginal artery, and the middle colic from above and the inferior hemorrhoidal from below maintain circulation to the left colon. (**REF.** 1—p. 1938)

489. E. The sudden onset of pain in the right chest with cough, shortness of breath, and hemoptysis on the sixth postoperative day is a classic presentation of pulmonary embolism. Subphrenic abscess does not appear as a sudden event. Atelectasis usually occurs in patients who are bedridden and have not been ambulated. It could be that acute myocardial infarction might produce right-sided pain, but the most common cause of the symptoms described is a pulmonary embolism. (**REFS.** 1—pp. 1737–1738; 2—p. 984)

490. C. The common femoral veins are the most common source of pulmonary emboli. Radioisotopic studies have indicated that thrombosis occurs most often in the smaller veins of the calf and the plantar plexus, but the ones that are likely to cause emboli usually arise from the common femoral veins. (**REF.** 1—p. 1731)

491. C. The history and findings are classic of acute arterial embolus. Symptoms of arterial thrombosis are slow and do not have a sudden onset. Deep venous thrombosis does not produce sudden severe pain in the leg. The embolus in this situation usually arises from the infarcted area in the left ventricle. Pain of dissecting aneurysm usually is in the chest and the abdomen, not in the leg. (**REF.** 2—p. 900)

492. C. A patient with an acute embolus should be operated on immediately. While waiting for the operation, the patient should be anticoagulated. Other methods of treatment outlined are not acceptable in the management of acute embolism. (**REF.** 2— pp. 900–901)

493. D. The x-ray shows the classic feature of a "double bubble." This is usually caused by duodenal atresia or annular pancreas. It also may be produced by peritoneal bands or intestinal malrotation. Congenital pyloric stenosis is not associated with a double-bubble appearance. Further, pyloric stenosis usually manifests itself 6–8 weeks after birth. (**REF.** 1—pp. 848, 876)

494. C. A duodenoduodenostomy is the choice of operation for either an atresia or for an annulus of the pancreas. Division of the annulus might result in a pancreatic ductal fistula. Gastrojejunostomy leaves the child at risk for anastomotic ulceration. A Billroth II or pyloromyotomy is not indicated. (**REF.** 2—p. 1347)

495. D. The x-ray shows a thin film of air under both domes of the diaphragm. This feature of pneumoperitoneum is most often the result of a perforated peptic ulcer. The second most frequent cause is a perforated diverticulum. This finding is not associated with myocardial infarction or any of the other conditions listed. (**REF.** 1—p. 799)

496. C. Closure of a perforated ulcer is the simplest and the safest operation. This patient has had a myocardial infarction and probably has pulmonary damage due to chronic smoking. In such a situation the minimum should be done. Laparotomy and drainage alone leaves the perforation untouched and might permit continued contamination of the peritoneal cavity. Surgical rather than conservative treatment always gives better results. (**REF.** 1— p. 799)

497. C. The lesion shown in Fig. 23.3 is the classic villous adenoma. There is no invasion of the tumor through the stroma or at the base. (**REFS.** 1—p. 1004; 2—p. 1193)

498. A. Since the lesion histologically appears benign, it can be adequately excised through a proctoscope. Proctectomy and abdominoperineal resection are only indicated when there is definite evidence of malignancy. Most rectal villous adenomas can be adequately excised through a proctoscope. Fulguration does not provide tissue for adequate examination of the detail. (**REF.** 2—pp. 1192–1194)

499. A. Some villous adenomas are associated with massive secretion of mucous and diarrhea. This massive mucous diarrhea is associated with hypokalemia, hyponatremia, hypochloremia, and dehydration. Hypocalcemia is not a feature. (**REF.** 1—p. 1004)

500. D. The swelling described in the left groin is typical of a varicocele. In addition, the intravenous pyelogram shows a mass in the left kidney and deformity of the left renal pelvis and calyces. Therefore, the answer is D. A left-sided varicocele in the young may be idiopathic, but the onset of a left-sided varicocele in the adult should raise the suspicion of a left renal tumor that has extended through the left renal vein and has blocked the left testicular venous drainage. (**REF.** 2—p. 1685)

501. D. In the further evaluation of a renal mass, selective abdominal arteriography is most valuable. This will not only indicate whether the lesion is avascular (such as a cystic lesion), but also can help differentiate benign from malignant renal tumors. (**REF.** 2—p. 1707)

502. B. Renal cell carcinomas are associated with increased red cell mass because of production of erythropoietin. Testicular tumors are associated with increased chorionic gonadotropin levels, while hepatic tumors produce elevated alpha-fetoprotein levels. VMA levels in urine are increased in pheochromocytomas and in neuroblastomas. Elevated serum acid phosphatase is a finding associated with prostatic cancer. (**REF.** 1—p. 1650)

503. B. The scintiscan of this 45-year-old female shows a non-functioning nodule in the right lobe of the thyroid. The ideal definitive management of this is by lobectomy. There is an increased incidence of malignancy in "cold" solitary nodules. Because of the risk of malignancy, suppression therapy should not be used, since this will delay the diagnosis. Fine needle aspiration cytology is a safe, effective, and often reliable method of making a diagnosis. (**REF.** 1—p. 602)

504. D. With a diagnosis of papillary carcinoma, the best treatment is near-total thyroidectomy and the administration of thyroxin. This tumor may be multicentric and hence it is necessary to go back and remove as much thyroid tissue as possible. The administration of thyroxin is to suppress secretion of TSH by the pituitary and thereby further suppress growth of any residual tumor. (**REF.** 1—p. 605)

505. C. Childhood irradiation of the face, neck, or the upper chest has been associated with a high incidence of thyroid cancer. Other factors listed are not carcinogenic for the thyroid. (**REF.** 1—p. 603)

506. B. The history of abdominal pain, diarrhea, and weight loss in a young female and the associated x-ray findings indicate a diagnosis of Crohn's disease. The x-ray shows multiple narrowed segments of the small bowel and one particularly in the ileum. Appendicitis is usually associated with acute onset and a short history. Carcinoid tumors do not produce diarrhea as much as chronic bowel obstruction. Amoebic disease affects the colon, and carcinoma of the small bowel is very uncommon. (**REF.** 1—pp. 914–927)

507. D. Endocarditis (of tricuspid and pulmonary valves) is seen in association with a carcinoid tumor secreting 5-hydroxytryptamine. All others are associated manifestations of Crohn's disease. (**REF.** 1—pp. 921–922)

508. C. Radical surgical treatment does not prevent recurrence. In fact, recurrence of Crohn's disease occurs frequently irrespective of the treatment undertaken. All others are correct. (**REF.** 1—pp. 924–927)

509. D. The early management of a severely injured patient demands that attention first be given to injuries that interfere with vital physiologic functions. Since hypoxia may be lethal within a matter of minutes, establishing an effective airway is the most important therapeutic priority. Then, exsanguinating hemorrhage should be rapidly controlled and shock resuscitation begun by administering an intravenous balanced salt solution and drawing blood for typing and cross-matching. Assurance of tetanus prophylaxis is important but of less priority than the establishment of an adequate airway and control of hemorrhagic shock. (**REF.** 2—p. 200)

510. C. Direct finger pressure on a bleeding wound or blood vessel is the safest, most effective means of temporarily controlling external hemorrhage. Arterial tourniquets may lead to tissue loss through occlusion of collateral circulation. Venous tourniquets, which are tight enough to obstruct venous return but loose enough not to occlude arterial flow, accentuate blood loss while increasing edema in the area of injury. Although superficial vessels that are easily visible may be clamped and ligated, unnecessary probing of a wound with a hemostat may lead to injury of nearby structures and enhance the risk of infection. Application of a gravitational pressure suit may aid in treating profound shock from major intra-abdominal hemorrhage, but has no major role in the control of external hemorrhage. (**REF.** 2—p. 200)

511. D. If a patient who has been exposed to smoke, especially within a closed space, begins to display signs of agitation and confusion, a diagnosis of acute carbon monoxide poisoning should be suspected. Specific treatment for this condition consists of administration of oxygen. Nonspecific treatment includes rapid fluid resuscitation when necessary, escharotomies of the abdomen and chest as needed to avoid inhibition of diaphragmatic and chest wall excursion, provision of a warm, dry environment to minimize oxygen demands, frequent monitoring of respiratory function, and the provision of humidified air to breathe. Because acute hypovolemia or head trauma may cause the same clinical findings as smoke inhalation, when a history of smoke exposure is present, oxygen should be administered immediately and then further workup for blood loss or closed head injury should be undertaken.

Sedation with morphine or with major tranquilizers of a patient who had been exposed to smoke can depress respiration and may interfere with further evaluation for other injuries. (**REF.** 2— p. 270)

512. A. The x-ray is a lateral view of the upper abdomen showing gallbladder with stones. The procedure was an oral cholecysto-gram. Since this is a lateral view and the shadows are in front, they cannot be renal stones. Osteoarthritis does not produce right upper quadrant pain alone. Most common cause of right upper quadrant pain in a middle-aged female is cholelithiasis with cho-lecystitis. The best way to visualize air in the portal system is an anterior–posterior view, not a lateral view. The x-ray also shows multiple filling defects in the gallbladder with central densities diagnostic of gallstones. (**REF.** 2—p. 1316)

513. E. Sclerosing cholangitis is a rare diffuse chronic inflamma-tion of unknown etiology and is not related to gallstones. All other conditions could be secondary to stones in the gallbladder that have migrated into the common duct. Cancer of the gallbladder is associated with stones in about 90–95% of patients, and although not all patients with gallstones develop cancer, the association is remarkable. (**REF.** 2—p. 1322)

514. D. The ideal management of cholelithiasis with chronic cho-lecystitis is a cholecystectomy and operative cholangiography. Most centers do a routine operative cholangiogram so that the presence of any stones in the common duct can be recognized and, further, the ductal anatomy is clear. Exploration of the duct is only required when there are stones or stricture of the common bile duct. In the past, cholecystectomy alone was done without operative cholangiography, but because of the reasons mentioned above, most surgeons now perform an operative cholangiography. Cholecystostomy is occasionally performed for acute cholecystitis when the patient is sick and the anatomy is not very clear. The treatment of gallstones with chenodeoxycholic acid has not been very successful. It only works in cholesterol stones and is not ap-plicable for mixed stones or very large stones, and patients do not tolerate the drug well. (**REF.** 2—p. 1327)

515. D. The upper gastrointestinal series demonstrates a large filling defect in the distal half of the stomach, and this is due to a cancer. Gastric ulcers usually have a base that lies outside the gastric contour. The patient does have an esophageal diverticulum, but this could not be the cause of the anorexia, weight loss, melena, and vomiting. (**REF.** 2—p. 1133)

516. D. Previous peptic gastric ulceration is not an etiologic factor for gastric cancer. For many years it was thought that cancer could arise from a benign peptic ulcer. This was a problem in understanding its etiology, and now it is believed that gastric cancers arise de novo and it is seldom that benign gastric ulcers become malignant. All other factors are associated with gastric cancer. (**REF.** 2—p. 1133)

517. C. The choice of operation is a radical distal subtotal gastrectomy. This would involve removal of the distal part of the stomach, the first part of the duodenum, the omentum, and the lymph nodes in the gastrohepatic ligament. If necessary, a splenectomy can also be added to the situation. A simple partial gastrectomy without removing the lymph node area is an inadequate operation. On the other hand, total gastrectomy carries a high mortality and does not improve the results. A gastrojejunostomy may be occasionally considered for relief of obstruction due to cancer, but is not a procedure of choice because it still leaves an ulcerated bleeding tumor in the stomach. A radical pancreaticoduodenectomy is usually performed for cancer of the second part of the duodenum, cancer of the head of the pancreas, or cancer of the terminal bile duct. (**REF.** 2—p. 1134)

518. C. The lesion shown is a large abdominal aortic aneurysm which is located infrarenally. Both kidneys are well-visualized, and there is no evidence of a renal tumor. An aortocaval fistula would be associated with a large bruit, congestive heart failure, and visualization of the inferior vena cava during the angiogram. A patient with aortoduodenal fistula will present with massive GI bleeding. Aortography is a useful technique in evaluation of abdominal aortic aneurysms. (**REF.** 1—pp. 1830–1837)

519. E. Hypertension is associated in about 40% of patients with abdominal aortic aneurysms. Involvement of renal vessels is very uncommon and is only seen in 1–2%. Concomitant aneurysms of the popliteal and femoral vessels are also very uncommon. The risk of distal emboli does exist, but this manifestation is also very uncommon. (**REF.** 2—p. 949)

520. C. Ischemic colitis is the complication that should be considered in the immediate postoperative period. Aortoduodenal fistula do not manifest that early, and renal failure with uremic ulceration is very uncommon in elective abdominal aortic surgery. On the other hand, ischemic colitis is a significant problem and occurs if at least one of the internal iliac vessels is not left open. (**REF.** 2—p. 954)

References

10. Anesthesiology

1. Miller R.D. (Ed): *Anesthesia*, 2nd Edition, Churchill Livingstone, New York, NY 1985

2. Stoelting R.K. and Dierdorf S.F. (Eds): *Anesthesia and Co-Existing Diseases*, Churchill Livingstone, New York, NY, 1983

11. Emergency Medicine

1. Barkin R.M. and Rosen P.: *Emergency Pediatrics*, C.V. Mosby, St. Louis, MO, 1984

2. Behrman R.E. and Vaughan III V.C.: *Nelson Textbook of Pediatrics*, 12th Edition, W.B. Saunders, Philadelphia, PA, 1985

3. Haddad L.M. and Winchester J.F.: *Clinical Management of Poisoning and Drug Overdose*, W.B. Saunders, Philadelphia, PA, 1983

4. Roberts J.R. and Hedges J.R.: *Clinical Procedures in Emergency Medicine*, W.B. Saunders, Philadelphia, PA, 1985

5. Rosen P., Baker F.J., Braen G.R., Dailey R.H., and Levy R.C.: *Emergency Medicine, Concepts and Clinical Practice*, C.V. Mosby, St. Louis, MO, 1983

6. Schwartz G.R., Safar P., Stone J.H., Storey P.B., and Wagner D.K.: *Principles and Practice of Emergency Medicine*, 2nd Edition, W.B. Saunders, Philadelphia, PA, 1986

7. Wyngarden J.B. and Smith L.H.: *Cecil Textbook of Medicine*, 17th Edition, W.B. Saunders, Philadelphia, PA, 1985

8. Zuidema G.D., Rutherford R.B., and Ballinger W.F.: *The Management of Trauma*, 4th Edition, W.B. Saunders, Philadelphia, PA, 1985

12. Family Medicine

1. Ballenger J.J.: *Diseases of the Nose, Throat, Ear, Head, and Neck*, 13th Edition, Lea & Febiger, Philadelphia, PA, 1985

2. Fanaroff M.B. et al. (Eds): *Behrman's Neonatal Perinatal Medicine (Diseases of the Fetus and Infant)*, 3rd Edition, C.V. Mosby, St. Louis, MO, 1983

3. Gilman A. et al.: *The Pharmacological Basis of Therapeutics*, 7th edition, Macmillan, New York, NY, 1985

4. Kaplan H.I.: *Comprehensive Textbook of Psychiatry*, 4th Edition, Volume 1, Williams & Wilkins, Baltimore, MD, 1984

5. O'Brien R. and Chafety M.: *The Encyclopedia of Alcoholism*, Facts on File, New York, NY, 1982

6. Pritchard J.A. et al. (Eds): *Williams Obstetrics*, Appleton-Century-Crofts, Norwalk, CT, 1984

7. Schwartz S.I. et al.: *Principles of Surgery*, 4th Edition, McGraw-Hill, New York, NY, 1985

8. Wyngaarden J.B. and Smith L.H.: *Loeb Textbook of Medicine*, Vol. 2, W.B. Saunders, Philadelphia, PA, 1985

13. Internal Medicine

1. Hurst J.W., Logue R.B., Rackley C.E., Schlant R.C., Sonnenblick E.H., Wallace A.G., and Wenger N.K.: *The Heart*, 6th Edition, McGraw-Hill, New York, NY, 1986

2. Rakel R.E.: *Conn's Current Therapy*, W.B. Saunders, Philadelphia, PA, 1986

3. Williams W.J., Beutler E., Erslev A.J., and Lichtman M.A.: *Hematology*, 3rd Edition, McGraw-Hill, New York, NY, 1983

4. Wyngaarden J.B. and Smith L.H.: *Cecil Textbook of Medicine*, 17th Edition, W.B. Saunders, Philadelphia, PA, 1985

14. Medical Ethics

1. Abrams A. and Buckner M.D.: *Medical Ethics*, MIT Press, Cambridge, MA, 1983

2. Engelhardt Jr. H.: *The Foundations of Bioethics*, Oxford University Press, New York, NY, 1986

3. Hiller, M.D.: *Medical Ethics and the Law*, Ballinger, Cambridge, MA, 1981

4. McCormick, R.A.: *How Brave a New World*, Doubleday, Garden City, NY, 1981

15. Neurology

1. Aminoff M. (Ed): *Neurologic Clinics, August 1985: Electrodiagnosis*, W.B. Saunders, Philadelphia, PA, 1985

2. Dalessio D.J.: Seizure disorders and pregnancy. *N Eng J Med.* 312:559, 1985

3. Gilroy J. and Meyer J.S.: *Medical Neurology*, Macmillan, New York, NY, 1979

4. Jankovic J. (Ed): *Neurologic Clinics Aug 1984: Movement Disorders*, W.B. Saunders, Philadelphia, PA, 1984

5. Kirshner H.S.: *Behavioral Neurology*, Churchill Livingstone, New York, NY, 1986

6. Lindsley D.F. and Holmes J.E.: *Basic Human Neurophysiology*, Elsevier, New York, NY, 1984

7. Medical Research Council: *Aids to the Examination of the Peripheral Nervous System*, Her Majesty's Stationery Office, London, 1976

8. Plum F. and Posner J.B.: *The Diagnosis of Stupor and Coma*, F.A. Davis, Philadelphia, PA, 1980

9. Swaiman K. (Ed): *Neurologic Clinics Feb 1985: Pediatric Neurology*, W.B. Saunders, Philadelphia, PA, 1985

10. Toole, J.F.: *Cerebrovascular Disorders*, 3rd Edition, Raven, New York, NY, 1984

11. Zimmerman E.A. and Nilaver G.: Neuroendocrinology. In *Current Neurology*, Vol. 3 Appel, S. (Ed), Wiley, New York, NY, 1981

16. Obstetrics and Gynecology

1. Brown E.R. and Nair V.: Laboratory identification of sexually transmitted diseases. *J Reprod Med.* 30:3, 1985

2. Danforth D.N.: *Obstetrics and Gynecology*, 5th Edition, Harper & Row, Hagerstown, MD, 1986

3. Herbst A.L et al.: DES exposed offspring. *Contemp OB/GYN.* 7, 1985.

4. Laube D.W.: Premenstrual syndrome. *Female Patient.* 11:1, 1986

5. Mann L.I. et al.: Common obstetric problems. *Female Patient.* 9:4, 1984

6. Micha, J.P.: Genital warts: Treatable warning of cancer. *Female Patient.* 9:10, 1984

7. Pritchard J.A., MacDonald P.C., and Gant N.F.: *Williams Obstetrics*, Appleton-Century-Crofts, Norwalk, CT, 1985

8. Nadelson C.C., and Notman, M.T.: Caring for the rape victim. *Female Patient.* 10:3, 1985

9. Semchyshyn S.: Preventing prematurity. *Female Patient.* 11:1, 1986

10. Speroff L.: Why mammography is effective. *Contemp OB/GYN.* 9, 1985

11. Sutherland J.E. and Gebhart R.M.: The protocol for periodic health examinations. *Female Patient.* 11:2, 1986

12. Wilson J.R., Carrington E.R., and Ledger W.J.; *Obstetrics & Gynecology*, 7th Edition, C.V. Mosby, St. Louis, MO, 1983

17. Ophthalmology

1. Henkind P., Walsh J.B., and Berger A.N. (Eds): Physicians Desk Reference for Ophthalmology, 14th Edition, Medical Economics Co., Oradell, NJ, 1986

2. Newell F.: *Ophthalmology Principles and Concepts*, 5th Edition, C.V. Mosby, St. Louis, MO, 1982

3. Scheie H.G. and Albert D.M.: *Textbook of Ophthalmology*, W.B. Saunders, Philadelphia, PA, 1977

4. Thorn G.W., Adams R.D., Braunwald E., Isselbacher K.J., and Petersdorf R.G. (Eds): *Harrison's Principles of Internal Medicine*, 8th Edition, McGraw-Hill, New York, NY, 1977

18. Otorhinolaryngology

1. Ballenger J.J.: *Diseases of the Nose, Throat, Ear, Head, and Neck*, 13th Edition, Lea & Febiger, Philadelphia, PA, 1985

2. DeWeese D.D. and Saunders W.H.: *Textbook of Otolaryngology*, 6th Edition, C.V. Mosby, St. Louis, MO, 1982

3. Karmody C.S.: *Textbook of Otolaryngology*, Lea & Febiger, Philadelphia, PA, 1983

19. Pediatrics

1. Behrman R.E., Vaughan III V., and Nelson W.E. (Eds): *Nelson Textbook of Pediatrics*, 11th Edition, W.B. Saunders, Philadelphia, PA, 1982

2. Fanaroff A. and Martin R. (Eds): *Behrman's Neonatal Perinatal Medicine*, C.V. Mosby, St. Louis, MO, 1983

3. *1986 Red Book: Report of the Committee on Infectious Diseases*, American Academy of Pediatrics, 1986

4. Rudolph A. and Barnett L. (Eds): *Pediatrics*, 16th Edition, Appleton-Century-Crofts, Norwalk, CT, 1977

20. Public Health and Preventive Medicine

1. Burton L.E. and Smith H.H.: *Public Health and Community Medicine*, 2nd Edition, Williams & Wilkins, Baltimore, MD, 1975

2. *CA-A Cancer Journal for Clinicians* 36(1), January/February 1986.

3. Friedman G.D.: *Primer of Epidemiology*, McGraw-Hill, New York, NY, 1980

4. Hanlon J.J.: *Public Health Administration and Practice*, 6th Edition, C.V. Mosby, St. Louis, MO, 1974

5. Johnson R.R.: *Elementary Statistics*, 2nd Edition, Duxbery Press, North Scituate, MA, 1976

6. Last J.M.: *Public Health and Preventive Medicine*, 12th Edition, Appleton-Century-Crofts, New York, NY, 1986

7. MacMahon B. and Pugh T.F.: *Epidemiology Principles and Practice*, Little, Brown, Boston, MA, 1970

8. Mausner J.S. and Kramer S.: *Epidemiology an Introductory Text*, W.B. Saunders, Philadelphia, PA, 1985

9. *Morbidity and Mortality Weekly Report.* 35:5, February 7, 1986

10. *Morbidity and Mortality Weekly Report.* 35:6, February 14, 1986

11. *New Directions in International Health Cooperation, A Report to the President*, U.S. Government Printing Office, Stock Number 040-000-00404-1, Washington, D.C., 1978

12. Turner C.E.: *Personal and Community Health*, 14th Edition, C.V. Mosby, St. Louis, MO, 1971

21. Psychiatry

1. American Psychiatric Association: *Diagnostic and Statistical Manual of Mental Disorders*, 3rd Edition, APA, Washington, D.C., 1980

2. Kaplan H.I. and Sadock B.J.: *Comprehensive Textbook of Psychiatry*, 4th Edition, Williams & Wilkins, Baltimore, MD, 1985

3. Kaplan H.I. and Sadock B.J.: *Modern Synopsis of Comprehensive Textbook of Psychiatry*, 3rd Edition, Williams & Wilkins, Baltimore, MD, 1981

4. Kolb L.C. and Brodie H.K.H.: *Modern Clinical Psychiatry*, 10th Edition, W.B. Saunders, Philadelphia, PA, 1982

5. Nicholi A.M. (Ed): *The Harvard Guide to Modern Psychiatry*, Belknap Press of Harvard, Cambridge, MA, 1978

6. Simons R.C. and Pardes H.: *Understanding Human Behavior in Health and Illness*, 2nd Edition, Williams & Wilkins, Baltimore, MD, 1981

22. Radiology

1. Cohen M., Grosfeld J., Baehner R., and Weetman R.: Lung CT for detection of metastases. *Am J Roentgenol*. 139:895–898, 1982

2. Goldberg B.B. (Ed): *Abdominal Ultrasonography*, 2nd Edition, Wiley, New York, 1984

3. Juhl J.H.: *Essentials of Roentgen Interpretation*, 4th Edition, Harper & Row, Hagerstown, MD, 1981

4. Kalifa G. (Ed): *Pediatric Ultrasonography*, Springer-Verlag, Berlin, 1986

5. Keats T.E. and Lusted L.B.: *Atlas of Roentgenographic Measurement*, 5th Edition, Year Book, Chicago, 1985

6. Oestreich A.E.: *Pediatric Radiology—Medical Outline Series*, 3rd Edition, Medical Examination, New Hyde Park, NY, 1984

7. Oestreich A.E. and Crawford A.H.: *Atlas of Pediatric Orthopedic Radiology*, Thieme, Stuttgart, 1985

8. Sauerbrei E.E. and Paloschi G.G.B.: The ultrasonic features of hypertrophic phyloric stenosis. *Radiology*. 147:503–506, 1983

9. Sherman J.L. et al.: Angiomyolipoma. *Am J Roentgenol*. 137:1221–1226, 1981

23. Surgery

1. Sabiston D.C.: *David-Christopher Textbook of Surgery*, 13th Edition, W.B. Saunders, Philadelphia, PA, 1986

2. Schwartz D.I. (Ed): *Principles of Surgery*, 4rd Edition, McGraw-Hill, New York, NY, 1984

PART III

The third and final part of *FLEX Review* corresponds to Day III of the Federation Licensing Examination (FLEX), a measure of what examining boards term "clinical competence." Like the exam itself, this portion of the review comprises three separate sections: therapeutics, pictorial, and patient management problems.

The 25 multiple-choice questions on therapeutics offer a multidisciplinary review of drug therapy. These questions are designed to test your knowledge of the appropriate use of therapeutic modalities in patient care. The answers, comments, and references for this and the following section begin on page 416.

The 30 multiple-choice questions in the pictorial section are intended to exercise your clinical interpretive skills. These questions are based on a variety of pictorial materials, including roentgenograms, chemistry profiles, patient photographs, pictures of various lesions, and graphs and diagrams of several kinds.

Ten patient management problems, two each in medicine, obstetrics and gynecology, pediatrics, and surgery, and one each in psychiatry and radiology, make up the final section. Detailed instructions for responding to these specially constructed problems are found on page 423. A response section follows the patient management problems. A pen for revealing the latent images is attached.

24

Therapeutics
Jared Zelman, M. D., F. A. A. F. P.

DIRECTIONS Each of the questions or incomplete statements below is followed by four or five suggested answers or completions. Select the **one** that is best in each case.

1. Verapamil may be used with all of the following medications EXCEPT
   A. concomitant use of lidocaine
   B. concomitant use of digitalis
   C. concomitant use of IV propranolol
   D. concomitant use of thyroid extract
   E. concomitant use of coumadin

2. Nitroprusside is the drug of choice in hypertensive crisis, EXCEPT in the following clinical situation:
   A. Aortic dissection
   B. Toxemia of pregnancy
   C. Hypertension with stroke syndromes
   D. Hypertension with pulmonary edema
   E. Hypertension with congestive heart failure and angina

3. All of the following drugs are useful in treating patients with PAT (paroxysmal atrial tachycardia) EXCEPT
   A. lidocaine
   B. procainamide
   C. digitalis
   D. verapamil
   E. propranolol

4. Regular insulin
   A. reaches its peak in 2–8 hours and has duration of 5–6 hours.
   B. reaches its peak in 1–2 hours and has a duration of 12–16 hours
   C. reaches its peak in 1–2 hours and has a duration of 5–6 hours
   D. reaches its peak in 2–8 hours and has a duration of 24–28 hours

5. The need for insulin is increased by all of the following EXCEPT
   A. pregnancy
   B. infections, fever, and sepsis
   C. "idiopathic spontaneous exacerbations"
   D. hypothyroidism
   E. deep x-ray therapy and ultraviolet-ray burns

6. Phenobarbital and other inducers of hepatic enzymes increase plasma levels of
   A. warfarin
   B. digitoxin
   C. quinidine
   D. dexamethasone
   E. none of the above

7. In which of the following antibiotics would aluminum ions, present in antacids, be more likely to form insoluble chelates and prevent absorption?
   A. Penicillins
   B. Tetracyclines
   C. Erythromycin
   D. Sulfonamides
   E. None of the above

DIRECTIONS: Each group of questions below consists of five lettered headings followed by a list of numbered words or statements. For **each** numbered word or statement, select the **one** lettered heading that is most closely associated with it. Each lettered heading may be selected once, more than once, or not at all.

Questions 8–12: Match the drug with its antidote.

   A. Acetaminophen
   B. Bromide
   C. Heavy metals
   D. Isoniazid
   E. Cyanide

8. BAL, penicillamine, disodium edetate

9. Pyridoxine

10. Amyl nitrite perles, sodium nitrite, sodium thiosulfate

11. Sodium chloride

12. N-Acetylcysteine

Questions 13–18: Match the drug with its antidote.

    A. Deferoxamine
    B. Atropine and Pralidoxime (2-PAM)
    C. Ethanol
    D. Oxygen
    E. Naloxone (Narcan)

13. Organophosphates

14. Iron

15. Carbon monoxide

16. Ethylene glycol

17. Narcotics

18. Methanol

DIRECTIONS: For each of the questions or incomplete statements below, **one or more** of the answers or completions given is correct. Select

    A if only *1, 2, and 3* are correct
    B if only *1 and 3* are correct
    C if only *2 and 4* are correct
    D if only *4* is correct
    E if *all* are correct

Questions 19–25:

19. Drugs that vasodilate both the arterial and venous systems include
    1. dopamine
    2. sodium nitroprusside
    3. minoxidil
    4. captopril

20. Dopamine is a catecholamine that
   1. primarily enhances myocardial contractility by stimulating alpha-adrenergic receptors
   2. At high doses (greater than 20 μg/kg per minute) can cause significant alpha receptor stimulation that may result in deleterious vasoconstriction
   3. decreases cardiac output at low doses (1–5 μg/kg per minute)
   4. dilates mesenteric, coronary, renal, and cerebral arteries

21. As a thrombolytic agent, streptokinase
   1. activates the fibrinolytic system indirectly by promoting the conversion of plasminogen to plasmin
   2. activates the fibrinolytic system directly by promoting the conversion of plasminogen to plasmin
   3. activates the fibrinolytic system in an exogenous fashion
   4. is a naturally occurring thrombolytic substance that directly converts plasminogen to plasmin

22. The role of the calcium channel blockers nifedipine and diltiazem in patients with acute congestive heart failure derives from their ability to
   1. enhance vascular tone
   2. reduce aortic outflow impedance
   3. only slightly decrease ventricular emptying
   4. increase myocardial oxygen supply

23. Hyperuricemia is associated with
   1. primary gout
   2. renal insufficiency
   3. alcoholism
   4. pseudogout

24. In prescribing gold injections for a patient with rheumatoid arthritis, one must periodically monitor
   1. white blood cell count
   2. renal function
   3. skin for rashes
   4. chest x-ray

Directions Summarized

A	B	C	D	E
1, 2, 3 only	1, 3 only	2, 4 only	4 only	All are correct

25. Drugs that may produce positive direct antiglobulin (Coombs') tests include
1. hydralazine
2. levodopa
3. phenytoin
4. quinidine

25

Pictorial
Jared Zelman, M. D., F. A. A. F. P.

DIRECTIONS: Each of the questions or incomplete statements below is followed by four or five suggested answers or completions. Select the **one** that is best in each case.

26. The patient in Fig. 25.1 is likely to have all of the following EXCEPT
    A. tachycardia
    B. goiter
    C. peptic ulcer disease
    D. heat intolerance
    E. skin changes

Fig. 25.1

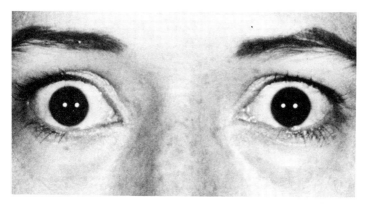

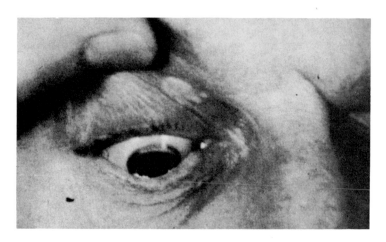

Fig. 25.2

27. The eyelid lesion seen in the patient in Fig. 25.2 should be approached as follows:
   A. Evaluate for a possible blood lipid disorder
   B. Biopsy
   C. Advise patient to stay away from the sun
   D. Treat with cryotherapy and examine genetalia for further lesions
   E. Treat total body with gamma benzene hexachloride (Kwell)

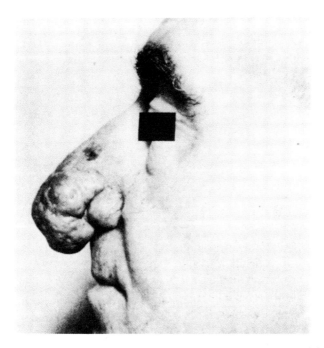

Figure 25.3 (Reprinted courtesy of Marie-Louise Johnson, M.D.)

28. The lesion in Fig. 25.3 is
    A. basal cell CA
    B. squamous cell CA
    C. rhinophyma
    D. fibrosarcoma
    E. acanthoma or ketoacanthoma

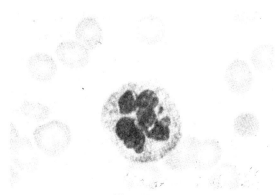

Fig. 25.4

29. The peripheral smear in Fig. 25.4 represents which disease?
    A. Iron deficiency anemia
    B. Sickle cell anemia
    C. Pernicious anemia
    D. Leukemia

30. The disease represented in Fig. 25.4 is caused by
    A. iron deficiency
    B. folate deficiency
    C. vitamin B_{12} deficiency
    D. pyridoxine deficiency

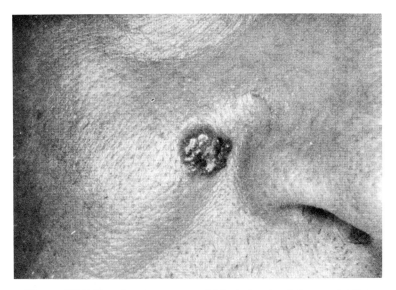

Figure 25.5 (Reprinted courtesy of Marie-Louise Johnson, M.D.)

31. Which of the following statements concerning the lesion in Fig. 25.5 is NOT true?
   A. Rarely seen in blacks or Orientals
   B. Men are more often affected than women.
   C. Metastasizes readily
   D. Is prevalent in the United States
   E. Ultraviolet light and oral inorganic arsenic exposure are associated with this lesion

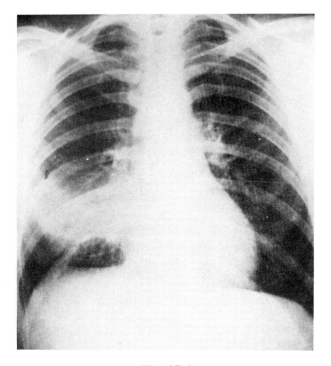

Fig. 25.6

32. Figure 25.6 shows
    A. partial pneumothorax
    B. right upper lobe pneumonia
    C. right middle lobe pneumonia
    D. right lower lobe pneumonia
    E. acute tuberculosis

33. Which of the following signs is depicted in Fig. 25.6?
    A. Trendelenberg sign
    B. Silhouette sign
    C. Chadwick sign
    D. Babinski sign
    E. None of the above

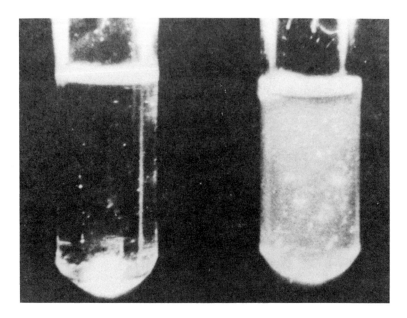

Fig. 25.7

34. The tube on the right in Fig. 25.7 would be LEAST likely
to be found in patients with
A. rheumatoid arthritis
B. septic arthritis
C. osteoarthritis
D. lupus arthritis
E. gouty arthritis

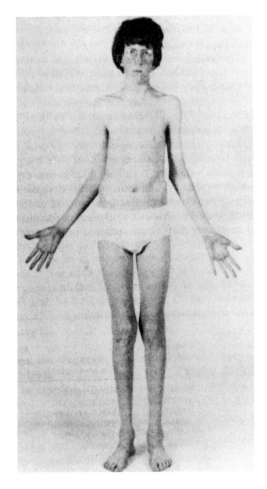

Fig. 25.8

35. Figure 25.8 depicts a 16-year-old boy with the Marfan syndrome. Which of the following would be LEAST likely to occur in this syndrome?
   A. Dislocated lens
   B. Inward displacement of the sternum
   C. Arachnodactyly
   D. High arched palate
   E. Autosomal recessive inheritance

36. About what percent of patients with this syndrome have cardiovascular abnormalities?
   A. Less than 1%
   B. 3–5%
   C. 10–15%
   D. 50%
   E. 90%

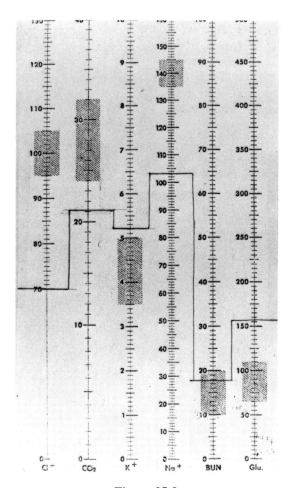

Figure 25.9

37. The chemistry 6 profile in Fig. 25.9 was obtained from a 60-year-old black male who had sustained multiple fractures, including a basilar skull fracture when a train collided with his truck. Other lab values were as follows:

Serum osmolality ...225.0 mOsmol/kg
Urine osmolality....595.0 mOsmol/kg
Spot urine sodium ..120.0 mEq/L
Serum sodium ......116.0 mEq/L
Serum chloride ..... 84.0 mEq/L
Serum BUN .... 9.0 mEq/L
Serum creatinine ..... 0.8 mEq/L
Serum uric acid....... 2.0 mEq/L

The patient most likely has hyponatremia which is
A. spurious
B. secondary to severe dehydration
C. secondary to inappropriate secretion of ADH
D. secondary to diabetes insipidus
E. secondary to Cushing's disease

38. General treatment of this disorder may include all of the following EXCEPT
A. hypertonic saline
B. hypertonic saline plus furosemide
C. fluid restriction
D. vasopressors
E. demeclocycline (Declomycin)

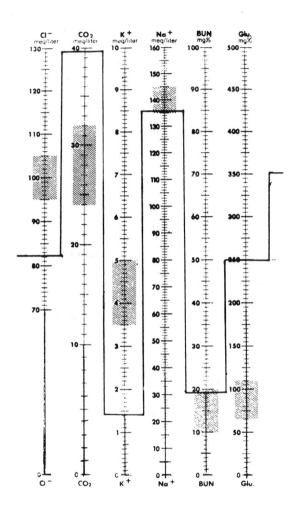

Figure 25.10

39. The chemistry profile in Fig. 25.10 was obtained from a 72-year-old white male who exhibited severe muscle weakness and suffered a respiratory arrest. Which of the following medications would the patient LEAST likely be taking?

A. A laxative such as Ex-Lax

B. A laxative such as Blackdraught

C. A diuretic such as hydrochlorothiazide

D. A diuretic such as Aldactone

E. A corticosteroid such as prednisone

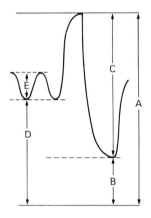

Figure 25.11

Questions 40–44: The following questions are related to normal lung volumes (refer to Fig. 25.11).

  40. Total lung capacity

  41. Vital capacity

  42. Functional residual capacity

  43. Tidal volume

  44. Residual volume

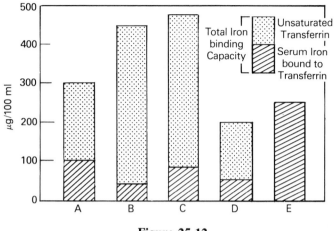

Figure 25.12

Questions 45–48:   Figure 25.12 depicts serum iron-binding capacity in various disorders.

45.   Which of the bars would most likely be normal?

46.   Which of the bars would be most likely to occur with infection, inflammation, or malignancy?

47.   Hemochromatosis or hemosiderosis would most likely be represented by which bar?

48.   Which of the bars would be most likely to occur with iron deficiency?

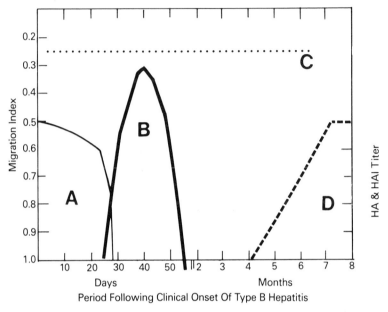

Figure 25.13

Questions 49–52: Figure 25.13 depicts immunologic events during the course of acute and convalescent phases of icteric hepatitis B infection.

49. Leukocyte migration inhibition (LMI) response

50. Antibody to HBsAg (anti-HBs)

51. Antibody to hepatitis B core antigen (anti-HBc)

52. Hepatitis B surface antigen (HBsAg)

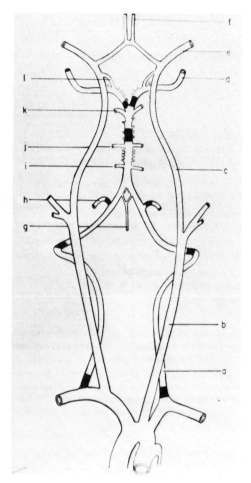

Figure 25.14

Questions 53–55: Figure 25.14 depicts arteries supplying the brain and the common sites of occlusive atherosclerotic disease in the vertebrobasilar system (solid black areas).

53. Posterior inferior cerebellar artery

54. Left vertebral artery

55. Posterior cerebral artery

Answers and Comments

24. Therapeutics

1. C. The concomitant use of verapamil with IV beta-adrenergic blocking agents is contraindicated. (**REFS.** 6—p. 46; 9—p. 110)

2. B. Nitroprusside is relatively contraindicated because of its potential side effects on the fetus, unless blood levels are carefully monitored. Diazoxide may be used, but may suppress uterine contractions. Hydralazine drip with magnesium sulfate has been the standard. Some authors use combinations of diazoxide with Lasix or Hydralazine with Aldomet, but nitroprusside has not gained favor. (**REFS.** 2—p. 30; 10—p. 883; 11—p. 194)

3. A. All the medications listed with the exception of lidocaine have been shown to effectively block the AV node and convert supraventricular tachycardia to a sinus rhythm. (**REF.** 11—p. 63)

4. C. Semilente has a rapid onset of action, peaking in 1–2 hours, with a duration of 12–16 hours. NPH is intermediate in onset, peaking in 2–8 hours, and having a duration of 24–28 hours. (**REF.** 8—p. 620)

5. D. The need for insulin is augmented by increased food intake and weight gain; reduction or cessation of physical exercise; withdrawal of oral hypoglycemic agents; and therapy with thyroid hormone and corticosteroids. (**REF.** 13—p. 94)

6. E. The actions of a number of drugs are inhibited by treatment with "inducing agents." Phenobarbital and other inducers of hepatic enzymes lower plasma levels of warfarin, bishydroxycoumarin, digitoxin, quinidine, dexamethasone, and metyrapone. (**REF.** 7—p. 400)

7. B. Aluminum ions, present in antacids, form insoluble chelates with the tetracyclines, thereby preventing absorption of these drugs. Ferrous ions similarly block tetracycline absorption. (**REF.** 7—p. 399)

8. C
9. D
10. E
11. B
12. A
13. B
14. A
15. D
16. C
17. E
18. C (All in **Ref.** 1—P. 19)

19. C. Both sodium nitroprusside and captopril vasodilate both the arterial and venous systems. Prazosin (Minipress) also dilates the arterial and venous beds. Dopamine is a vasopressor. Minoxidil is an arterial vasodilator. (**REF.** 3—p. 196)

20. C. Dopamine is a catecholamine that primarily enhances myocardial contractility by stimulating beta-adrenergic receptors. Low-dosage dopamine exerts some inotropic and chronotropic effects, which maintain hemodynamic benefits up to infusions of $20\mu g$/kg per minute. (**REF.** 5—pp. 101–104)

21. B. Streptokinase combines with plasminogen to produce an activator complex, and this catalyzes the conversion of circulating plasminogen to plasmin. It is the thrombolytic therapy of choice in acute myocardial infarctions. (**REF.** 4—pp. 51–56)

22. C. The calcium channel blockers inhibit calcium ion influx in smooth muscle cells, and this results in relaxation of vascular tone. As a result, they reduce aortic outflow impedance, allowing for better ventricular emptying and coronary artery vasodilation, which increases myocardial oxygen supply. (**REF.** 4—p. 190)

23. A. (**REF.** 12—p. 327)

24. A. (**REF.** 12—p. 140)

25. E. Other drugs that may produce positive direct antiglobulin (Coombs') tests include cephalosporins, methadone, methyldopa, and high doses of antibiotics. (**REFS.** 6—pp. 319–323;10—p. 1226)

25. Pictorial

26. C. The gastrointestinal manifestations of thyrotoxicosis include increased appetite, hyperdefecation, diarrhea, and, rarely, constipation and anorexia. Peptic ulcer disease is not a component of hyperthyroidism. (**REF.** 5—pp. 152, 154)

27. A. Palpebral xanthomas (xanthelasmas) are common in primary hyperlipoproteinemia, but may be transmitted as a familial trait in the absence of hypercholesterolemia. (**REF.** 5—p. 737)

28. C. (**REF.** 8—p. 2243, Fig. 555–1)

29. C. This shows a gigantic poly (macrocytic hypersegmented poly) in a patient with pernicious anemia. A few macrocytic red cells are noted, along with mild poikilocytes. (**REF.** 8—plate 2.E)

30. C. Pernicious anemia is a macrocytic anemia due to atrophic gastropathy, deficient intrinsic factor, and eventual vitamin B_{12} deficiency. (**REF.** 8— p. 897)

31. C. Basal cell epithilioma is the most common cancer of the skin. They very rarely metastasize; they are locally invasive. (**REFS.** 6—p. 835; 8—p. 2271)

32. C. The figure shows obliteration of the right heart border by pneumonia in the right middle middle lobe. (**REF.** 3—p. 56)

33. B. The figure depicts the silhouette sign. (**REF.** 3—p. 56)

34. C. In synovial fluid obtained from patients with rheumatoid arthritis, septic arthritis, and other inflammatory joint diseases, the mucin clot forms a flocculent precipitate or is friable, and the surrounding solution becomes cloudy (tube on right). (**REF.** 2—p. 61)

35. E. The Marfan syndrome is inherited as an autosomal dominant. (**REF.** 6— p. 574)

36. E. About 90% of patients with Marfan syndrome have cardiovascular abnormalities, some of which may be evident only with sensitive diagnostic modalities such as echocardiography. Weakness in the media of the aorta causes the most lifethreatening abnormality in the Marfan syndrome, progressive dilation, and dissecting aneurysm of the proximal portion of the ascending aorta. Clinical manifestations such as diastolic murmur or roentgenographic evidence of aortic dilatation may be detected in infancy or as late as in the fifth or sixth decades. The predilection for involvement of the ascending aorta is not surprising in view of the hemodynamic stresses that occur there. (**REF.** 6—574)

37. C. The patient described most likely has hyponatremia which is secondary to inappropriate secretion of ADH. (**REF.** 7)

38. D. Vasopressors would not be used in the treatment of this patient. (**REF.** 7)

39. D. The patient described would least likely be taking Aldactone, since this diuretic has potassium-retaining properties. (**REF.** 7)

40. A.

41. C.
42. D.
43. E.
44. B. (All from REF. 8—p. 373)

45. A
46. D.
47. E.
48. B. (All from **REF.** 6—p. 1850)

49. B. The immunologic events during the course of the acute and
50. D. convalescent phases of icteric type B hepatitis are shown
51. C. in the graph. They divided the sequence of events into
52. A. three phases. In the first phase, the acute hepatitis is associated with the presence of HBsAg in the serum and the appearance of anti-HBc. The second phase coincides with the disappearance of HBsAg and the appearance of cell-mediated immunity as indicated by a positive IMI test that disappears after 3–6 weeks. The third phase begins with the appearance of anti-HBs approximately 2 weeks to 2 months after the disappearance of HBsAg. Not all patients develop detectable anti-HBs. (**REF.** 4—p. 126)

53. H.
54. A.
55. D. (All in REF. 1—p. 1186)

References

24. Therapeutics

1. Bryson P. D: *Comprehensive Review in Toxicology*, Aspen Systems, 1986

2. Burrow G. N., and Ferris T. F.: *Medical Complications during Pregnancy*, 2nd Edition, W. B. Saunders, Philadelphia, PA, 1982

3. *Emergency Medicine Reports*, Vol. 5, No. 25, summer/fall 1984

4. *Emergency Medicine Reports*, Vol. 6, No. 7, winter/spring 1985

5. *Emergency Medicine Reports*, Vol. 6, No. 13, winter/spring 1985

6. Hansten P. D.: *Drug Interactions*, 5th Edition, Lea and Febiger, Philadelphia, PA, 1985

7. Isselbacher K. J. et al.: *Harrison's Principles of Internal Medicine*, 10th Edition, McGraw-Hill, New York, NY, 1980

8. Mazzaferri E. L. (Ed): *Textbook of Endocrinology*, 3rd Edition, Medical Examination/Elsevier, New York, NY, 1986

9. McIntyre K. M. and Lewis A. J. (Eds): *Textbook of Advanced Cardiac Life Support*, American Heart Association, 1983

10. Rosen P. et al.: *Emergency Medicine, Concepts and Clinical Practice*, C. V. Mosby, St. Louis, MO, 1983

11. Tintinalli J. E. et al.: *Emergency Medicine, A Comprehensive Study Guide*, American College of Emergency Physicians, McGraw-Hill, New York, NY, 1985

12. Turner R. A. and Wise C. N.: *Textbook of Rheumatology*, Medical Examination/Elsevier, New York, NY, 1986

13. Waife S. O.: *Diabetes Mellitus*, 8th Edition, Lilly, Indianapolis IN, 1979

25. Pictorial

1. Anon: *J Family Practice*. 1978(June 6)

2. Arthritis Foundation: *Syllabus, Revised Clinical Slide Collection on the Rheumatic Diseases*, Arthritis Foundation, Atlanta, GA, 1981

3. Felson B.: *Chest Roentgenology*, W. B. Saunders, Philadelphia PA, 1973

4. Krugman S., Ward R., and Katz S.: *Infectious Diseases of Children*, 8th Edition, C. V. Mosby, St. Louis, MO, 1981

5. Mazzaferri E. L.: *Textbook of Endocrinology*, 3rd Edition, Medical Examination/Elsevier, New York, NY, 1986

6. Petersdorf R. G. et al. (Eds): *Harrison's Principles of Internal Medicine*, 10th Edition, McGraw-Hill, New York, NY, 1983

7. Pieroni R. E.: Unpublished observations

8. Wyngaarden J. B. and Smith L. H. (Eds.): *Cecil Textbook of Medicine*, 17th Edition, W. B. Saunders, Philadelphia, PA, 1985

26

Patient Management Problems

Instructions

The objective of the patient management problem is to test the reader's skill and judgment in dealing with patient care situations. These types of problems attempt to place the reader in the position of the clinician and to provide him/her with realistic feedback of the consequences of each decision he/she makes.

A brief history is provided for each patient. After the patient history, a series of management stages is presented (A–1, A–2, etc.) The reader is presented with numerous courses of action or inquiries within each stage, and may select a course of action in any sequence within a particular stage.

For each course of action chosen, there are corresponding responses in the response section. Use the enclosed special pen to develop the concealed image information. Apply the pen LIGHTLY, from left to right, after the number of the response, to visualize the response (which ends at the asterisk*) corresponding to the course(s) of action that were chosen. Utilize the feedback received to determine whether additional choices should be made *within* the stage or move on to the next stage. Once a stage has been left, *do not* go back to a previous stage.

The reader is faced with three types of courses of action: those that should be done, those that should be avoided, and those that are optional. The selection of incorrect actions and the failure to select correct actions are both penalized in the scoring system (see page 449). Optional selections are not penalized.

The individual cases (patients) are classified by letters A–J. All ten should be completed before totaling your score.

The answers, discussions of the problem, and references for each case begin on page 449.

Note: To assure full usage of the latent image pen, please recap when not in use.

Internal Medicine
Michael A. Baker, M.D., F.R.C.P.(C), F.A.C.P.

Patient A

A 47-year-old man is admitted to hospital with a history of having vomited "coffee grounds" material. Three months previously he was hospitalized elsewhere for a painful right leg and was discharged on medication, which he is currently taking. He has had some epigastric distress in recent days, but this has not been relieved by eating. On cursory examination, he is diaphoretic, has a pulse of 100/minute, and is slightly pale.

A–1. Initial management should include
    1. start intravenous
    2. subcutaneous morphine
    3. nasogastric tube
    4. send blood to blood bank
    5. intravenous furosemide
    6. take blood pressure
    7. intravenous dopamine

A–2. Additional important points in the history should include
8. bleeding with previous surgery
9. recent foreign travel
10. identification of medication
11. amount of alcohol ingested
12. family history of seizures
13. symptoms in right leg
14. color of bowel movements

A–3. The following laboratory tests should be done urgently
15. arterial PO_2
16. prothrombin time
17. hematocrit
18. platelet count

Records are obtained from his previous hospital admission, documenting a deep vein thrombosis with suspected pulmonary embolism. He was discharged on Coumadin (warfarin) but did not return for follow-up. Prothrombin time is 50 seconds (control 12.5) and hemoglobin is 11 gm/100 ml. Blood pressure is 95/65.

A–4. At this point you should do the following:
19. Calculate blood volume
20. Give prednisone 100 mg IV
21. Liver function studies
22. Gave vitamin K_1
23. Give IM diazepam
24. Start arterial line to monitor blood pressure
25. Give stored plasma
26. Monitor urine output

After 4 days in hospital his hemoglobin is stable at 10.5 gm/100 ml, and the prothrombin time is 15 seconds (control 13). His blood pressure is 125/80 and he has had melena stools for 2 days.

A–5. Further investigation should include
27. chest x-ray
28. urinalysis
29. gastroscopy
30. venogram
31. serum iron
32. barium enema
33. reticulocyte count
34. daily prothrombin time

A–6. Therapy should now include
35. cryoprecipitate
36. heparin
37. iron
38. cimetidine

Patient B

A 67-year-old man is brought to your office by his wife. She states that he has become progressively confused over the past few days. In addition, he has been coughing a great deal, especially after smoking his frequent cigarettes. He is a thin patient with a ruddy complexion and shows some distress from rapid respirations.

B–1. Additional history should include
1. presence of sputum
2. smoking history
3. chest pain
4. appetite
5. pruritus
6. previous similar episodes
7. weight loss

On careful examination, the patient is noted to have slightly elevated jugular venous pressure, cyanosis of the tongue and mucous membranes, poor breath sounds in all pulmonary areas, pitting edema of the ankles, and a fever of 38 °C. He is admitted to hospital.

B–2. Investigation at this point should include
   8. blood counts
   9. transtracheal aspiration
   10. arterial blood gases
   11. chest x-ray
   12. serum electrolytes
   13. pulmonary function studies
   14. sputum culture
   15. urinalysis
   16. CAT scan
   17. ECG
   18. patient's weight

Laboratory results within the first hour show the following: hemoglobin 16.5 gm/100 ml, white count 15,000/mm^3; PO$_2$ 55 mm Hg, PCO$_2$ 59 mm Hg, pH 7.0. The sputum is purulent and shows mixed flora on Gram stain. A "bedside" x-ray is obtained that shows hyperaeration and increased bronchovascular markings, but is not of sufficient quality to interpret further.

B–3. The best management should now include
   19. phlebotomy
   20. 100% O$_2$ by nasal prongs
   21. diuretics
   22. digitalis
   23. infusion of bicarbonate
   24. oral penicillin
   25. bronchodilator inhalation
   26. 24% O$_2$ by Venturi mask
   27. intravenous ampicillin

After 7 days in hospital the patient is much improved, but remains somewhat confused. Furthermore, weakness in the left arm has become evident. Laboratory results show: PO$_2$ 92 mm Hg, PCO$_2$ 45 mm Hg (both on room air), sodium 128, potassium 4.0, chloride 89, CO$_2$ 25 (all in mEq/L). An x-ray is now obtained in the radiology department and shows a small "coin" lesion in the right middle lobe.

B–4. Investigations should now include
   28. sputum cytology
   29. chest tomograms
   30. lung scan
   31. brain scan
   32. phlebotomy
   33. serum calcium
   34. serum alkaline phosphatase
   35. serum LDH
   36. urine hemosiderin
   37. urine and serum osmolality
   38. urine pH

Obstetrics and Gynecology
Raymond E. Probst, M. D.

Patient C

A 28-year-old white female, gravida 1 para 0, is admitted with a complaint of amenorrhea and galactorrhea of 4 years duration. She desires to become pregnant.

C–1. Based on this information, you would want to inquire about
1. onset of menses
2. regularity of menses
3. nausea
4. frequency of urination
5. history of medication taken
6. decrease in size of breasts
7. headache
8. change in vision

C–2. You would then proceed as follows:
9. CBC
10. IVP
11. Serum prolactin
12. T_3 and T_4
13. 17-Ketosteroids and ketogenic steroid
14. Pelvic pneumogram
15. Brachial arteriogram
16. Smear of colostrum
17. Pregnancy test
18. Serum testosterone

C–3. Based on this information, you would then proceed with the following:
19. Hysterogram
20. Carotid arteriogram
21. Pneumoencephalogram
22. Sella turcica tomogram
23. Visual fields

C–4. You then advise the following:
24. Clomiphene
25. Pergonal
26. Cyclic medroxyprogesterone
27. CAT scan
28. Laparoscopy
29. Ovarian wedge resection
30. Adrenal angiography
31. Transsphenoidal craniotomy
32. Transtemporal craniotomy
33. Bromocriptine methylate

Patient D

A 26-year-old white female, p 2–0–0–2, 38 weeks pregnant enters the hospital because of epigastric pain, swelling, and a feeling of being dizzy.

D–1. Based on this information, the following is of value:
  1. Complete physical
  2. Fetal heart rate
  3. Pelvic exam
  4. Fetal ECG
  5. Alpha-fetoprotein

D–2. Based on this information, you would want to obtain
  6. CBC
  7. urinalysis
  8. BUN
  9. uric acid
  10. blood cultures
  11. electrolytes

D–3. You then proceed as follows:
  12. Absolute bed rest
  13. Force fluids
  14. Diuretics
  15. Intake and output
  16. Magnesium sulfate
  17. Pitocin induction

After several hours of induction, the patient's blood pressure rises to 190/110 and she has a grand mal seizure. It is also noted that she is now bleeding from the gingiva, and has areas of ecchymosis on her body.

D–4. The following information is now necessary:
  18. T_3 and T_4
  19. Type and cross-match packed cells
  20. Type and cross-match whole fresh blood
  21. Fibrinogen
  22. Chest x-ray
  23. Prothrombin time
  24. Partial thromboplastin time
  25. Creatinine
  26. CBC
  27. Protamine sulfate
  28. Fibrin split products
  29. Platelet count

D-5. Based on this information, you would advise
  30. Apresoline hydralazine hydrochloride drip IV
  31. rupture membranes
  32. direct fetal monitoring
  33. fetal scalp pH
  34. packed cells given
  35. whole blood given
  36. L/S ratio
  37. expeditious delivery

Pediatrics
Raymond M. Russo, M.D., F.A.A.P.

Patient E

A well-developed, 14-month-old child is admitted to the hospital for moderate dehydration with abdominal distention, hypospadias, and undescended testes that cannot be palpated. Symptoms include anorexia, vomiting, and mild diarrhea (twice daily). This is not the first hospital admission for dehydration; two previous stays were required at age 11 months and 13 months.

E-1. Initial investigation should include
1. CBC
2. urinalysis
3. electrolytes, BUN, glucose
4. blood pH and bicarbonate
5. chest x-ray
6. flat and upright x-ray of abdomen
7. stool cultures
8. blood culture
9. urine culture
10. stool pH and reducing substances
11. upper GI series and barium enema

E–2. Initial management and subsequent investigation should consist of

12. one-third to one-half isotonic NaCl solution until urine is voided
13. the addition of intravenous KCl and Na bicarbonate after voiding
14. daily weights
15. chart intake and output
16. trimethobenzamide HCl 15 mg/kg/day to control vomiting
17. give ampicillin 200 mg/kg/day IV
18. order a buccal smear
19. measure urinary 17-ketosteroids
20. obtain surgical consult
21. radiographic bone age determination

The patient has failed to respond to therapy and remains dehydrated. Vomiting persists, although there is no diarrhea. Sodium values have remained low and potassium values elevated; acidosis persists.

E–3. Further management should include

22. daily monitoring of electrolytes
23. change intravenous fluids to isotonic saline with KCl and Na bicarbonate
24. give hypertonic NaCl solution to correct hyponatremia
25. restrict potassium
26. measure urinary pregnanetriol
27. obtain a contrast x-ray of urogenital sinus
28. measure plasma renin
29. administer hydrocortisone 10–50 mg/kg/day
30. initiate desoxycorticosterone 0.5–3 mg/day

The patient has now responded well to therapy and is no longer vomiting, and is not acidotic or dehydrated.

E–4. Further long-range management should include
    31. treatment with hydrocortisone
    32. treatment with desoxycorticosterone
    33. treatment with added NaCl
    34. monitoring of bone age
    35. monitoring of urinary 17-ketosteroids and pregnanetriol
    36. consider clitorecession and vaginoplasty
    37. consider testicular prothesis and testosterone administration
    38. arrange for exploratory laparotomy to rule out adrenal cortical tumors
    39. consider subtotal adrenalectomy at puberty

Patient F

An 11-year-old male of Mediterranean ancestry is admitted with severe pain in both lower extremities, low-grade fever, jaundice, pallor, and hepatomegaly. He has had many previous admissions for jaundice and has required periodic transfusions. He underwent splenectomy 1 year prior to this admission.

F–1. Initial investigation should include
    1. CBC
    2. bilirubin—direct, indirect, and total
    3. liver profile
    4. urine for bile and urobilinogen
    5. stool for occult blood
    6. blood culture
    7. chest x-ray
    8. x-ray of both extremities
    9. skull x-ray
    10. bleeding—clotting and clot retraction time
    11. Coombs' test

F–2. Immediate therapy should include
    12. transfusion with packed red cells
    13. chelation therapy with desferoxamine
    14. penicillin G, 1.2 million U IM daily
    15. acetaminophen 300 mg every 6 hours for relief of pain

F–3. In light of the results obtained, the following additional in vestigation should be undertaken:
  16. Hemoglobin electrophoresis
  17. Serum iron and total iron-binding capacity (TIBC)
  18. Erythrocyte osmotic fragility
  19. Liver biopsy
  20. Partial thromboplastin time
  21. Thromboplastin generation test

The patient has not responded and continues to have leg pain over the midtibial regions bilaterally. He has occasional temperature elevations and is pale and weaker than usual. A generalized lymphadenopathy was noted for the first time.

F–4. Subsequent management should consist of
  22. codeine phosphate 30 mg every 4 hours *prn* for pain
  23. bone marrow determination
  24. determination of urinary formiminoglutamic acid (FIGLU) after histamine loading
  25. administration of folic acid 10 mg daily
  26. administration of iron 6 mg three times a day
  27. administration of vitamin B_{12}, 15 μg daily IM
  28. orthopedic consultation
  29. lumbar puncture
  30. repeat bacterial cultures of blood, urine, CSF, nose, and throat
  31. radiographic survey of the skeletal system

F–5. At this point, the patient will require the following therapy:
  32. Vincristine 1.5/mg/m^2 IV once weekly for 4–6 weeks
  33. Prednisone 40 mg/m^2 orally every day for 4–6 weeks
  34. Methotrexate 200 mg/m^2 orally once weekly
  35. Cyclophosphamide 200 mg/m^2 orally once weekly
  36. Transfusions with packed red cells as determined by complete blood counts
  37. Prophylactic penicillin G
  38. Administration of vitamin B_6, 10 mg daily

Psychiatry
Edward H. Liston, M. D.

Patient G

A 30-year-old married white woman presents with a 3-week history of gradually progressive symptoms of increased activity, pressured speech, labile mood with irritability and euphoria, decreased sleep, and racing thoughts. She is brought in by police for resisting arrest for reckless driving and suspicion of being intoxicated. On examination she is loquacious, is noted to be overtly seductive, claims to be a "goddess from the love planet," and reports auditory hallucinations of "music of the spheres." When questioned about the reality of her hallucinations, the patient suddenly becomes accusatory, yells profanities, and threatens you with physical harm. She denies that she is ill, that she has been using alcohol or drugs, or that she has had any prior psychiatric problems. Her husband, however, reports that she has had similar but less severe symptoms on two other occasions in the past 5 years. Prior to the onset of this illness the patient had been functioning well at home and at work. There is no known history of trauma or loss of consciousness. Physical examination is unremarkable.

G-1. For immediate management you decide to
1. refer patient to a crisis intervention clinic
2. release patient to custody of police until legal charges are dealt with
3. arrange immediate voluntary hospitalization
4. hospitalize patient involuntarily if necessary
5. arrange for admission to a general medical unit for medical clearance.

G-2. Your differential diagnosis includes
6. bipolar disorder
7. major depressive episode with mood incongruent psychotic features
8. paranoid schizophrenia
9. histrionic personality disorder
10. toxic organic mental disorder

G-3. Laboratory studies that you order at this point are
11. thyroid function tests
12. dexamethasone suppression test
13. toxic blood screen
14. liver function tests
15. CT scan of the head
16. renal function tests

G-4. Following hospital admission the patient remains hyperactive, hypersexual, and verbally assaultive, and has attempted to strike a staff member. You consider the following immediate interventions:
17. Neuroleptic medication
18. Intravenous lithium chloride
19. Carbamazepine
20. Seclusion and restraint

G-5. You elect to treat the patient with lithium carbonate. You should

21. monitor the patient's 24-hour urine lithium concentration
22. attempt to achieve a serum lithium concentration of at least 2.0 mEq/L
23. anticipate that between 900–2100 mg of lithium carbonate per day will be required for a therapeutic response
24. plan to discontinue lithium immediately upon resolution of symptoms

G-6. Complications of lithium therapy of which you should be aware include

25. goiter
26. thyrotoxicosis
27. pigmentary retinopathy
28. renal tubular dysfunction
29. cholestatic jaundice

G-7. Following recovery from the acute episode the patient announces her plan to become pregnant. In counseling this patient you include the following points:

30. The risk of her offspring developing major affective disorder is 15–20%
31. The risk of her offspring developing schizophrenia is approximately 1%
32. It is important to continue maintenance therapy with lithium throughout her pregnancy
33. Lithium must be discontinued at least during the first trimester of pregnancy
34. Amniocentesis to assess fetal chromosome color-blindness homogeneity will help to clarify morbidity risk
35. Breast feeding should not be used if the patient is taking lithium postpartum

Radiology
Alan E. Oestreich, M.D.

Patient H

A 5-year-old girl with a past history of several respiratory infections and occasional abdominal pain now presents with a 12-hour history of severe abdominal cramping. On physical examination there is a sensation of a mass in the right side of the abdomen.

H–1. Based on this information, the following imaging studies would be of value:
1. Abdominal ultrasound
2. Plain film of the abdomen
3. Hysterosalgingogram
4. Barium (or water-soluble contrast) enema
5. Fluoroscopy of the diaphragm
6. Doppler examination of the aorta
7. Thorotrast hepatography
8. Intravenous cholangiogram

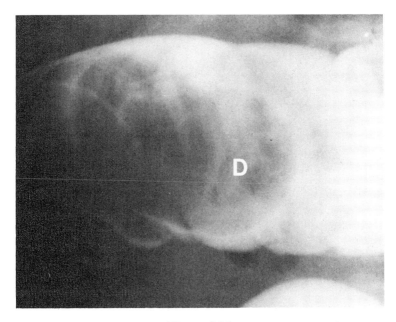

Figure 26.1

H–2. A barium enema was obtained (Fig. 26.1) which showed a left-convex filling defect (D) in the proximal transverse colon. One should next consider

9. needle biopsy of "D" under fluoroscopic control
10. attempt to treat by use of further barium
11. laparotomy if barium enema cannot resolve the problem
12. stop the enema; wait 24 hours to see if "D" resolves
13. proceed directly to upper gastrointestinal contrast study

H–3. Since the patient's age is 5 years, the following tests are appropriate to rule out associated diagnoses if the immediate symptoms were resolved by the radiologic enema:

14. Urinalysis
15. Sweat chloride
16. Magnetic resonance imaging of spine
17. Head circumference
18. Chest radiograph
19. Physical examination search for palpable nodes
20. Technitium scan of abdomen
21. Open biopsy of the pancreas
22. Upper gastrointestinal series with small bowel follow-through
23. CT of the abdomen

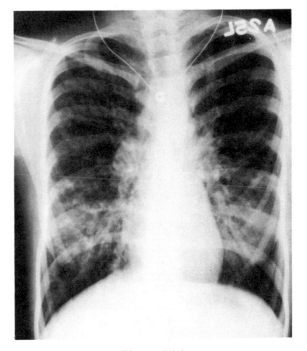

Figure 26.2

H–4. Figure 26.2 is a chest radiograph of the same patient 9 years later. The following steps are important in the long-term management of the patient's primary disease:
24. Prompt treatment of congestive heart failure
25. Methotrexate for weight gain
26. Splenectomy
27. Monthly head circumferences
28. Chest radiograph for acute chest pain
29. Pancreatic enzyme replacement with meals
30. Vitamin C for periosteal reaction along bones
31. Yearly lymphangiogram
32. Pulmonary postural drainage as needed
33. Salt restriction in hot climates

Surgery

M. D. Ram, M.D., M.S. (Surg.), Ph.D., F.R.C.S. (England, Edinburgh, and Canada), F.A.C.S.

Patient I

A 60-year-old man was brought to the emergency room with a history of hematemesis and passing out of 6 hours duration. He vomited on three occasions and the vomitus contained bright red blood. He also had melena once. He was known to have had epigastric discomfort for the last 2–3 years. He was an alcoholic until recently, but at present takes only one or two drinks a week.

On examination he was pale, sweaty, and was not in acute pain. Pulse was 110/minute, BP 100/60 mm Hg, respiration, 30/minute. The abdomen was slightly protuberant and the liver and spleen were palpable. The patient was not jaundiced.

I–1. Initial investigations should include
1. CBC
2. electrolytes, glucose, urea
3. serum LDH, transaminases, bilirubin
4. sedimentation rate
5. serum albumin, globulin, and alkaline phosphatase
6. chest x-ray
7. ECG
8. typing and cross-matching of blood
9. serum calcium and phosphorus
10. serum amylase

I–2. Immediate steps in management include
    11. upper GI endoscopy
    12. colonoscopy
    13. barium swallow
    14. nasogastric suction
    15. iced saline gastric lavage
    16. intravenous fluids
    17. blood transfusion
    18. parenteral hyperalimentation
    19. Foley catheter in bladder
    20. gastric hypothermia with balloon

The barium swallow revealed esophageal varices. Liver function studies revealed serum albumin of 3.0 g, bilirubin of 2.0 mg/100 ml, slightly elevated transaminases, and a BUN of 40 mg/100 ml.

I–3. Further steps in the management include
    21. Sengstaken-Blakemore tube
    22. intravenous Pitressin infusion
    23. selective arterial catheterization and Pitressin infusion
    24. selective arterial catheterization and gelfoam embolization
    25. needle biopsy of the liver

The patient stopped bleeding and made a steady recovery. However, over the next 3 months he was readmitted twice with similar minor episodes.

I–4. Further management may include
    26. transesophageal injection of sclerosing agents into the varices
    27. portocaval shunt
    28. splenectomy
    29. vagotomy and drainage along with ligation of varices
    30. distal splenorenal shunt

Following operation the patient went into hepatic coma, renal failure, and developed ascites.

I–5. Further management includes
   31. oral lactulose
   32. neomycin by mouth
   33. exchange transfusions
   34. parenteral hyperalimentation
   35. peritoneal dialysis
   36. hemodialysis
   37. diuretics
   38. peritoneal venous shunting
   39. salt restriction
   40. auxiliary liver transplantation

Patient J

A 55-year-old black female was admitted with a 3-week history of right upper quadrant abdominal pain, nausea, and yellowish discoloration of urine. She lost about 10 lb. Her history included having five children, constipation, and bleeding per rectum. On examination she was slightly obese and not in acute distress, and clinically no abnormality could be found except for some degree of jaundice.

J–1. Initial evaluation will include
   1. complete blood count
   2. SMA–6
   3. serum transaminases and LDH
   4. serum bilirubin
   5. serum alkaline phosphatase
   6. serum acid phosphatase
   7. serum amylase
   8. serum proteins
   9. prothrombin time
   10. partial thromboplastin time
   11. sickle cell preparation
   12. urine for urobilinogen
   13. urine for bile pigments
   14. blood cultures
   15. hepatitis antigen

J–2. Initial orders will include
16. normal saline IV
17. low-fat diet
18. antibiotics by parenteral route
19. parenteral hyperalimentation
20. vitamin B complex

J–3. Over the next 2 days she became more jaundiced. Radiologic studies indicated are
21. plain x-ray of abdomen
22. oral cholecystogram
23. intravenous cholangiogram
24. ultrasound study of abdomen
25. upper GI barium study
26. barium enema
27. endoscopic retrograde pancreatocholangiography
28. percutaneous transhepatic cholangiography
29. intravenous pyelography
30. CAT scan

J–4. Investigations reveal an obstruction of the common bile duct probably caused by stones. Further steps in management may include
31. oral administration of vitamin K
32. bowel preparation with antibiotics
33. cholecystectomy with operative cholangiography
34. choledochoduodenostomy
35. sphincteroplasty
36. Whipple's operation
37. choledochojejunostomy using a Roux-en-Y loop
38. gastrojejunostomy
39. choledocholithotomy and closure over a T-tube
40. splenectomy

Scoring System

The scoring system for the patient management problems is designed to reward correct selections and to penalize incorrect selections. Incorrect selections due to omission and commission are both subject to penalty. That is, selecting incorrect actions and not selecting correct actions are both penalized. Selecting or not selecting actions that are optional does not affect your score.

For each correct selection you receive one point, and for each incorrect selection you receive minus one point. Your final score is determined by taking the sum of the total positive points obtained and the total negative points obtained and then dividing by the total number of positive points possible times 100. This gives you the percentage correct (Proficiency Score) in the patient management section.

$+$ = 1 positive point $(+1)$
$-$ = 1 negative point (-1)
0 = optional (no points)
$X1$ = Total Positive Points Obtained
$X2$ = Total Negative Points Obtained
Z = Total Positive Points Possible = 199

$$\text{Proficiency Score (\%)} = \frac{X1 + (-X2)}{Z} \times 100$$

Patient A

SCORING

A-1.	A-2.	A-3.	A-4.	A-5.	A-6.
1. +	8. +	15. −	19. 0	27. 0	35. −
2. −	9. 0	16. +	20. −	28. 0	36. −
3. +	10. +	17. +	21. 0	29. +	37. +
4. +	11. +	18. 0	22. +	30. −	38. +
5. −	12. 0		23. −	31. 0	
6. +	13. +		24. −	32. −	
7. −	14. +		25. +	33. +	
			26. +	34. +	

DISCUSSION

The onset of "coffee-grounds" vomiting is a clear indication of upper gastrointestinal bleeding and leaves no question as to the emergent nature of the management. Excessive sweating, with rapid pulse and pallor, indicates rapid recent blood loss, which is confirmed when the blood pressure is ordered and found to be 100/70. An intravenous line is started with a wide-bore needle because of impending shock and a nasogastric tube aspiration confirms blood in the stomach and removes peptic secretions and clots.

After controlling access to intravenous fluids, the history of painful leg is explored and the medication is determined to have been Coumadin, given for treatment of deep vein thrombosis. Patients who are bleeding must be questioned for previous bleeding history, family history of bleeding, and medication history. Alcohol is a frequent instigating or aggravating cause of bleeding and GI ulceration and in this patient may be an important factor. The prothrombin time checks the anticoagulant effect of Coumadin as well as the effect of the alcohol on production of coagulation factors in the liver. The platelet count is checked to determine the effect of alcohol on short-term suppression of platelet production.

Since the patient is bleeding and has a prolonged prothrombin time, vitamin K_1 is given, but does not act for 24–72 hours. To cover the immediate defect, plasma is infused. Fresh plasma is not necessary, since stored plasma contains the vitamin K-dependent factors (II, VII, IX, X). Arterial punctures and intramuscular injections should be avoided in patients on anticoagulants.

After the patient is stable it is important to determine the cause of the upper GI bleed. Gastroscopy reveals healing erosions caused by the alcohol. The elevated reticulocyte count indicates adequate iron stores for the short term at least. Although he has had a recent deep vein thrombosis, further anticoagulants are contraindicated at present. Iron therapy is continued for 2–3 months to replenish stores. Cimetidine should aid healing of erosions.

REFERENCES

1. Wintrobe M. M. et al.: *Clinical Hematology*, 8th Edition, Lea and Febiger, Philadelphia, PA, 1981, p. 1056

2. Wyngaarden J. B. and Smith L. H.: *Cecil Textbook of Medicine*, 17th Edition, W. B. Saunders, Philadelphia, PA, 1985, pp. 835–837

Patient B

SCORING

B-1.	B-2.	B-3.	B-4.
1. +	8. +	19. −	28. +
2. +	9. −	20. −	29. +
3. +	10. +	21. 0	30. −
4. +	11. +	22. 0	31. +
5. 0	12. 0	23. −	32. −
6. +	13. −	24. −	33. +
7. +	14. +	25. +	34. +
	15. 0	26. +	35. 0
	16. −	27. +	36. −
	17. +		37. +
	18. +		38. 0

DISCUSSION

This patient has chronic bronchitis and emphysema of the "blue bloater" type. He becomes progressively confused over several days because of exacerbation of bronchitis by bacterial infection, leading to cyanosis. He is a long-term cigarette smoker and this has helped to create the current problems. His thin physique leads you to inquire about appetite and weight loss. The production of sputum and the occurrence of several previous episodes helps steer subsequent investigation and management.

The presence of right heart failure, secondary to hypoxia and possibly increased pulmonary vascular resistance, is noted on physical examination. Central cyanosis, respiratory distress, and fever indicate serious illness and direct subsequent management. Arterial blood gases are critical to patient assessment, but pulmonary function studies would be superfluous and difficult at this stage.

Hypoxia and hypercapnea lead you to treat with low-dose oxygen, using an open mask. Digitalis is unlikely to relieve the right heart failure and diuretics would be optional. Intravenous ampicillin is used until definitive cultures are returned.

After recovery from the acute episode, the residual confusion can no longer be blamed on hypoxia. A "coin" lesion in this setting is highly suspicious of carcinoma of the lung and this is confirmed on sputum cytology. A brain metastasis is suggested by the localized neurologic finding and is confirmed by scan. The hyponatremia suggests inappropriate ADH secretion, which is investigated by the serum and urine osmolality.

REFERENCE

1. Wyngaarden J. B. and Smith L. H.: *Cecil Textbook of Medicine*, 17th Edition, W. B. Saunders, Philadelphia, PA, 1985, pp. 399–403

Patient C

SCORING

C-1.	C-2.	C-3.	C-4.
1. +	9. 0	19. 0	24. 0
2. +	10. 0	20. −	25. 0
3. 0	11. +	21. +	26. 0
4. 0	12. +	22. +	27. 0
5. +	13. +	23. +	28. −
6. 0	14. 0		29. −
7. +	15. +		30. −
8. +	16. 0		31. +
	17. 0		32. −
	18. 0		33. +

DISCUSSION

This patient represents a case of amenorrhea galactorrhea due to a pituitary microadenoma. An extensive endocrinologic workup is used to ascertain if the patient has an ovarian estrogen failure or an absence of preovulatory release of LH. She is found to have a microadenoma of the pituitary, and wishes to become pregnant; the tumor is removed surgically transsphenoidally. She is then placed on bromocriptine and becomes pregnant.

REFERENCES

1. Danforth D. N.: *Obstetrics and Gynecology*, 5th Edition, Harper & Row, Hagerstown, MD, 1986, p. 889

2. Richard R. M.: Amenorrhea/galactorrhea and pituitary tumors. *Contemp Ob/Gyn.* 13(5):169–202, 1979

Patient D

SCORING

D-1.	D-2.	D-3.	D-4.	D-5.
1. +	6. +	12. +	18. −	30. +
2. +	7. +	13. −	19. 0	31. +
3. +	8. +	14. −	20. +	32. +
4. +	9. +	15. +	21. +	33. +
5. 0	10. 0	16. +	22. +	34. 0
	11. +	17. +	23. +	35. −
			24. +	36. +
			25. +	37. +
			26. +	
			27. +	
			28. +	
			29. +	

DISCUSSION

The patient discussed in this case has developed severe preeclampsia. After the rudimentary tests are done she seems to be under control and labor is induced. She then develops disseminated intravascular coagulation during convulsions and this is shown by the elevation in split products. Fresh whole blood is administered and the fetus is delivered.

REFERENCES

1. Danforth D. N.: *Obstetrics and Gynecology*, 5th Edition, Harper & Row, Hagerstown, MD, 1986, pp. 446–464

2. Richart R. M.: Amenorrhea/galactorrhea and pituitary tumors. *Contemp Ob/Gyn.* 13(5):169–202, 1979

Patient E

SCORING

E-1.	E-2.	E-3.	E-4.
1. +	12. +	22. +	31. +
2. +	13. +	23. −	32. +
3. +	14. +	24. −	33. +
4. +	15. +	25. −	34. +
5. 0	16. −	26. +	35. +
6. +	17. −	27. +	36. +
7. +	18. +	28. +	37. −
8. 0	19. +	29. +	38. −
9. +	20. −	30. +	39. −
10. +	21. +		
11. −			

DISCUSSION

A child presenting with vomiting, dehydration, and abdominal distention would have to be investigated for the presence of acidosis and severe electrolyte disturbance. In addition, the possibility of an infectious etiology of the gastrointestinal or genitourinary tract would also have to be considered. Therefore, obtaining a CBC, urinalysis, electrolyte, BUN, and cultures would be consistent with good clinical management. A chest x- ray for an occult infection in the lung, which may not have produced cough symptoms or auscultatory findings, is optional. Abdominal distention is common with gastroenteritis and other acute disturbances of the gastrointestinal tract, and, in the absence of fever, paralytic ileus, or signs of localizing abdominal tenderness, an abdominal x-ray would not be indicated. Disaccharidase deficiency, which can present this way, especially in light of two previous admissions for a similar problem, would also be a justifiable consideration.

The presence, however, of ambiguous genitalia where testes cannot be palpated and the failure of ordinary measures to rehydrate the child and correct acidosis must also make one think of the adrenogenital syndrome. The use of potassium in the IV fluids after urine has been voided is correct, but not enough to correct electrolyte deficits. Similarly, the use of trimethobenzamide would not be indicated for control of a child this ill. Monitoring weight and intake/output is simply good clinical practice in managing dehydrated children. The use of ampicillin, despite the lack of clear evidence of infection, should be descried in this situation. A surgical consult is not warranted.

The investigation for ambiguous genitalia should include a buccal smear, which indeed was chromatin-positive, giving a clear indication that the genotypic sex was female, not male. At this point, the possibility of adrenogenital syndrome with virilization in a female child was greatly strengthened. Virtually confirmatory evidence was obtained with the finding of an elevated urinary 17-ketosteroid determination, since the hyperfunctioning adrenal cortex will result in increased excretion of 17-ketosteroids. Values greater than 2 mg/24 hours in children less than 8 years of age are abnormally high.

The change to isotonic and hypertonic sodium choloride solutions will not by themselves correct the hyponatremia until the underlying defect is corrected. In this case, sodium chloride is rapidly lost in the urine. Restriction of potassium is not indicated, and, in the face of possible total body potassium depletion despite an elevated serum rise, could be dangerous.

Measuring urinary pregnanetriol gives additional evidence of adrenogenital syndrome, since it is frequently elevated. Occasional rises in plasma renin may also be seen. The constellation of elevated 17-ketosteroids, pregnanetriol, serum renin, and salt-losing defect makes 21-hydroxylase deficiency the most likely form of adrenogenital syndrome. The x-ray of the urogenital sinus adds considerably more to the evidence that this is a virilizing process in a female child. The good response to hydrocortisone, which helps turn off the increased corticotropin from the pituitary gland, is indicative of adrenal hyperplasia rather than an adrenal cortical tumor, which is not suppressed as readily. This is the reason for monitoring 17-ketosteroids and pregnanetriol for the several weeks it takes hydrocortisone to be fully effective. If these levels did not decrease, the need to rule out a tumor would become imperative. The use of desoxycorticosterone is necessary to control the loss of sodium in the urine.

Once the diagnosis has been established and the acute phase under control, consideration must be given to long-term management. Hydrocortisone, desoxycorticosterone, and additional dietary salt are life-long requirements needing periodic dose adjustment to serve the individual needs of the growing child. In addition, the bone age should be evaluated periodically to gauge the success of therapy in limiting virilization. Lack of success here can lead ultimately to short stature. Since the child is genetically female and young enough to not have made a conclusive sexual self-identity, attention should be directed to making her a phenotypic female as well. Surgery can accomplish this. After the age of 3, when sexual self-identification takes place, this may not be indicated. There is no reason for exploratory surgery to rule out adrenal tumors, since suppression was achieved with therapy. Adrenalectomy is not advocated in the treatment of adrenogenital syndrome.

REFERENCES

1. Kempe C. H., Silver H. K., and O'Brien D.: *Current Pediatric Diagnosis and Treatment*, 7th Edition, Lange Medical, Los Altos, CA, 1982, pp. 696–698

2. Russo R. M. and Gururaj V. J.: *Practical Points in Pediatrics*, 4th Edition, Medical Examination, New York, NY, 1985, pp. 376–378

Patient F

SCORING

F-1.	F-2.	F-3.	F-4.	F-5.
1. +	12. −	16. +	22. +	32. +
2. +	13. −	17. +	23. +	33. +
3. 0	14. −	18. +	24. +	34. −
4. +	15. −	19. −	25. −	35. −
5. 0		20. −	26. −	36. +
6. +		21. −	27. −	37. +
7. 0			28. −	38. −
8. +			29. +	
9. +			30. +	
10. 0			31. +	
11. 0				

DISCUSSION

The presentation of a child of Mediterranean origin with pallor, jaundice, hepatomegaly, and a past history of splenomegaly and multiple transfusions should lead to little confusion in making a presumptive diagnosis of thalassemia of the beta variety. This child did present with additional symptoms of low-grade fever and severe bone pain in the lower extremities that warrant additional diagnostic speculation. A febrile response to past transfusions is not unlikely in patients frequently receiving donor blood. In addition, it is known that splenectomized thalassemia patients are at much greater risk for developing pneumococcal septicemia. For this reason, a blood culture is warranted. Marrow hyperplasia, commonly encountered in thalassemia major, of the erythroid series can also be a source of local bone pain. The presence of pain in both legs leads one away from osteomyelitis as a cause, since it would be unusual to have bilateral involvement.

The presence of jaundice and pallor can be expected with a diagnosis of thalassemia major, and little is added by doing a liver profile measuring bilirubin or urine bile and urobilinogen except as a benchmark for future comparison and to rule out the unlikely possibility of infectious processes involving the liver. Cirrhosis is a long term complication in thalassemia victims, and increasing levels of direct-reacting bilirubin or increasingly abnormal liver function studies can be expected after many years. Although no harm is done, it is probably a bit of wasted effort to look for occult blood in the stool on this indication. There is little reason to suggest blood loss.

The skull x-ray is useful for demonstrating typical bony changes: the "hair on end" appearance of the cortex and thickened maxillofacial bones. Similarly, long-bone x-rays will demonstrate osteoporosis and thin cortices—all indications of erythroid marrow hyperplasia. Hyperplasia is the result of the increased demand for erythrocytes to carry oxygen. In addition, an x-ray study is indicated to rule out other possible causes of bone pain. There does not appear to be an overly compelling reason to obtain a chest x-ray. Occult pulmonary infection in this age group is not likely and the information obtained, i.e., cardiac enlargement, is to be expected in thalassemia major. However, it serves also for later comparison, since another long-term risk is cardiac failure. The bleeding, clotting, clot retraction times, and the Coombs' test would also be wasteful of the laboratory's time and needlessly costly to the purchaser of health care services.

Immediate therapy included none of the options listed, since the symptomology had not been adequately investigated at this point. A transfusion of packed red cells was not indicated, because the hemoglobin was high for a child with thalassemia major. Transfusions usually are not required until the hemoglobin falls below 5–6 gm/100 ml. There was insufficient evidence of the need for chelation therapy with desferrioxamine, since the urinary excretion of iron was not yet determined, nor the serum iron or iron-binding capacity. Penicillin has been recommended on a prophylactic basis to prevent pneumococcal sepsis in a splenectomized thalassemic patient. However, in the course of determining an etiology for low-grade fever in a child who is not very acutely ill and has no other sign of infection, this is not indicated as a therapy. Acetaminophen is a reasonably effective analgesic useful for the leg pains the child complained of, but is probably unwise to use in the face of possible liver disease.

The second set of diagnostic tests does indeed establish the diagnosis beyond reasonable question. The hemoglobin electrophoresis is the *sine qua non* for determining beta-thalassemia major. The serum iron and total iron-binding capacity are useful in gauging the need for chelation therapy. Erythrocyte osmotic fragility is also a useful red cell measure in thalassemia. The liver biopsy is unwarranted, however, since little can be learned from it, and it is an invasive procedure not without some risk. The partial thromboplastin time and thromboplastin generation test add nothing to the diagnosis and are indicated in the coagulopathies, not the hemoglobinopathies.

The development of a new finding such as generalized lymphadenopathy as well as the continued leg pain and temperature spikes should serve to notify the physician that there is more to explain. Leg pain is not unheard of in thalassemia major and is explained on the basis of erythroid hyperplasia of the marrow. It is known that marrow hyperplasia may be a response to deficiencies in essential erythrocyte building elements. It is also known that a highly proliferative marrow has a great demand for folic acid. Administration of folic acid could be helpful in decreasing erythroid hyperplasia and thus the leg pains. However, the etiology of generalized lymphadenopathy cannot be explained on this basis; therefore, the clinician must seek other explanations. At this time, a bone marrow aspiration would be indicated to reach this explanation. In the present case, aspiration revealed a second disease process: an acute leukemia complicating a long-standing illness. This is illustrative of the need to search for new illnesses presenting against a background of chronic disease.

Administering folic acid to leukemia patients is like adding fuel to fire. It provides the necessary substrate for cellular proliferation and has the opposite effect of folic acid antagonists used in chemotherapy against leukemia. Thus, folic acid would be absolutely contraindicated in the present case even though it is useful in uncomplicated cases of thalassemia major.

Iron administration is also contraindicated, since there is no demonstrable need for iron and since hemosiderosis is a long-term danger in thalassemia. Vitamin B_{12} would not be indicated either and an orthopedic consultation would accomplish little. A lumbar puncture to rule out central nervous system leukemia should be done. Repeat cultures for bacterial organisms are indicated in view of the continued temperature spikes and a double reason (thalassemia and leukemia) for increased susceptibility to infection. A skeletal survey is useful in determining whether osteolytic leukemic lesions are present.

At this point, induction therapy to effect a remission in the leukemic process is indicated. Both prednisone and vincristine are effective induction drugs and are warranted. Transfusion needs are likely to grow in view of the combined diseases and thus should be closely monitored. It would appear to be reasonable to institute prophylactic penicillin therapy, since pneumococcal susceptibility would not be decreased, but probably enhanced by the leukemic process.

One would not want to attempt induction of remission with either methotrexate or cyclophosphamide. These are useful drugs in maintaining, but not in inducing remission. Again, the use of vitamin B_6 or folic acid would be contraindicated.

REFERENCES

1. Kempe, C. H., Silver, H. K., and O'Brien D.: *Current Pediatric Diagnosis and Treatment*, 7th Edition, Lange Medical, Los Altos, CA, 1982, pp. 372–375, 389–391, 896–900

2. Russo R. M. and Gururaj, V. J.: *Practical Points in Pediatrics*, 4th Edition, Medical Examination, New York, NY, 1985, pp. 300–301

Patient G

SCORING

G-1.	G-2.	G-3.	G-4.	G-5.	G-6.	G-7.
1. −	6. +	11. +	17. +	21. 0	25. +	30. +
2. −	7. −	12. 0	18. −	22. −	26. −	31. 0
3. +	8. −	13. +	19. −	23. +	27. −	32. −
4. +	9. 0	14. 0	20. +	24. −	28. +	33. +
5. −	10. +	15. 0			29. −	34. −
		16. +				35. +

DISCUSSION

The patient's presentation is that of a relatively acute psychotic disturbance with poorly controlled impulses, potentially dangerous behavior, and little or no insight into the nature or seriousness of her illness. Initial management calls for immediate admission to a psychiatric hospital; referral for outpatient care or release to the police would be inappropriate and possibly negligent. Voluntary hospitalization, as with most patients, is preferable, but there should be no hesitation to seek involuntary detention, since the patient's illness involves potential danger to herself or others and indicates that she may at present be gravely disabled.

The clinical picture of elevated, expansive, and irritable mood, hyperactivity, pressured speech, racing thoughts, grandiosity, decreased sleep, and hypersexuality is typical of a manic episode (bipolar disorder, manic) and the past history of similar episodes indicates that it is recurrent. The history is not suggestive either of major depression or schizophrenia. The presence of mood congruent psychotic features (delusions and hallucinations) is consistent with either mania or paranoid schizophrenia. However, the latter tends to be ruled out by the brief duration of illness and by the absence of such symptoms as thought control or broadcasting, auditory hallucinations of voices, incoherent and markedly illogical thinking, inappropriate or flattened affect, and deterioration in functioning. The patient may have an underlying personality disorder, but that cannot be determined from the information at hand

and is of relatively minor importance with respect to immediate management. An organic mental disorder secondary to intoxication or other cause is a possibility to consider in the differential diagnosis, although the 3-week history argues against this, as does the normal physical examination.

Laboratory investigation should include thyroid function tests because of the need for baseline studies in anticipation of treatment with lithium salts, as well as for the (unlikely) possibility that the syndrome is secondary to hyperthyroidism. Renal function tests are also indicated for baseline, pre-lithium assessment. A toxic blood screen is appropriate in this patient because the clinical picture could be secondary to the effects of substances such as cocaine, amphetamine, or phencyclidine. The result of this screen might also be important in this case from a legal perspective in view of the patient's arrest. The dexamethasone suppression test may be useful in confirming the diagnosis of major depression in some patients, but has little or no clinical utility in acute mania. There is no reason from the history and findings to suggest the need for liver function tests, nor is there any indication of pathology likely to be demonstrable on CT scan.

The treatment of choice for this patient is lithium salts. However, since there is a latency of several days before lithium begins to manifest reduction in symptoms, the psychotic aspects of the patient's illness may require early treatment with neuroleptic medications as well, and overtly dangerous behavior may require seclusion and restraint. Carbamazepine may be useful in some cases of lithium-resistant mania, but should not be used until lithium resistance or intolerance has been established. Lithium is not available in parenteral form; such use in any case would be potentially dangerous because of the risk of producing sudden toxic blood levels. Lithium concentration is monitored in blood, not urine. The target concentration for a typical manic patient is in the range of 0.5–1.5 mEq/L; levels in excess of 2.0 mEq/L tend to result in excessive side effects or toxicity and are rarely necessary for therapeutic effect. Satisfactory blood levels can usually be achieved by administration of lithium carbonate in a dosage range of 900–2100 mg/day in divided doses. The exact requirements are a function of volume of distribution and excretion rate and must be determined for each individual by monitoring serum lithium concentration every few days at the outset of treatment and by observing the patient carefully for side effects or toxic manifestations. With the resolution of the acute mania, lithium must not be discontinued, although a decrease in dosage is usually necessary to effect maintenance levels of 0.4–0.8 mEq/1. In the case of this patient with a prior history of two manic or hypomanic episodes and the current one of severe mania, prophylactic use of lithium should be continued indefinitely. Complications of lithium therapy include hypothyroidism, with or without goiter, and renal tubular dysfunction, manifested symptomatically by polyuria and polydipsia. Hyperthyroidism is not known to be a complication of lithium treatment, nor are pigmentary retinopathy (seen with thioridazine) or cholestatic jaundice (seen with some phenothiazines).

Genetic and pregnancy counseling in this case is important. The patient should be apprised of the 15–20% morbidity risk for each of her children developing bipolar illness. (The risk for their developing schizophrenia is no higher than the 1% expected for the general population.) No current biologic markers are available to determine actual morbidity risk for affective disorder. Lithium must be discontinued at least during the first trimester of pregnancy because it is teratogenic. If the patient were to remain asymptomatic, lithium should also be withheld for the second and third trimesters. Following delivery, lithium maintenance therapy may be resumed, but breast feeding should not be attempted, because lithium is secreted in breast milk.

REFERENCES

1. Kaplan H. I. and Sadock B. J.: *Comprehensive Textbook of Psychiatry*, 4th Edition, Williams & Wilkins, Baltimore, MD, 1985, pp. 39–40, 821–833, 1315–1318, 1576–1582

2. American Psychiatric Association: *Diagnostic and Statistical Manual of Mental Disorders*, 3rd Edition, APA, Washington, D.C., 1980, pp. 181–193, 205–224, 313–315

Patient H

SCORING

H-1.	H-2.	H-3.	H-4.
1. +	9. −	14. 0	24. +
2. +	10. +	15. +	25. −
3. −	11. +	16. 0	26. −
4. +	12. −	17. 0	27. 0
5. 0	13. −	18. +	28. +
6. 0		19. +	29. +
7. −		20. +	30. −
8. −		21. −	31. −
		22. +	32. +
		23. +	33. −

DISCUSSION

This child has acute symptoms raising the possibility of intussusception, even though most cases of intussusception occur before 2 years of age. Other possibilities should include appendicial abscess, constipation, and ovarian abnormality, including acute torsion. Abdominal ultrasound has value for appendicial abscess, ovarian abnormality, and diagnosis of intussusception; plain abdominal radiograph often shows paucity of gas in the right lower quadrant in each of those conditions, as well as showing stool in constipation. The intussusceptum may be directly shown indenting gas on plain film; plain film would rule out pneumoperitoneum or severe small bowel obstruction. Intravenous cholangiography is rarely indicated today for any cause.

On the barium enema (Fig. 26.1) "D" represents the intussusceptum. Current practice is to attempt hydrostatic reduction of intussusception during contrast enema, unless the child is too sick or has signs of severe obstruction, peritonitis, or pneumoperitoneum. Reduction is successful in the majority of cases, avoiding emergency surgery, which is the only alternative. Reduction is complete if contrast flows freely into the distal ileum after the intussuscepted ileum is pushed through the ileocecal valve. The child would then be observed about 24 hours for possible recurrence.

Since the likelihood of a primary "cause" of intussusception increases past 2 years of age, consideration should be given to cystic fibrosis (by measurement of sweat chloride) in view of the history of frequent respiratory infections. Other primary causes are Meckel diverticulum (if not shown at surgery, one may use a technitium Meckel scan), lymphoma (search for nodes; small bowel contrast study), lipoma (CT of the abdomen), and other small bowel abnormalities. Cystic fibrosis changes in the pancreas can be recognized by ultrasound; open biopsy of the pancreas is contraindicated.

Figure 26.2 shows peribronchial thickening, dilated bronchi, and prominent central pulmonary arteries, with a relatively small heart, all of which indeed suggest cystic fibrosis as her diagnosis. For cystic fibrosis, prompt treatment of any acute congestive heart failure, as well as any pneumonia, is important. Although portal hypertension following multinodular biliary cirrhosis may occur, splenectomy is generally not advisable, especially since protection against infection would be further impaired. Acute chest pain may result from pneumothorax, which has an increased incidence. Pancreatic enzyme replacement with meals is important to prevent impaction of thick stool. Periosteal reaction along bone in advanced lung disease is from hypertrophic pulmonary osteoarthropathy (not scurvy). The bronchiectasis and its complications are treated with postural drainage, inhalation of mucolytic agents, bronchodilators, and expectorant drugs. Increased salt loss in cystic fibrosis is treated with prophylactic sodium chloride in hot climates, *not* salt restriction.

REFERENCES

1. Singleton E. B., Wagner M. L., and Dutton, R. V.: *Radiology of the Alimentary Tract in Infants and Children*, 2nd Edition, W. B. Saunders, Philadelphia, PA, 1977, pp. 257–267

2. Juhl J. H.: *Essentials of Roentgen Interpretation*, 4th Edition, Harper & Row, Hagerstown, MD, 1981, pp. 856–859

3. Ziai M, ed.: *Pediatrics*, 3rd Edition, Little, Brown, Boston, MA, 1984, pp. 279–281

Patient I

SCORING

I-1.	I-2.	I-3.	I-4.	I-5.
1. +	11. +	21. +	26. 0	31. +
2. +	12. −	22. +	27. +	32. +
3. +	13. +	23. 0	28. −	33. 0
4. 0	14. +	24. −	29. −	34. −
5. +	15. +	25. −	30. +	35. −
6. +	16. +			36. −
7. +	17. +			37. −
8. +	18. −			38. 0
9. −	19. +			39. +
10. −	20. 0			40. −

DISCUSSION

The differential diagnosis of upper gastrointestinal bleeding in this patient is fairly straightforward. The most common causes are bleeding esophageal varices and bleeding duodenal and gastric ulcers. Other less frequent causes are bleeding from ulceration in hiatus hernia. Mallory-Weiss tears of the gastroesophageal junction, and acute gastritis. This patient is a known alcoholic and continues to drink. In addition, the distention of the abdomen and hepatosplenomegaly are strong pointers toward portal hypertension. His history is not suggestive of peptic ulceration. Initial evaluation requires measurement of a complete blood count and basic electrolytes, glucose, and urea. Studies on liver enzymes and bilirubin are important in assessment of liver function. Sedimentation rate has no particular value in the immediate management, but is an optional study. Serum proteins, alkaline phosphatase, chest x-ray, and ECG are again essential in the preoperative evaluation of an elderly gentleman, and in addition are of prognostic value in terms of liver function. Serum calcium, phosphorus, and amylase have no value in this situation and are unnecessary.

Although there is a presumptive diagnosis of bleeding varices, one should exclude other conditions, and upper endoscopy would be helpful. On the other hand, colonoscopy is not indicated in the immediate management of a patient with upper GI bleeding. A barium swallow might demonstrate varices or peptic ulceration. Insertion of a nasogastric tube for monitoring bleeding and also to implement iced saline gastric lavage is useful. Intravenous fluids and, if necessary, blood transfusions are necessary in the resuscitation and management of this patient. On the other hand, in an acute bleed, there is no indication for parenteral hyperalimentation. Further, in the patient who already possibly has a sick liver, intravenous administration of amino acids might result in hepatic failure. A Foley catheter is useful in management of fluid balance and assessment of renal perfusion. Gastric hypothermia was used in the past with variable results, but has no consistent benefit; therefore, it is optional.

The most valuable steps in the management of this patient are intravenous. Pitressin infusion and the use of Sengstaken-Blakemore tube. Intravenous Pitressin reduces splanchnic arterial flow and thereby produces portal hypotension and this might reduce the bleeding from the varices. Similarly, the Sengstaken-Blakemore tube is of value because the baloons produce tamponade by direct pressure on the esophageal varices. On the other hand, selective arterial catheterization and Pitressin infusion have no greater advantage than peripheral intravenous Pitressin infusion, but may be used when the arterial catheter is already in place during a diagnostic study. Arterial catheterization and gelfoam embolization is of no value in this situation because the bleeding is from multiple dilated varices. There is no indication for needle biopsy of the liver, since the problem at this stage is an emergency bleeding and not one of managing the liver.

In the elective management of patients with recurrent hemorrhage from bleeding varices, the choice of procedure currently is either a portocaval shunt or a distal splenorenal shunt. Both have strong advocates. Transesophageal injection of sclerosing agents into the varices has been practiced, with variable results. In the hands of those who are experienced, this is considered relatively simple and gives good results, but the results are not consistently obtained by everybody. On the other hand, splenectomy alone or vagotomy and drainage along with ligation of varices have no place in the management of esophageal varices. Both procedures will result in recurrent variceal hemorrhage.

The problems of this patient's management at this stage are very complicated and the prognosis is poor. In a patient who has hepatic failure, renal failure, and ascites, the mainstay of treatment is essentially supportive. Ammonia intoxication should be reduced, and toward this purpose, oral lactulose and oral neomycin are advocated. Lactulose lowers pH in the colon and reduces ammonia production by colonic organisms. Neomycin is effective in reducing bacterial flora in the colon and in the same way reduces ammonia production. The use of large exchange transfusions has had some variable success, and in centers where large amounts of blood are available it may be tried. However, this might result in bleeding problems of a disseminated nature. Parenteral hyperalimentation is not indicated, because the additional nitrogen load on the liver might result in further deterioration of the patient's condition. Management of the patient with renal failure along with hepatic failure is very, very difficult. Peritoneal dialysis is difficult to manage because of the ascites. Hemodialysis, by adding additional strain on the circulatory system, often worsens the patient's condition. Diuretics have been of no value. Salt restriction is useful to reduce further ascites. Some authors have recommended peritoneal venous shunting in this situation, but the exact indications for peritoneal venous shunting in hepatorenal syndrome are not clear. Auxiliary liver transplantation was recommended in the early years of liver transplantation, but the addition of this major operative procedure often results in a fatal outcome and is no longer practiced.

REFERENCES

1. Sabiston, D. C. (Ed): *Davis-Christopher Textbook of Surgery*, 13th Edition, W. B. Saunders, Philadelphia, PA, 1986, pp. 828–829, 1100–1112

2. Schwartz, S. I. (Ed): *Principles of Surgery*, 4th Edition, McGraw-Hill, New York, NY, 1984, pp. 1045–1050, 1278–1284

Patient J

SCORING

J-1.	J-2.	J-3.	J-4.
1. +	16. 0	21. +	31. −
2. +	17. +	22. −	32. −
3. +	18. −	23. −	33. +
4. +	19. −	24. +	34. +
5. +	20. 0	25. +	35. 0
6. −		26. +	36. −
7. −		27. +	37. 0
8. +		28. +	38. −
9. +		29. 0	39. +
10. −		30. +	40. −
11. 0			
12. +			
13. +			
14. −			
15. +			

DISCUSSION

The history and findings in this patient warrant a complete workup for a differential diagnosis of jaundice. The fact that she was multiparous and the jaundice was associated with abdominal pain leads to a strong suspicion of stones as a cause of jaundice. However, at age 55, one also has to think of a possible carcinoma. In addition, it is a possibility that this black female could have hemolytic jaundice due to sickle cell disease, which is producing multiple stones.

Initial evaluation would include the routine blood counts and blood chemistries. Elevations of transaminases and LDH would indicate a hepatocellular variety of jaundice as against an obstructive one. Serum bilirubin and alkaline phosphatase would be elevated in obstructive jaundice and measurements are indicated in the evaluation of this patient. On the other hand, elevated serum acid phosphatase is a feature of prostatic cancer. Serum protein levels and prothrombin time would indicate the degree of hepatic dysfunction due to the obstructive jaundice. Prothrombin synthesis is impaired in prolonged obstructive jaundice. On the other hand, partial thromboplastin time has no value in this particular situation. Since the patient is a black female, it is desirable to do the sickle cell preparation, although this has no immediate bearing on the management of the jaundice. When there is complete obstruction, there is no urobilinogen in the urine. On the other hand, bile pigments, which are not normally present in urine, may be present in obstructive jaundice. Blood cultures are not indicated since the patient does not have any evidence of sepsis. A hepatitis antigen study is desirable, since she might have had some blood transfusions in the past.

In the initial management of this patient, it is important that a low-fat diet be prescribed, since jaundiced patients do not tolerate fatty foods. The need for intravenous fluids, however, is not so very clear unless the patient is dehydrated and then one might want to hydrate her intravenously. There is no indication for antibiotics, since the patient does not have any evidence of cholangitis. Similarly, at this stage there is no indication for parenteral hyperalimentation. The use of vitamin B complex is optional, although as long as the patient is taking some food by mouth, she is unlikely to be short of vitamin B complex.

A plain x-ray of the abdomen shows stones in about 20% of instances and may be helpful in the diagnosis. On the other hand, oral cholecystography and intravenous cholangiography are useless in jaundiced patients, since the biliary tract is not visualized by these techniques. Ultrasound study of the abdomen would indicate dilated ducts, and it also might point to stones in the gallbladder or common bile duct. In addition, if there is a lesion in the head of pancreas, the ultrasound study might delineate this mass well. An upper GI barium study and a barium enema are routinely performed to exclude a primary malignancy in the GI tract and a possible secondary in the liver causing the jaundice. In addition, the upper GI will reveal alterations in the duodenal outline in patients who might have ampullary carcinoma or carcinoma of the head of pancreas. Both endoscopic retrograde cholangiopancreatography (ERCP) and percutaneous transhepatic cholangiography (PTC) are very worthwhile and would help pinpoint the diagnosis in this patient. The PTC is more often of help to the surgeon than the ERCP. Also, ERCP is not available at all institutions, but when available, it is worth obtaining. Intravenous pyelography is not of direct help in the evaluation or management, but is an optional study just to be sure that the renal tract is normal. In recent years the investigation of jaundice has included computer-assisted axial tomography. This technique would very well reveal dilatation of the ducts, stones, and possible carcinoma of the head of pancreas or of the ampulla of Vater, and is very useful in the further management.

Prior to the operation, the patient should receive vitamin K parenterally. There is no benefit in giving vitamin K orally, because it is not absorbed in the absence of bile salts in the GI tract. Bowel preparation with antibiotics is not indicated in patients who are to undergo surgery for jaundice. Whatever operation might be performed, it would only involve the duodenum or the small bowel, and the colon would not be involved directly. The preliminary step for most procedures is a cholecystectomy with operative cholangiograms. Even when there is definitive knowledge of stones in the bile duct, preexploration cholangiography is useful to outline the anatomy of the bile ducts and to define the number and location of the stones. Following this, an attempt is made to remove the stones and close the common duct over a T-tube. A week or 10 days after the operation, a second cholangiogram is done to make sure that there are no retained stones. In patients who have multiple stones with dilated ducts, choledochoduodenostomy or sphincteroplasty has been used to prevent recurrence of obstruction due to stone formation. When biliary enteric anastomosis is performed, choledochoduodenostomy is much more popular, although some surgeons still do a choledochojejunostomy. The latter operation requires creation of another intestinal anastomosis and this is not desirable. There is no place for Whipple's operation in the treatment of patients with jaundice due to common duct stones. The operation is only indicated in patients with carcinoma of the head of pancreas or of the ampulla. Similarly, gastrojejunostomy is not indicated in this situation. Splenectomy is not usually combined with common duct exploration at the same time because the operation is further prolonged. In this patient, it is not indicated.

REFERENCES

1. Sabiston D. C. (Ed): *Davis-Christopher Textbook of Surgery*, 13th Edition, W. B. Saunders, Philadelphia, PA, 1986, pp. 1132–1134

2. Schwartz S. I. (Ed): *Principles of Surgery*, 4th Edition, Mc-Graw-Hill, New York, NY, 1984, pp. 1051–1058, 1322–1324

Responses

For each course of action you choose, there are corresponding responses in this section. You will use the enclosed special pen to develop the concealed information. Apply the pen LIGHTLY, from left to right after the number of the response, to visualize the response (which ends at the asterisk*) corresponding to the course(s) of action that you choose.

Sample Responses (Visualize All 3)

1.

2.

3.

Patient A

A-1. 1.

2.

3.

4.

5.

6.

7.

A-2. 8.

9.

10.

11.

12.

13.

14.

A–3. 15.

16.

17.

18.

A–4. 19.

20.

21.

22.

23.

24.

25.

26.

A–5. 27.

28.

29.

30.

31.

32.

33.

34.

A–6. 35.

36.

37.

38.

END OF RESPONSES FOR PATIENT A

Patient B

B–1. 1.

2.

3.

4.

5.

6.

7.

B–2. 8.

9.

10.

11.

12.

13.

14.

15.

16.

17.

18.

B–3. 19.

20.

21.

22.

23.

24.

25.

26.

27.

B–4. 28.

29.

30.

31.

32.

33.

34.

35.

36.

37.

38.

END OF RESPONSES FOR PATIENT B

Patient C

C–1. 1.

2.

3.

4.

5.

6.

7.

8.

C–2. 9.

10.

11.

12.

13.

14.

15.

16.

17.

18.

C–3. 19.

20.

21.

22.

23.

C–4. 24.

25.

26.

27.

28.

29.

30.

31.

32.

33.

END OF RESPONSES FOR PATIENT C

Patient D

D–1. 1.

2.

3.

4.

5.

D–2. 6.

7.

8.

9.

10.

11.

D–3. 12.

13.

14.

15.

16.

17.

D–4. 18.

19.

20.

21.

22.

23.

24.

25.

26.

27.

28.

29.

D–5. 30.

31.

32.

33.

34.

35.

36.

37.

END OF RESPONSES FOR PATIENT D

Patient E

E–1. 1.

2.

3.

4.

5.

6.

7.

8.

9.

10.

11.

E–2. 12.

13.

14.

15.

16.

17.

18.

19.

20.

21.

E–3. 22.

23.

24.

25.

26.

27.

28.

29.

30.

E–4. 31.

32.

33.

34.

35.

36.

37.

38.

39.

END OF RESPONSES FOR PATIENT E

Patient F

F–1. 1.

2.

3.

4.

5.

6.

7.

8.

9.

10.

11.

F–2. 12.

13.

14.

15.

F–3. 16.

17.

18.

19.

20.

21.

F–4. 22.

23.

24.

25.

26.

27.

28.

29.

30.

31.

F–5. 32.

33.

34.

35.

36.

37.

38.

END OF RESPONSES FOR PATIENT F

Patient G

G–1. 1.

2.

3.

4.

5.

G–2. 6.

7.

8.

9.

10.

G–3. 11.

12.

13.

14.

15.

16.

G–4. 17.

18.

19.

20.

G–5. 21.

22.

23.

24.

G–6. 25.

26.

27.

28.

29.

G–7. 30.

31.

32.

33.

34.

35.

END OF RESPONSES FOR PATIENT G

Patient H

H–1. 1.

2.

3.

4.

5.

6.

7.

8.

H–2. 9.

10.

11.

12.

13.

H–3. 14.

15.

16.

17.

18.

19.

20.

21.

22.

23.

H–4. 24.

25.

26.

27.

28.

29.

30.

31.

32.

33.

END OF RESPONSES FOR PATIENT H

Patient I

I–1. 1.

2.

3.

4.

5.

6.

7.

8.

9.

10.

I–2. 11.

12.

13.

14.

15.

16.

17.

18.

19.

20.

I–3. 21.

22.

23.

24.

25.

I–4. 26.

27.

28.

29.

30.

I–5. 31.

32.

33.

34.

35.

36.

37.

38.

39.

40.

END OF RESPONSES FOR PATIENT I

Patient J

J–1. 1.

2.

3.

4.

5.

6.

7.

8.

9.

10.

11.

12.

13.

14.

15.

J–2. 16.

17.

18.

19.

20.

J–3. 21.

22.

23.

24.

25.

26.

27.

28.

29.

30.

J–4. 31.

32.

33.

34.

36.

37.

38.

39.

40.

END OF RESPONSES FOR PATIENT J